W0081999

Prepare to Defend Yourself
. . . How to Age Gracefully & Escape with Your Dignity

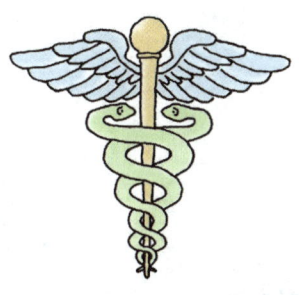

*This book's publication is supported by the
Texas A&M School of Rural Public Health, whose mission is
to improve the health of communities through education,
research, service, outreach, and creative partnerships.*

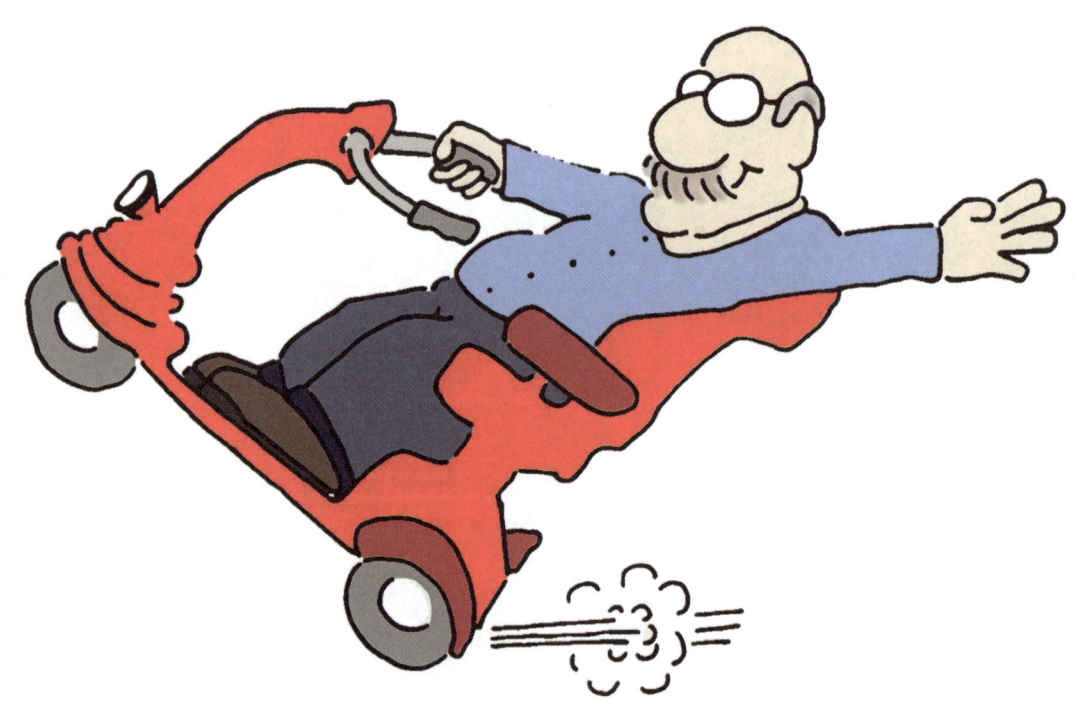

Prepare to Defend Yourself

. . . How to Age Gracefully & Escape with Your Dignity

MATTHEW MINSON, MD

TEXAS A&M UNIVERSITY PRESS • COLLEGE STATION

Copyright © 2016
by Matthew Minson
All rights reserved
First edition

This paper meets the requirements
of ANSI/NISO Z39.48-1992
(Permanence of Paper).
Binding materials have been
chosen for durability.
Manufactured in
the United States of America.

LIBRARY OF CONGRESS CATALOGING-IN-PUBLICATION DATA

Names: Minson, Matthew, 1961– author.
Title: Prepare to defend yourself ... how to age gracefully & escape
with your dignity / Matthew Minson, MD.
Other titles: How to age gracefully & escape with your dignity
Description: First edition. | College Station: Texas A&M University Press,
[2016] | Includes bibliographical references and index.
Identifiers: LCCN 2015038052| ISBN 9781623494124 (pbk.: alk. paper)
| ISBN 9781623494131 (ebook)
Subjects: LCSH: Older people—United States—Life skills guides. | Older people—
Medical care—United States. | Older people—United States—Economic conditions.
| Older people—United States—Conduct of life.
Classification: LCC HQ1064.U5 M565 2016 | DDC 646.790973—
dc23 LC record available at http://lccn.loc.gov/2015038052

THIS BOOK IS DEDICATED TO:

MY MOTHER

—WHO INTRODUCED ME

TO THE MAGIC OF WORDS,

DR. WILLIAM RAUB

—WHOSE STANDARD OF SCHOLARSHIP

AND SERVICE I CAN ONLY HOPE TO MATCH,

CLIFFORD LANE '59—

THE TRUEST AGGIE,

AND, AS ALWAYS, KELLI

—WITHOUT WHOM…

CONTENTS

The Pursuit of Happiness

INTRODUCTION

If you have read my first book, *Prepare to Defend Yourself . . . How to Navigate the Healthcare System & Escape with Your Life*, then you know I am a sucker for a good historical anecdote. You also probably recall that I started writing these books because of the potential a system can have for underserving or even abusing an individual. I was originally inspired, or more accurately stated, I was angered when I saw an older woman being led to believe she needed to pay an outstanding bill that was already covered by her insurance. Right after that, my own wife almost became the victim of three successive and critical medical mistakes. It was a wakeup call. I realized I needed to do something to help people become better, more empowered healthcare consumers.

That is how the first book came to be.

Now, while I was writing the book, I was fortunate to have an amazing group of readers—a book club composed of seniors—who were almost brutal in their criticism and comments. In fact, you could say I suffered the paper cut equivalent of the Prussian Saber Club at their hands, but the result was great. Their contributions were candid, valuable, insightful, and right-on.

The one thing they continuously recommended was that I expand the topic beyond a discussion of health care to include aging issues. This made sense. If you look at the overarching target and scope of the US

Department of Health and Human Services, you see included in the department's title the words "health *and* human services."

Health, absent the supporting Human Services, is like talking about light bulbs without acknowledging the importance of the power grid, like Edison without Nikola Tesla, jam without bread, Abbott without Costello. You get the idea.

So while considering history and the idea of human services, it occurred to me that the ideology I wanted to communicate had already been addressed by the Founding Fathers—a bunch of people much more eloquent than me—and it was actually summed up in three simply stated but marvelously complex concepts.

It was a hot July day in the late 18th century.

Philadelphia.

The city was sweltering. All the odors and raw qualities of an early American city, without the luxuries of plumbing, air conditioning, and electricity, were at their greatest, most offensive effect. People moved a little slower in a kinetic self-defense, and dogs panted in the shade of the Philadelphia State House. Inside, a tall, lanky, redheaded man listened as a short, thick, passionate man championed the concepts of his recently drafted proposal for independence. The other members of the Continental Congress sweated and in a final, critical step voted to adopt the declaration.

Among the many things in contention was the wording of what everyone in the small building believed was critical to advance from mere survival to the more elevated state of truly living. It was not a new concept. With a nod to Thomas Paine, the *Rights of Man* (humanity) have probably been in the heart and soul, if not the mind, of our ancestors since they first emerged from the cave. Only in the last century, however, had those rights been communicated in the Epicurean philosophy, which taught the pursuit of happiness as autarchy. That, they believed, translated as self-sufficiency and thus freedom. The English philosopher *and physician* John Locke originally labeled it "life, liberty, and the pursuit of property [estates]."

More recently, it had been adapted to address a greater concept that was facilitated by "owning property." The economies of the world in those days were based on agriculture, and properly maintained and productive property assured wealth, stability, security, and the luxury of advancing from a struggle for existence to a contemplation of the more philosophical. It advanced people from mere survival to truly living.

As John Adams is reported to have said when queried by the French as to his favor of the arts, "I must see to the obtaining of Liberty, so that my sons can study engineering and mathematics . . . then their sons will have the privilege of studying music and art."

In a word, it is the idea of *happiness*, that elusive and universally sought quality of our existence that promises fulfillment, satisfaction, and spiritual enrichment.

And so those sweating men included in their manifesto an adjustment of language to espouse "life, liberty, and the pursuit of happiness."

They have been some of the most cherished words in the American consciousness ever since.

The Life part seems pretty self-evident.

You breathe in… you breathe out… you repeat.

As long as you can.

As we all know, however, it is much more complicated than that. That idea describes survival. Life or, more appropriately, living is an involved and spectacular constellation of actions, experiences, values, and thoughts. Hopefully it amounts to fulfillment. Getting there often requires personal liberty, autonomy, and self-determination and leads ideally—if we are particularly fortunate—to happiness.

Earlier, I stated that as I was preparing for this book, I realized that the template was already provided.

The section of the book titled "Life" will include not just the idea of staying alive, but things you can do to maximize the maintenance and quality of your health, as well as some uniquely senior applications to nutrition, activity, behavior, and then what to prepare for as your health inevitably must decline. Provided tools will assist with recommended activities, nutrition guides, resources, and more.

"Liberty" will address the concepts of independent living and how to self-assess when it is time to transition from single or solitary living to aging in place and more. Resources for self and partner assessment of what and when it is time will accompany this. We'll examine independent versus congregate living and the strata of assisted living arrangements, including nursing assistance and nursing homes, and how to be a good

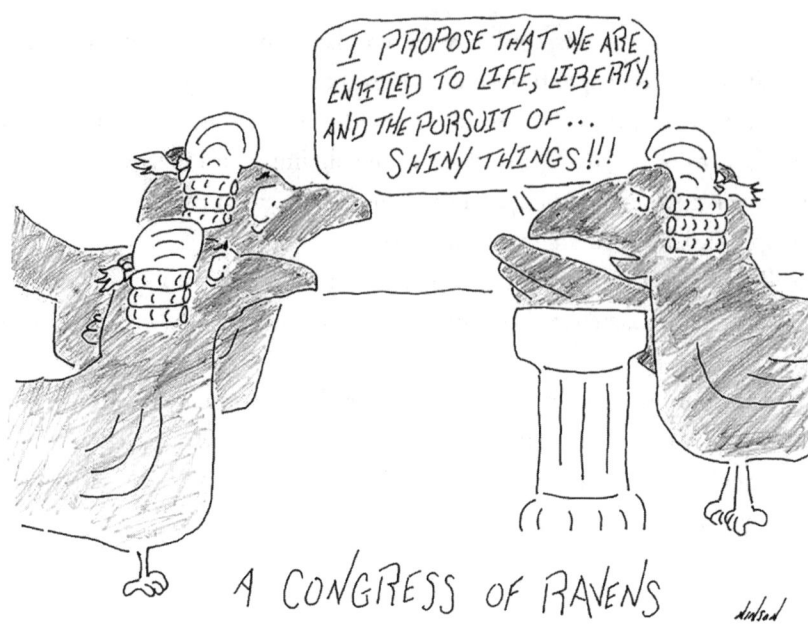

A CONGRESS OF RAVENS

consumer with the aid of nonprofits, government agencies, advocacy organizations, and more.

"Liberty" will also cover the importance of staying informed and where reliable information is available about legislative and political activities that will affect the lives of seniors. As money assures a certain independence, sources of aid for less affluent seniors will also be covered along with tools, lists, and contacts.

Finally, with an admitted bias toward the standard contributors to "the Pursuit Happiness," we will cover love, sex, and end-of-life issues. In particular, the chapter on the end of life—SPOILER ALERT: all biographies end the same way—covers steps everyone should take to protect their surviving loved ones and to assure that their wishes will be followed.

I have also added one other heading—"Safety and Security"—in the chapter on preventing abuse. Certainly it could be included in the section on happiness or life, but as it contributes to all three, I will dedicate a specific section to physical and personal security and describe advocacy organizations as well as federal, state, and local regulatory agencies and programs established to support seniors.

As I conducted the research for this book, it occurred to me that it was

Congress—first the Continental Congress, which gave us the Declaration of Independence, and later the Constitutional Congress—that articulated these principles that we "still hold dear." I also learned that humans are not the only animals that group up into congresses. Among those others are salamanders, baboons, and ravens. Somehow that seems oddly appropriate. With that in mind, I had to wonder what the congress of ravens might consider its ideal principles.

Regardless of all that, it was surprising to me that there really is so much that contributes to the human experience and that with advancing age the necessity to assure that it is properly defended is critical. The purpose of this book is to do just that, to provide you with the tools and information necessary to become your own advocate.

So, let's get started, and, as always . . .

Be well,
Matthew Minson, MD

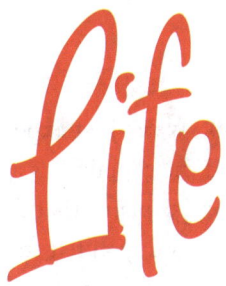

Do not go gentle into that good night,
Old age should burn and rave at close of day;
Rage, rage against the dying of the light . . .

Dylan Thomas

I really like the idea expressed in that poem, and it seems a perfect way to start off this exploration of aging. Granted, Thomas's communication to his father was about the last scene of the last act of life, but I like to consider it as a call to action about the whole concept of aging.

What I also like about the spirit of the poem is that it doesn't accept the inevitable *process of aging* with a tone of surrender and acquiescence. It also does not deny the nature of aging or what it means, but it takes it on fiercely. It says up front that you don't have to be passive about it. In fact, it advocates just the opposite: that we all should take on aging with a kind of defiant and vigorous mindset, even though there are some inevitables.

For many, growing old is forbidding, even terrifying, and fraught with difficulty. For many others, growing old is a dynamic time of accomplishment, gratification, reflection, and reward and, yes, fraught with difficulty.

Oddly enough, the same can be said for every age and phase of life. The purpose of this book is to give you the tools and resources that will help shift your experience toward the latter.

For that reason, I want to keep the beautiful, powerful words of that poem in mind as we start.

"Folks, from the flight deck, we've just experienced a problem . . ."

You are on an airliner, and the captain has come on over the speaker and in a tight, drawling second explains that the plane has suffered engine failure. Even before he said a word, you felt the disturbing lurch and drop of the aircraft followed by that awful emptiness of an amusement-park ride as everything falls away beneath your seat.

You know… *something* is wrong.

You also suddenly wish you had paid more attention to the safety video and had actually read that goofy laminated card in the seat back in front of you when the flight attendant asked.

The facemasks and airbags drop from the panel above you, and all of a sudden one consideration becomes paramount: the preservation of life. You want to stay alive.

That is one way of looking at life. It certainly fits in with Maslow's famous hierarchy of needs. In the world of disaster medicine and humanitarian assistance where a significant portion of my medical practice occurs, survival certainly comes into play.

Now, before we go any further, consider this conversation:

"We want to do whatever is necessary to give her the best life possible."

It could have been said by two parents talking about a newborn that has a medical condition requiring surgery. It could be any conversation about any loved one. In the case I am about to relate, it involved two children and their mother as they considered the options of a progressive debilitating illness. In counsel with them, I assumed I knew what those words meant, but then it occurred to me that I was making a pretty big assumption. It was also a concept I would be revisiting soon enough as I contemplated some decisions regarding my own parent's adjustment to living arrangements just a few years later.

In each of the theoretical situations I referred to above, the one quality that was common to each group was the subject's health. So it makes sense that we dedicate a little time to thinking about what the word *health* really means.

Think about it. You can be in the worst, most calamitous situation possible—plane crash, hospital admission, whatever—you can have your house swallowed by a sinkhole at the very moment that an errant twister sucks up every amphibian in a local pond and then deposits them on your head in a veritable plague of frogs, while at the same time, a fiery meteorite crashes down on your prized bed of petunias—and as sure as you're born, some nitwit will offer the most offensive consolation statement ever.

He'll say, usually with some big smile, "Well, at least you have your health!"

If you are like me, you'll have to stifle the urge right then to exhibit how vigorous your health is by socking him squarely in the head.

I almost hate to say it, but he is right. Health is important stuff when you consider it in the grand scheme of "life."

Now as we get started, you should understand that I am also making a distinction between the terms *health* and *health care*. While there is some overlap (health care is a component of health, and, in fact, good health care contributes to the prevention of disease and addresses illness early to maintain health), the true concept of health is a much greater enterprise.

"Health" has a number of definitions. The World Health Organization defines it as "a state of complete physical, mental, and social well-being and not merely the absence of disease or infirmity." Webster likes "the condition of being of sound body, mind, or spirit."

There are a bunch of other definitions, but these are a good start at understanding the idea of health.

So what determines if someone is healthy? A number of factors, obviously. Some are super apparent. Others are more abstract. According to the Centers for Disease Control and Prevention (CDC), the determinants of health are "the factors that contribute to a person's current state of health. These factors may be biological, socioeconomic, psychosocial, behavioral, or social in nature. Scientists generally recognize five determinants of health of a population."

So what are the big five determinants of *your* health? For the purposes of our exploration in this book, they are biology and genetics, behavior, physical environment, social or psychological environment, and access to healthcare services.

The Big Five

Biology and genetics
Behavior
Physical environment
Social environment
Health services

CHAPTER 1

BIOLOGY AND GENETICS

WHY THE GENE POOL NEEDS
A LIFEGUARD!

If you ever took a biology course, you know the story of Gregor Mendel, the friar that discovered and articulated the principles of genetics. While farmers and herdsmen had known for centuries that selective breeding produced desired results in livestock and plants, he was the first to describe the dominant and recessive traits and how they worked.

Genetics is the fixed determinant that affects our health. Think about it. You can change your jeans, but not your genes, right? Genetics determines our sex and the illnesses and issues that follow. It also reflects racial inheritance, which carries certain potential for some medical conditions. African Americans and sickle cell predisposition, thalassemias in Jewish populations, or differing racial response to certain antihypertensive regimens serve as some obvious examples. Genetics can also provide for certain illness potentials regardless of race or ethnicity, and while that is important for all ages, it is ever more critical as we age.

Take familial hyperlipidemia, for example. This is a condition that is inherited and causes fatty plaque deposits to occur earlier and more heavily in those with the condition than it does for people who do not have the gene. Why does this matter? Well, you've heard of cholesterol, triglycerides, and "bad fats"? You may have even heard your healthcare provider express concern. It's because these fats can build up (as plaques) and block blood flow to vital organs, like your heart. So unless you don't mind early debilitation and death, you might want to address certain behaviors and avail yourself of access to health care to monitor or take therapeutic and preventative action as needed.

For an aging person this takes on even more importance. Why?

Well, in the spirit of the first book in the series, let's look at the human in terms of the review of bodily systems and consider how each of them changes as you pass the age of fifty. To help with that, keep in mind the words of that great 20th-century philosopher, Popeye, whose famous line "I am what I am" could have been the perfect introduction to this first chapter.

Now, I know I could write this chapter without using any "medical" terms, but that wouldn't be useful to you. Your healthcare providers will surely use technical language—probably most of the time. So with that in mind, when I use a term, I'll explain what it means so that they don't have to. This will make your future conversations with your provider less introductory and more substantial in informing and serving your health.

Metabolism: Welcome to Science Class

Aside from genetics, at the heart of everything biological are the qualities and changes in our *metabolism*, the fire of our physical engine. This affects all aspects of our bodies. Metabolism ranges from the way we assimilate and burn nutrients to our physical composition, including the fat-versus-muscle balance. This latter aspect can change dramatically even when there are no readily evident changes in the shape or structure of what we see in the mirror. That also leads us to the basic building unit of our body, the cell.

In *Metaphysics* the Greek critic, philosopher, physicist, and zoologist Aristotle said, "The whole is greater than the sum of its parts." Conceptually, that is going to be something you will want to keep in mind as we explore this entire section. At the most basic level, we are simply a collection of cells—specialized, synchronous, and synergistic, we hope.

Some cells have a high turnover rate, originating, living, and then dying in a relatively short period of time. This generally applies to cells with more accelerated or dynamic metabolic function. In a sense, the more rapidly the "machinery" of a cell has to work, the sooner it tends to wear out. Think skin, blood cells, mucus membranes (the moist tissue lining the mouth), the lining of the gastrointestinal tract... stuff like that.

A classic illustration of this is the red blood cell. Red blood cells carry oxygen from the lungs to the various cells of the body via an iron atom incorporated in the molecule hemoglobin. They originate in the red blood cell nursery of the bone marrow and take about seven days to mature. I always imagine an extremely chaotic puberty for red blood cells, but I guess that is necessary considering that they only live about 120 days. That said, you really do have all new red blood cells every four months or so, so the next time someone looks at you at lunch and says, "What's different about you?" you can answer, "Well, I have all new erythrocytes, and I just bought this tie."

Anyway, that's rapid turnover.

Other cells are much more permanent. They are usually less metabolically dynamic and have more of an "infrastructural" function. To put this in context, the following helps illustrate what I mean in terms of the differences of cell life spans:

- Brain cells of the cerebral cortex (the gray matter) are, for the most part, with you from birth.
- Brain cells of the visual cortex (the cells in the back of the brain that process input from the eyes) are also with you from birth.
- Some brain cells of the cerebellum (the structures at the base of the brain) are slightly younger than you are.
- Intercostal muscle cells (between the ribs) are about 15 years old.
- Gastrointestinal *lining* cells are about 5 days old.
- Other gastrointestinal cells can be about 15 years old.

Old cells eventually die, sometimes because they are programmed to do so (genetics), sometimes because of injury (including toxins or other environmental insults), and at other times due to a disease process. Genetically programmed death is called apoptosis. There are a number of factors that affect this triggered end of life. Since a cell replicates by division, some cells reach a maximum number of divisions. This is determined by an organelle or structure known as a *telomere*. Telomeres move the cell's genetic material in preparation for cell division. Each time a cell divides, the telomere shortens. Eventually, it becomes too short and the cell can no longer divide.

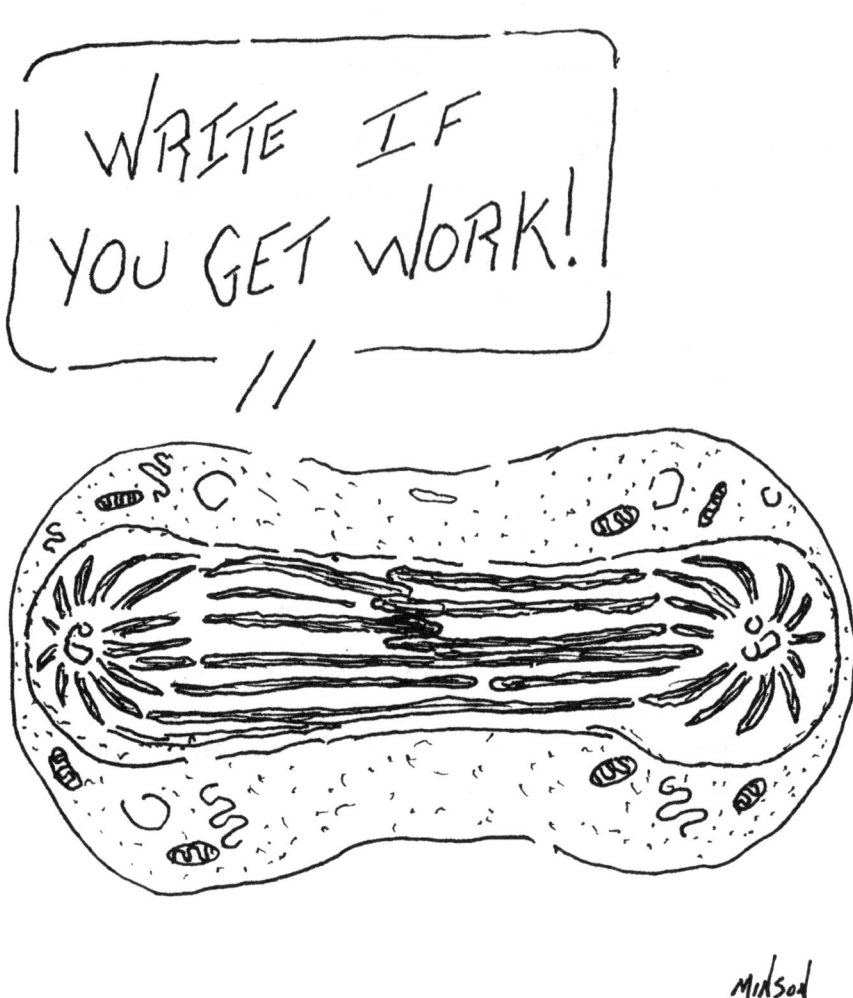

Now, while I am taking the fatalistic view that cell death—and in the long run, our death—is inevitable, there are groups that advocate that this may not always have to be the case.

ENTER, SENS

In 2013 in the *Time* Tech Exclusive "*Google vs. Death,*" Larry Page announced Calico, a new Google firm focusing on the challenges of health care, aging, and associated diseases. Arthur D. Levinson, chairman and former CEO of Genentech, chairman of Apple, and director of Hoffmann-La Roche, was announced as CEO and a founding investor with an intention to focus on early-stage, proof-of-concept research as a nonprofit in conjunction with the Strategies for Engineered Negligible Senescence (SENS) Research Foundation.

Loosely interpreted, that describes an effort to slow the aging process at the most basic, cellular level. Among the many areas of focus, they are looking at the factors affecting telomeric performance.

But as I said earlier, there are many other factors that impact a cell's lifespan. Injuries that kill cells may result from external factors, like burns or other trauma, or it may be due to byproducts of normal metabolism. Some of these byproducts are known as free radicals. Now, I always think that sounds like something you might find on the Berkeley campus of my medulla oblongata, but that's just me. Free radicals are given off when cells produce energy. This occurs in a cellular structure called the mito-chondria, which is commonly known as the powerhouse of the cell.

When I am dealing with a student and we are discussing an illness or pathology, I usually start off by asking, "What three basic things does a cell need to function?" I'm pretty predictable, so most have the quick answer, "Oxygen, fuel, and water."

SOME GUYS LIKED A BIG NUCLEUS, SOME WENT GAGA OVER GREAT MITOCHONDRIA, BUT JOEY HAD ALWAYS BEEN A SUCKER FOR A GREAT SET OF PSEUDOPODS

That is remarkably simplistic, but it is actually true. Nowhere in the body is the illustration of that principle more apparent than when you consider the brain. The basic operative cell of the brain is called a neuron. A neuron, and thus the brain, requires a constant, balanced supply of oxygen, water, and fuel to keep you thinking and making sense, especially when you are writing a book about aging issues.

The other day a patient reported that she had been at lunch and had begun slurring her words and appeared to not comprehend what her husband was saying to her. By the time she and I were speaking, the symptoms had abated, and her sense of humor—which was pretty good—had returned, as she added the phrase "even more than usual" to the admission that she had not comprehended her husband.

Of course, the possibility of a stroke was considered, but to the credit of the EMS personnel that responded, tests for other factors such as blood sugar levels (fuel) and an evaluation of her oxygenation and an electrocardiogram were obtained. She was actually suffering from an abnormal, intermittent slowing of the heart rate—an arrhythmia known as bradycardia—and that caused an abnormally low blood pressure and thus inadequate delivery of blood flow to the brain. This is called hypoperfusion, and for the very demanding human brain, even that momentary interruption of oxygen, fuel, and water delivery had caused a major shutdown of function.

So what happened? Happily, the condition was recognized and treated in time, and the patient recovered.

So that's it! Cells matter, and as they go, so do we. Taking the concept a little further, similar groups of cells constitute the different types of tissues and organs. Organs work in coordination as systems affecting the body overall, and that leads us back to the consideration of aging effects on different systems and tissues as you rocket past the age of fifty. One thing to keep in mind is that a decline in one organ system's function, whether due to an aging process, injury, or disease, can affect the function of another. For example, if atherosclerosis (fatty buildup) narrows the blood flow to, say, the kidneys or the eyes, then the kidneys will function less effectively and eyesight will be affected. This can then lead to other problems, like metabolic waste buildup—due to kidney failure—affecting the liver or poor eyesight that then leads to an injury.

You get the idea.

Speaking of sensory things, I am reminded of something another patient told me. He had altered the philosophical serenity mantra, commonly attributed to Reinhold Niebuhr, that says "God grant me the serenity to accept the things I cannot change; the courage to change the things I can; and the wisdom to know the difference."

His changes were "God grant me the senility to forget the people I never liked anyway; the good fortune to run into the ones I do; and the good eyesight to tell the difference."

His good-natured philosophy aside, most organs do tend to function less well as we age for the reasons I have already described. Just remember, this is not always because of cell loss or death. In healthy older people, the brain, for example, does not lose that many cells. Losses generally occur more commonly due to insults like a stroke or due to degenerative processes such as Alzheimer's or Parkinson's disease.

The Musculoskeletal System

One of the first systems that tends to show age-related changes is the musculoskeletal system. By that I am referring to muscles, tendons, ligaments, joints, and bones.

HOW BONES CHANGE AFTER 50

Almost everyone is aware that when bones become decalcified and thin, a condition known as osteoporosis occurs. This condition is associated with genetics—there's an increased likelihood due to inherited traits—and, in women, hormonal changes after menopause. Even if someone does not fully develop osteoporosis, both older men and women experience some loss of bone density and strength. That is where the increased risk of fracture lies. This is especially true of certain load-bearing joints and the articulating areas, like where the thighbone or femur angles into the socket of the hip or pelvis, or like the bones in the wrist (the radius and ulna) or the vertebra (bones of the spine).

This makes sense when you consider the likelihood of a fall onto the hands and knees or the dreaded fractured hip and the increased statistical prevalence and risk of that happening as we get older. Of course, other bony structures are just as vulnerable.

When osteoporotic changes take place in the spine, they can cause different problems. Remember what I said about one system affecting another? If degeneration occurs in the upper part of the spine (the cervical spine), the head tends to tip forward, making swallowing and mobility of the head difficult. If the changes take place in the thoracic, or chest, area, then breathing, movement, and posture may be impacted. If the occurrence is in the lower, or lumbar, area, then sitting, rising, and walking may become painfully affected.

But bones are not the only issue. The smooth lining between the bones that keeps them from abrading, or grinding, as they articulate, or touch, is provided by a structure called cartilage. Additionally, there is a tissue called the synovium that lines the joint and secretes a lubricating fluid known as synovial fluid. As we age, our cartilage thins and can be less effective at lubricating and protecting the bony interaction. If this gets bad enough, then a condition known as osteoarthritis (osteo means bony) occurs.

Finally, *ligaments*, which bind joints together (bone to bone), and *tendons*, which allow muscles to attach to bones, tend to lose their flexibility and strength as we age. This reduces range of motion and flexibility. Because the blood supply to these types of structures is lower compared to highly metabolic tissues, they also tend to heal more slowly when they are injured. On top of that, the cells in these structures are less metabolically active, so some of their inherent architecture and resilience is lost and thus injury is more likely to happen.

HOW MUSCLES CHANGE AFTER 50

Now, what I am about to say really bugs me, personally. Admittedly it's an ego thing. Around the age of 30, the amount of muscle tissue (mass) and strength begin to decrease, and the decrease continues throughout the rest of our lives. For most people muscle, mass and strength decline no more than 10–15 percent during our lifetime. This does not just apply to those big bulky muscles that we see flexing, enlarging, and inspiring envy at the gym.

The heart is also a muscle with unique properties, as are the tiny muscles of the eye or the smooth muscle of the gastrointestinal tract.

There is a really funny quote by Jarod Kintz that always comes to mind when I talk about the tiny muscles of the eye. He said "I consider conversations with people to be mind exercises, but I don't want to pull a muscle, so I stretch a lot. That is why I'm constantly either rolling my eyes or yawning."

I've tried using that in really boring settings, but I just can't seem to sell it. Maybe you will have better luck.

Anyway, this decline in muscular integrity occurs for a number of reasons, not the least of which are youthful injury, general health, diet, maintenance activities, and decreasing levels of certain hormones like testosterone. Now this last point may sound like I am speaking exclusively about men, but I'm not. Both women and men have circulating levels of "male and female" hormones. The differences are related to a bunch of factors like their underlying health, receptor tissues, and the amounts of those hormones.

In my youth I was something of an athlete with, at best, mediocre skills. Like many, my ambitions far exceeded my talent. As a result, I often overextended and I sustained some injuries. Fortunately, I am not a tobacco user and have never been a drug or alcohol abuser. Well, actually, that is a lie. I am notoriously dependent on caffeine, but other than that, I'm clean.

Anyway…

Now, as I am aging, I find that exercise has taken on less of an ambitious, vain tone and is more a maintenance mechanism for survival and quality of life. Now days when I exercise, I spend the time I should have indulged in my youth in stretching exercises and am even more focused on balancing cardiovascular work with strength training. Also, the cooling-down or postworkout period is as important as the exertional effort. I find that this often has a great deal to do with reducing and guarding against further injury and exacerbation of inflammation in arthritic joints.

Regarding injury, the human body has a fairly nifty mechanism for refilling injured or inactive tissue spaces, and three components are generally in play: calcium, fat, and collagen or scar tissue. The deposition of those materials and the chemical reactions in our bodies to those types of injuries are referred to, at least initially, as inflammation. Obviously, certain diseases can affect this sort of reaction.

So what can you do to maintain the integrity of your musculoskeletal system? A number of things. The most immediate that comes to mind has to do with behavior, which will be covered in the next chapter. Remember, our description of health included five things: genetics, behavior, physical and psychosocial environment, and access to health care. We will get to all of them.

The Eyes

The eyes are really amazing structures. The windows to soul and all that aside, they are our primary means for interacting, interpreting, and engaging with our world. Considered structurally, they are impressive interactions of specialized structure, muscle, and neurological tissues. The cornea (external layer), the lens, and the retina translate light and motion into the brain's interpretation of what we think of as *sight*.

I mentioned earlier the example of the interrelationship between the circulatory system and the eyes. In fact, when a healthcare provider looks at the back for your eye with an ophthalmoscope (that weird light) he or she is really getting a good look at the blood vessels, too. This can reveal early indications that diseases of the circulatory system are occurring. As we age, certain changes tend to occur to the eyes, regardless of the blood supply.

These changes include vision itself and the adjustments of vision or accommodation. Accommodation sounds very genteel, I know, but in medicine it refers to the ability of the muscles of the eye to "reshape" the eye so that it can adjust and focus on something from near to far and back again. For most people somewhere around the age of 40, certain changes in the ability to read in low light—not that anyone of any age should do that—and to read "up close" tends to diminish. Likewise, the ability to adjust to changes in distant-to-near and close-to-far vision is reduced. There are a number of reasons for that. Some are related to age and include properties of the eye and properties of components of the eye. So let's take them by composition of the eye.

The lens of the eye becomes stiffer after 50. This actually begins at 40 and progresses. Obviously, this affects the way the muscles of the eye change its shape to allow sharper focus. This is especially applicable to close-in focus becoming more difficult. This condition is known as presbyopia. That always sounds like a religious denomination to me, albeit one with extremely large-print hymnals, or like a condition exclusive to Protestants. It's not. It is an equal-opportunity disorder. How's that for fairness?

This condition explains the massive sales of "readers" among the over-50 set. If you are particularly unfortunate and have an astigmatism, or an irregularity in the curvature of the eye, your presbyopia may require bifocal lenses or glasses with variable-focus capability.

At the same time that the lens is becoming stiffer, it also starts to get denser and darker. Think about looking through a clear, transparent window versus stained glass. For that reason, more light—three times the amount, in fact—is generally necessary for a 50- or 60-year-old to see letters on a page with the same clarity experienced by a 20-year-old.

Repeat after me: "Lousy kids with their working eyes and funny taste in clothes."

The pupil is a small circular (in most people) black spot in the center of the colored part of the eye, which is called the iris. That is, of course, unless you are W. C. Fields. His eyes were mostly colored, a sort of pinkish bloodshot color, in fact. For most healthy people, however, just the iris has color. There is a small muscle surrounding the pupil that regulates the entry of light to the interior of the eye. Like all muscles, it tends to react with a little less vigor and speed as we age. This may result in decreased efficiency in adjustments to light changes. As a result of that, focus and vision may be compromised—think entering and exiting tunnels—or going in and out of the house. This is important to remember when driving or when tricky footing or slick surfaces in shadow and light environments may be encountered.

Yes, all you skiers, I am talking to you!

Functionally, the most involved part of the eye is the retina, a group of specialized cells on the concave-shaped back of the eye. This is where the external function of the eye transitions to the neurological, or brain-oriented, function of vision. It is where the receptor cells, known as rods and cones, are located. They "trigger" based on light (the rods) and color (the cones) into electrical impulses that move along the optic nerve to be interpreted in the back part of the brain as images.

So when you see something, it is because light is passing through the pupil to "project" onto the retina like those overhead projectors that anyone that attended junior high in the seventies will remember. Then a bunch of cells fire off signals that are carried by a big nerve to the brain, which makes sense of it all.

You *see* what I mean? Sorry, I couldn't resist writing that.

As we age, the number of rods and cones and some other elements are reduced. This affects a number of things, including depth perception. It also explains why certain color combinations, like black letters against a blue background, may be more difficult to see.

Just for what it's worth, as we age, some people will see occasional dots or specks that cross or float across their field of vision. These dark specks or *floaters* can be normal, but if they suddenly change or increase or begin interfering with vision, you should see your healthcare provider immediately. Similarly, if you start seeing flashes of light or experience any sudden changes in vision, seek emergency care.

The Ears

According to the National Institutes of Health (NIH), it is estimated that one-third of individuals between 65 and 75 have some degree of hearing loss. Just like with the eyes, the ears are often best considered with their composition in mind. The external ear is everything you can see from the outside and includes the canal down to the eardrum, or tympanic membrane. The most common cause of hearing loss associated with the external ear is due to earwax or *cerumen* blockage. I hope you aren't reading this over lunch, by the way.

Now I know what you are probably thinking. Earwax? Holy Hopping Catfish, how embarrassing, that's terrible. It's true, though. Cerumen buildup is very common and often so gradual that is not detected until the "wax" has hardened and become impacted. You shouldn't jump to the conclusion that this is an indication of some failure of hygiene. It can be due to abnormalities of the external ear and canal, so you shouldn't necessarily be embarrassed. The good news is that it is extremely easy to correct and only requires a simple physical examination by a healthcare provider to detect.

The tympanic membrane is where the first action of hearing occurs. Sound waves carried on the air encounter the membrane and move or vibrate it, depending on the frequency of the sound wave. Think of this like a drum head or an old woofer on a stereo speaker.

The area of the ear from the tympanic membrane to the sensory organ of hearing, the cochlea, is known as the middle ear. The middle ear contains three tiny bones commonly known as the hammer, anvil, and stirrup, which move or articulate with the action of the tympanic membrane and translate the energy or force to the cochlea.

Issues that lead to hearing loss associated with the middle ear include injuries to the eardrum such as trauma, like ruptures, punctures, or infections. Other disease processes can impede the function of the tiny bones and can also reduce hearing and the differentiation of the range of sounds.

Everything else, from the cochlea to the otic nerve, which carries electrical information to the brain for interpretation, constitutes the inner ear. Just like in the eye, where the retina provides the transformation of external representations of vision (light, shape, and movements) to electrical signals processed by the brain, sound is transformed to electrical stimuli that are interpreted by the brain. Within the cochlea are thousands of tiny hairlike structures that help translate sound vibrations through nerve cells into corresponding electrical signals that are transmitted to your brain. The vibrations of different sounds affect these tiny "hairs" in different ways, causing the nerve cells to send different signals to your brain. That's how you distinguish one sound from another.

Deafness and hearing impairments that occur due to compromise of the inner ear, nerves, or brain are generally known as *sensorineural deafness*. Broadly speaking, this is different from conditions that affect the middle and external ear, which are generally known as conductive (conduction) deafness. Often the causes of sensorineural deafness are exposure to loud noises, disease, illness, toxicities, or certain drug side effects.

As we age, some hearing loss occurs regardless of exposure to noise, though that certainly is the most common cause. The most common change is the loss of range or presbycusis.

When I was a boy, the very old husband of a married couple that had been together for half a century pointed out that he had lost the ability to hear the upper range of sound while his wife had seemingly lost the lower register.

"That way," he said, "I can't hear her when she rants and she can't hear me when I growl."

He attributed it to divine wisdom. His wife said it proved that God was a woman.

No matter who or what is responsible, certain sounds and frequencies become more difficult to detect. An example may be in the sharpness or brightness of music. This inevitably leads to some difficulty with communication as words may also be harder to understand. Oddly enough, one of the more common features of presbycusis is that consonants tend to drop while the vowels of the word remain. This is thought to be due to the fact that consonants are generally higher-pitched while vowels are of a lower register. Additionally, difficulties differentiating sound also occur. This usually presents as the inability to hear something you normally can when there is background noise. If, for example, you can't understand words you normally can when you are in a noisy restaurant, then sound differentiation may be the problem.

If you are noticing that everyone you talk with seems to be mumbling or you can't seem to understand people when out in public venues, then it might be worth getting an inexpensive audiogram and seeing your healthcare provider. The easiest way to do this is just explain to your healthcare provider that you want one. They'll refer you, or you could just look up an audiologist and arrange it on your own.

The Nervous System

I have already covered two of the bigger sensory elements with the discussion of vision and hearing, and it is worth repeating that all of our biological systems are interdependent. Just like the musculoskeletal function is tied to blood flow, an intact auditory apparatus without an intact nerve is nothing. With that in mind, I am going to eventually include smell and taste along with some other generalities in an overview of the nervous system's function.

Arguably, this part of our body is one of the most complex. It is responsible for personality and almost every one of our functions on a daily basis. Keeping that complexity in mind, you can imagine that a lot can go wrong. So it helps for you to know how it works.

Classically, structurally, the nervous system is thought of as the brain and spinal column or cord. This is the central nervous system, but there is an additional part that connects the rest of the body to the central nervous system. This is known as the peripheral nervous system. The peripheral nervous system includes the nerves that fire to facilitate muscle contraction and that carry signals of sensation and pain from the skin, muscles, and organs to the spinal cord and then to the brain. With that in mind, functionally, the nervous system can also be distinguished by the terms *somatic* or *motor* and autonomic nervous systems.

The autonomic nervous system is further divided into the sympathetic and parasympathetic nervous system. Sounds very emotional, I know, but stay with me.

The main function of the sympathetic nervous system is to mobilize the body's response under stressful circumstances. Thus, the sympathetic nervous system initializes the "fight or flight" response of the body. The sympathetic system innervates many different organs of the body, such as the eyes, lungs, kidneys, gastrointestinal tract, heart, and so on. It causes an increase in the heart rate and in the rate of certain hormones and secretions. One such secretion is a chemical known as renin from the kidneys. There is also stimulation of the release of glucose from the liver, which is released into the blood so as to make it available for use by the body. Remember what I said about fuel? Well, glucose is the primary fuel for a cell. You need that when it's a matter of "fighting or flighting."

The parasympathetic nervous system is the part of the autonomic nervous system that is responsible for the "rest and digest" or steady-state phase of the body. The nerves of this system send fibers to cardiac muscles, smooth muscles like the bladder and intestines, and to glandular tissues as well. The parasympathetic nervous system is also responsible for bringing about an increase in salivation, tear production, urination, digestion, and defecation. The basic parasympathetic system involves functions and actions that do not require an immediate reaction to the surrounding environment. So it is just the opposite of "fight or flight."

To better illustrate this, imagine you are a caveman. If that is not palatable, imagine I am a caveman. That is probably more fitting anyway. So I am sitting in my luxurious, split-level, ranch-style troglo-minium after a successful mammoth hunt, about to eat a delicious mammoth burger. With respect to Fred Flintstone, I couldn't actually be eating a brontosaurus burger since the brontosaurus was already extinct, but if that works better for you, go with that.

In anticipation of my little feast, my parasympathetic system kicks in, preparing to help me assimilate all those yummy mammoth nutrients. As such, my pupils constrict, and my salivary glands begin to secrete since mammoth is a particularly dry dish unless cooked just perfectly. My blood pressure happily lowers, my heart beats at a normal resting rate, and blood shunts away from my muscles and respiratory tract toward my stomach and gastrointestinal tract. As the first morsels of mammoth burger are swallowed, my gallbladder starts to contract to help with digestion.

All is right in my little cave-dwelling world. And then . . .

A pair of glowing eyes appear at the entrance, and I hear a guttural growl. It's my old nemesis the saber-toothed cat, Wendell. He's the same one that ate my brother, Og, last week, and he's not here to take my mammoth burger.

Before I can take another bite, my sympathetic nervous system takes over. My pupils dilate so I can better see where I left my Neanderthalian Nikes (historians, forgive me), since I am probably going to have to run for it. I stop making saliva and my heart rate increases, driving up my blood pressure to supply my heart, my lungs (my bronchial tubes dilate as well), and, of no lesser importance, despite what you may think of me in my caveman persona, my brain. My muscles then become enlarged with blood flow as I prepare to hurl my mammoth burger at Wendell. All the digestive activity comes to a stop, and in an effort to lower the payload should I have to make a run for it, my bowel empties on its own.

How exciting.

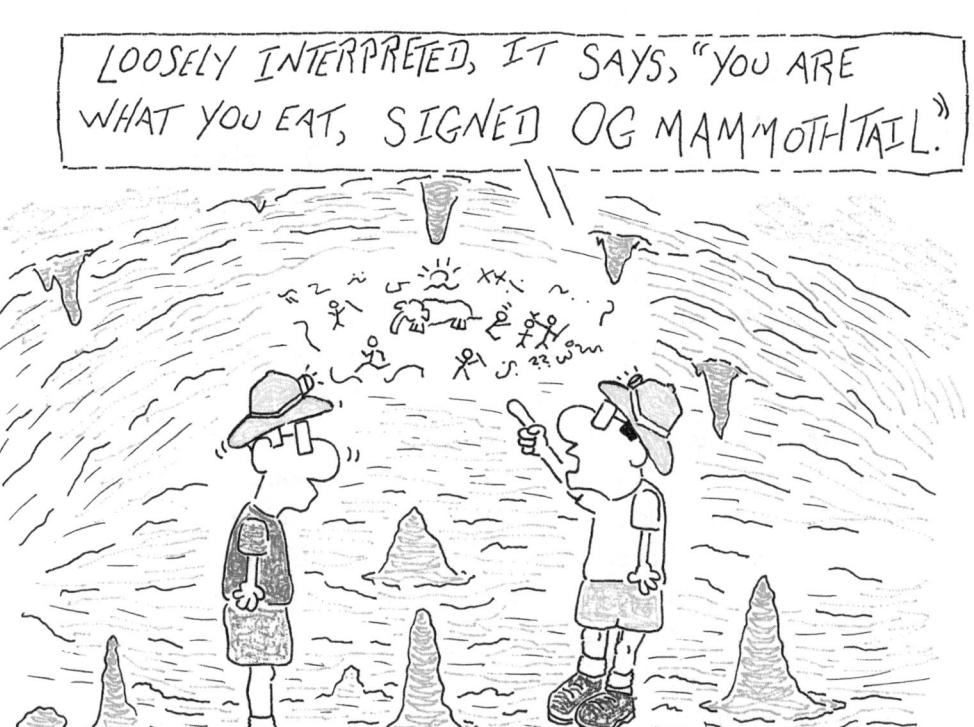

Needless to say, I bet you will remember how the sympathetic and parasympathetic nervous systems balance against each other from now on, huh?

Oh, and by the way, at the same time, upstairs in the brain, other actions undergo a symphony of electrical impulse and hormonal and chemical releases like serotonin, which affects mood, and dopamine, which affects movement and coordination so I can more effectively make my escape.

So, anyway, that's the nervous system.

HOW THE NERVOUS SYSTEM CHANGES AFTER 50

To some degree, the number of brain cells decrease in all of us as we age. Luckily, the brain compensates, at least partially, by making new connections among remaining cells, and new nerve pathways may generate. Fortunately, we start out with many more brain cells than we need in our lifetime, a situation known as redundancy.

With respect to every Spring Breaker on the planet, that doesn't mean it's okay to waste any of them.

In the story earlier about me as Og Mammothtail's brother, I mentioned the chemical or neuroendocrine transmitters. As we age, the levels and availability of those compounds decrease in some cases while increasing for others. Synapses, the spaces between nerve endings (think of the firing of spark plugs), also function less efficiently. Overall blood flow tends to decrease, and so the brain tends to function less effectively.

I can feel it even as I am typing.

At about the age of 60, the number of cells in the spinal cord also begins to decrease. This usually does not cause a change in strength or balance, but if certain disease processes occur, these changes can aggravate them.

Other senses such as taste and smell change as well. As with the ears and eyes, the structure of the organs affects the neurological function of vision and hearing. So it is with the tongue, the palate, and the nose. One interesting note: this loss of sensitivity actually leads some people to over-salt their food in attempt to overcome blandness. This often makes the control of hypertension or high blood pressure even more challenging.

The Teeth and Gums

Teeth are pretty fascinating things. You can use them to do all kinds of useful stuff. Some, like the incisors, are effective at tearing open potato chip bags and can even open beer bottles, though that tends to void the warranty. It also makes your dentist simultaneously unhappy and ecstatic, as he or she chastises you for being a nitwit and envisions the potential of sending you a large bill. They are also really good at (and probably better suited to) tearing off a hunk of mammoth or baked potato, whereas the canines, the more prominent of the frontal teeth, are extremely important to vampires. I'm kidding, of course. The canines are vestigial defensive structures according to anthropologists, so except for feral children, they are best considered like the incisors for tearing and cutting mammoth burgers or your favorite veggie wrap.

Premolars, including the bicuspids—or "the next group of teeth back," as I like to think of them—are good at breaking things into smaller morsels. Then the big boys or molars are the kings of the daily grind, pulverizing the food prior to swallowing.

What they all have in common is a critical link to your overall health. Since I have talked about everything else in terms of composition, I'll do the same here.

Basically, teeth can be considered in terms of the root and the crown. The crown is, as you would expect, the part above the gum line. The root is below, but it also has a communicating component within the crown. The crown is composed of three parts: the enamel, the dentin, and the pulp. Enamel, which covers the tooth, is one of the hardest compounds on the planet. This stuff can make a diamond look like a wimp, and yet over a lifetime even enamel can deteriorate. Underneath the enamel is a substance called dentin. And you thought that was a cinnamon-flavored gum.

Dentin is a mineralized, almost bone-hard, porous material. Cementum is a similar substance that binds the tooth, and the pulp is the chamber at the center that contains the nerve endings and blood vessels, which continue down into the root and beyond. That is really important, because it illustrates how integrated our teeth are to our circulatory system, nervous system, and the rest of the body, and thus, our overall health.

Given how that echoes everything else I've described by anatomical system, you are probably seeing a theme here. Everything relies on something else. It is all connected. Like the energy of the universe or the fundamental concept of *Star Wars*, it is all one big system. So whether you prefer Yoda, or Buddha for that matter, everything—at least in the body—is one big continuum of energy and function. So with that in mind, I can't talk about teeth without also including the gums and the mouth. Now, I like to garden, so I always see the gums and the soft moist tissues of the mouth like the garden bed—made up of tissues instead of earth, but with water, nutrients, and the like—and the teeth are kind of like the crop. The gums are also highly vascular, meaning enriched with a lot of blood vessels and very delicate. They are sensitive to injury, insult, and neglect. Like many other parts of the body, they require a lot of care. Bacteria, toxins like tobacco, acidic foods, and more take their toll and can result in degeneration and disease if not properly and regularly addressed. In particular, I am talking about the onset of inflammatory conditions. Inflammation and infection of the gum is called gingivitis. This inflammation can lead to deterioration, and a disease of the teeth is called . . . surprise, decay. We think of this as the dentist telling us we have a cavity. Cavities are known as caries. Cavities can occur anywhere that the tooth is exposed along the gum line. Ironically, as we age, more of the tooth becomes exposed. There are several reasons for that.

HOW TEETH AND GUMS CHANGE AFTER 50

I've spent a lot of time talking about the teeth and supporting structures for a reason. It's often been said that eyes are windows to the soul. If that is the case, then I would offer that the teeth are the entryway. All you have to do is take a look at every famous list of "turn-ons and turn-offs" and you'll see what I mean. Outside of puppies, kittens, and positive attitudes, good teeth reign supreme. I think there is an evolutionary reason for that. A bunch of studies of nonverbal communication show that the way something is communicated is just as important as what is communicated in making an impact. The smile and the emotional effect of that are, rightly or wrongly, integral. If you've ever watched an old western or pirate movie, you'll know that all the really cool cowboys and pirates have good teeth.

The bad guys . . . well, there you go.

And it goes without saying, we all want to be cool pirates.

One of the biggest changes as we age is the decreased ability of the mouth to produce saliva. This drying promotes the process of bacterial growth and the formation of plaque, hard bacterial deposits that adhere to the tooth and act like little acid factories that continue to wear on the enamel. Add to that the lack of regular brushing and flossing and you get a perfect setup for degeneration and disease. Some of the things you should look for are persistent bad breath, discoloration, and a retreating gum line. Think Austin Powers and you get the idea. Now, I know I am dedicating some real attention to teeth and the mouth, but that's because they really are great indicators of systemic problems. Changes to the circulatory system, immune system, nutritional status, reflux disease, hygiene, and more are easily shown in the teeth and mouth. So what do you say?

Put your money, or at least some effort, where your mouth is, and let's all just try to remain really cool pirates.

The Cardiovascular System

The heart has always had a certain mythology and romanticism about it. I guess the reasons are obvious. It's the organ that reassures us by its constant, faithful pumping. It shows changes with our emotions and skips a beat at just the right moment with just the right person. We identify it as the organ that exemplifies who we "really" are. So everybody knows it's important. Not to minimize the work of every romantic in history, but my celebration of its importance here is slightly more, well, practical.

Even with such a clinical orientation in mind, the magnificence of the heart and the circulatory system is no less impressive. A hollow-chambered muscular structure the size of your fist starts a coordinated, sequential, electrical firing well before we are born, and its end is the defining act at the end of life. During the interval it varies with the requirements of everything from fight or flight to the anxious reactions of a first kiss.

Take our caveman scenario, for example. When Wendell the sabertoothed cat was contemplating making me his next meal, sudden outflows of my neuroendocrine system along with the sympathetic track began to fire. This stimulated the electrical system in my heart, causing it to beat faster to provide increased blood flow to certain parts of my body. This would really help whether I needed to throw my mammoth burger or run like crazy. See, it's all connected. Sounds really Yoda-like, doesn't it?

The heart's cardiac muscle fibers themselves are unlike muscle fiber anywhere else in the body, able to sustain constant activity without rest. To that end, and much like the brain, the heart is pretty unforgiving when blood flow is interrupted or blocked. The most common example of that is when a coronary artery is plugged by a plaque, as in the condition known as atherosclerosis, or by a clot associated with coronary artery disease.

I have already indicated how important blood flow is to every other system in the body. The delivery of the three critical elements of fuel, oxygen, and water depend on it. For that reason, the heart and blood vessels need to be considered together. Basically, the components of the circulatory system are divided by those parts that deliver oxygenated blood to the tissues and those that return deoxygenated or depleted blood back to the heart.

The outflow from the heart passes through a monster-sized J-shaped blood vessel known as the aorta. From there, blood goes through a bunch of branches that carry it to different parts of the body. As the arteries narrow, they are called arterioles, and then they shrink to tiny vessels known as capillaries. This is where the little oxygen-carrying structures called hemoglobin offload oxygen to the cells and pick up carbon dioxide and metabolic waste products for the return trip.

On the way back, capillaries become veinules, then veins, then bigger veins like the vena cava, Latin for "hollow vein". This is like the return version of the aorta and feeds the deoxygenated blood into the heart. It is pumped from there to the lungs where the carbon dioxide is exchanged for oxygen, and the whole thing starts again.

I had a patient, a plumber, who was having problems with varicose veins and some other problems, including fatty plaque formations in his arteries that affected the circulation in his legs. Knowing what that meant, I was concerned that he might also have some vascular (blood vessel) issues elsewhere in his body. He was a really smart guy, and after hearing my long, drawn-out description of the circulatory system and how the blood vessels were all so interconnected, he said, "So, it's just like the plumbing in the house? If you have problems in the basement, you probably have problems upstairs and in the attic, too."

The man was a genius.

Since I mentioned atherosclerosis and we are considering genetics and biology, I wanted to devote a little bit of time to consideration of this condition. Now what we are going to talk about happens on the arterial side of the circulatory system. Each artery is composed of an interior layer called the "intima" or endothelium—personally, I wish it were called the IN-dothelium, but no Latin-speaking anatomist asked me. This is a really delicate layer. Surrounding it is a layer called the media (thank goodness, that sort of makes sense). The media is a ring of muscle that is important in things like high blood pressure (when it goes wrong) and maintaining proper blood flow (done right) to the other organ systems. The outer layer of connective tissue is called the externa.

I have nothing really interesting to say about the externa. So… moving on….

THE CIRCULATORY SYSTEM

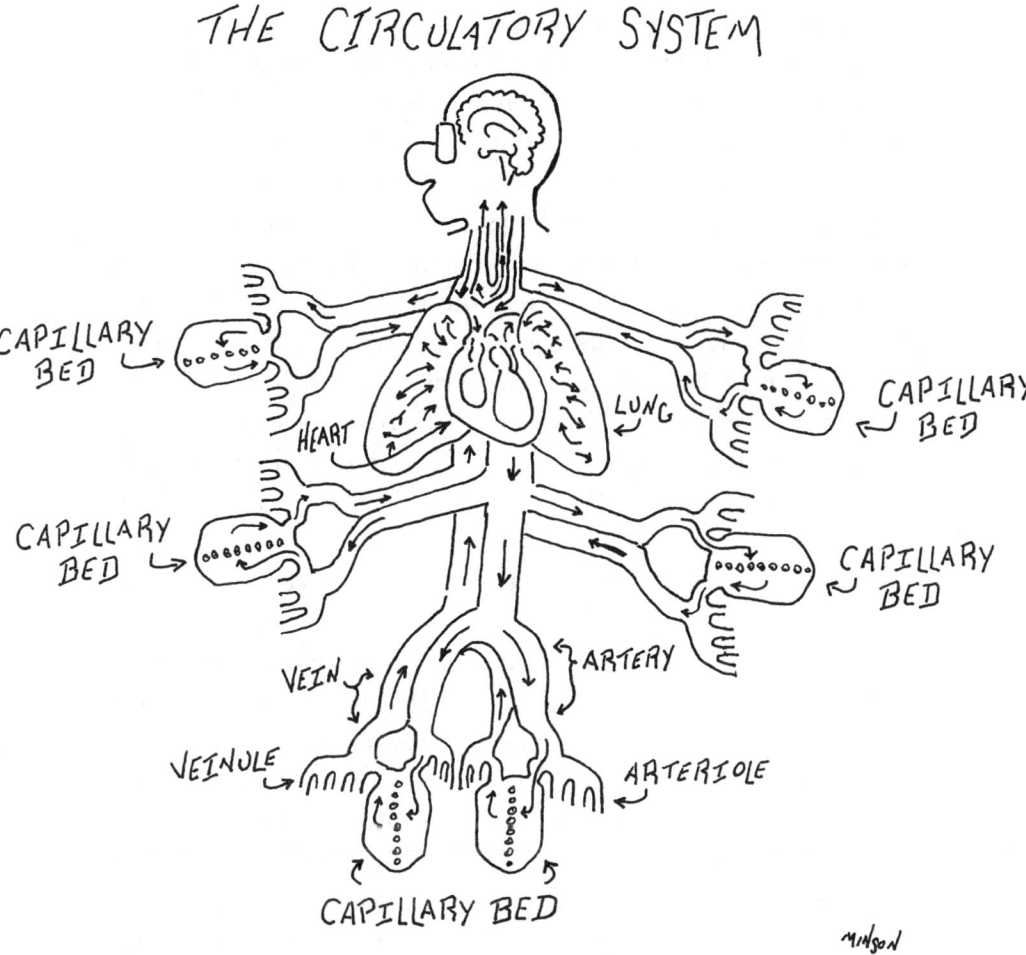

CAPILLARY BED

CAPILLARY BED

HEART

LUNG

CAPILLARY BED

CAPILLARY BED

VEIN

ARTERY

VEINULE

ARTERIOLE

CAPILLARY BED

MINSON

When there is damage to the endothelium due to high blood pressure, drug use, smoking, or other conditions, deposits of "bad" cholesterol and fat can form. The body reacts with an inflammatory response of white blood cells that try to cover the deposit. Over time this can accumulate to become a buildup—like an arterial speed bump—of cellular material, fat, and other "stuff" (not an actual scientific term) to become a plaque. If this keeps going, and generally it will, the speed bump or plaque gets bigger and bigger and the internal diameter of the artery gets narrower and narrower. If it gets big enough or tears loose and forms a clot, blocking the artery, no blood flow can get through.

At this point you don't need me to tell you, this is bad. If it happens in certain metabolically sensitive or needy tissues or systems, like the brain or the heart, then a stroke or heart attack (a myocardial infarction or M.I.) occurs. Now, you may hear a number of terms used by your healthcare provider for atherosclerotic disease (athero—you know what that means, sclerotic—narrowing or limiting), such as "hardening of the arteries" or, depending on the area in the body, peripheral vascular disease or coronary (heart) artery disease and finally cerebro (cerebro=brain) vascular disease. In most people, atherosclerotic disease becomes an issue in middle age; however, for some others, due to genetic conditions (remember familial hyperlipidemia?), it may present much earlier. If people in your family have a history of cardiovascular events or deaths due to heart attack or stroke in their 30s or 40s, you should make certain to inform your health-care provider and request early testing.

HOW THE CARDIOVASCULAR SYSTEM CHANGES AFTER 50

For most people, the issues described in the discussion of atherosclerosis begin to manifest around the age of 50. Hopefully most discover their issues due to cholesterol and lipid values on laboratory examinations arising from routine annual physical examinations with their primary care providers before they show symptoms. In the "Access to Health Care" chapter I'll discuss alternative methods to monitoring those numbers and values if access to a healthcare provider is a challenge.

In any case, as we pass the age of 50, certain physiological or inevitable changes occur, other than just the accumulation of plaque. For one thing, the efficiency of the heart as a muscular pump decreases. The heart's blood-pumping chambers don't fill as quickly as when we are younger, and the muscular contraction of the big pumping chambers or ventricles is less powerful. If you've ever been on a treadmill at a gym or looked at physical fitness tables, you may have noticed that maximal heart rates during exercise decrease as you age. Now you know the reason for that. This doesn't mean that everyone experiences these changes the same way. In fact, the more physically fit and active a person is, the less likely and impactful these changes are. Proper maintenance and effort can even delay these declines.

Well beyond the heart, the dynamic flexibility of the arteries—remember, this also depends on the nervous system and smooth muscle integrity—decreases so that changes in posture can cause sudden drops in blood pressure. This often manifests as dizziness or even a loss of consciousness or "blacking out" when you stand up suddenly. The term for this is *orthostatic* hypotension (hypo-low). Less blood flow goes to the brain and, well, you already know what that does.

This same sort of thing can occur when an individual valsalvas. This is a medical term for holding your breath as you bear down. Think about how a person compensates during constipation or that weird game some weird kids played during recess when they held their breath and contracted their abdominal muscles until they passed out, and you get the idea. Certain other changes, such as the ability of the artery to accommodate high pressures or increased blood flow when the heart pumps greater volume, also have effects, such as overall increased arterial "tone." Remember that part about the arterial media layer being smooth muscle? Well, when the artery "tries" to compensate continuously or—due to other factors—the tone of the muscle increases, then the arterial pressure can increase. This is one kind of high blood pressure, but it isn't the only kind.

If you recall the description of the aorta-artery-arteriole-capillary-veinule-vein-vena cava-heart circuit, you will remember that the venous side of the circuit is responsible for returning blood to the heart.

The veins don't have the same architecture as the arteries. They don't have as much muscle and the like built in. They utilize the contraction of muscles in the extremities and the pressure and momentum of the blood flow, along with small one way valves in the closed circuit system, to get the blood back around to the heart. Why is this useful information as we consider aging? Again, it goes back to overall health and physical fitness. If the blood collects and remains in the veins, they can distend, becoming unsightly and, even more important, dangerous. Think varicose veins. That's what we are describing. In some cases, when blood stagnates badly enough, it can form a clot. This is called a thrombus. If it is in a big vein of certain depth, it can be very dangerous. If you have ever heard the term deep venous thrombosis (DVT), then you know what we are talking about here. The most common place for this to occur is in the lower leg or calf, though it can happen elsewhere. If it breaks loose and moves to the heart and lungs, it can cause a condition known as a pulmonary embolus. This can actually be quite deadly.

So the heart and blood vessels change as we age. That's inevitable. No matter how hard we try, no matter how fit we continue to be, some decrease in performance is going to happen. This explains why there aren't many 60-year-old NFL rookies of the year or why the heavyweight boxing champion of the world has yet to be a 90-year-old. I'm still holding out hope that eventually Sylvester Stallone will rise from his nursing home as Rocky to take the title again, but even I will admit that's going to be a real challenge to the literary constant of the willful suspension of disbelief. Still, it might be worth watching when it comes on cable.

The Pulmonary System

If you thought the circulatory system was involved, then buckle up, because the pulmonary system is unmatched in its interesting complexity. Now, I know you are about to put the book down when I say that, but it is really crazily interesting so you might want to at least give it a look.

We've all heard the childhood chestnut "in with the good air, out with the bad."

Well, fundamentally that is exactly right. The way that happens involves the airway, the structural pipes, which are divided into the upper and lower airway and muscular and nervous system. The upper airway conducts "good" air through the mouth and nose to the larynx and trachea where the vocal cords and larger "pipes" are. From there, the airway is considered the lower airway. By the way, those pipes are ringed with stiff cartilage and smooth muscle that play a role in the amount of air that passes. The vocal cords exist right about where you feel the hard structure on the front of your neck between the chin and top of the breastbone. This is called the thyroid cartilage (often commonly known as the Adam's apple), in case you were wondering.

Air continues to the right and left bronchial tubes, which then divide into smaller bronchioles. These end in tiny sacs called alveoli, where the "air" exchange takes place with the bloodstream. Remember the description of the tiny blood vessels called capillaries? Well, for purposes of discussion, here is one place they come into play. These little air sacs are very thin and allow oxygen to cross their membrane into the bloodstream via the capillaries. At the same time, carbon dioxide, a metabolic waste product from the tissues that is carried to the heart and lungs by the veins, crosses from the capillaries to the alveoli. So, "in with the good air, out with the bad" really does apply here, except it's in with the oxygen, out with the carbon dioxide. So, now you know how it works. Obviously the airway needs to be clear and open. The lung tissues need to be very elastic, able to expand and contract. And the air sacs need to remain clear.

In something as complicated as this, a lot of things can go wrong. The airway can be blocked by something, like a piece of food. Thank you, Dr. Heimlich!

Farther down, there can be problems with constriction and restriction of the bronchial tubes, which we see with asthma, bronchitis, or chronic obstructive pulmonary disease (COPD). Remember the smooth muscle that makes arteries constrict? Well, that same smooth muscle is here too.

Finally, the alveoli have to be kept clear of fluid, which often accumulates in pneumonia, or other material that could increase the anatomical distance that oxygen and carbon dioxide have to pass for a proper exchange. The other muscles that affect the function of the lung are the diaphragm and the muscles between the ribs. Any failure or decreased function of any of these and the lungs cannot properly engage in respiration. This often results in a person feeling easily fatigued or short of breath.

So there you go. The Pulmonary System 101. Pretty painless, huh?

HOW THE PULMONARY SYSTEM CHANGES AFTER 50

In a healthy person—that is, one who doesn't smoke, engage in bad health habits, or suffer from a genetic or clinical disorder like cystic fibrosis—the pulmonary system should have adequate function to last you to the end of your life. That said, the efficiency of this very dynamic system does decline. This occurs in many ways.

Over time the lung tissue becomes less flexible, decreasing the amount of air that can be used for oxygen–carbon dioxide exchange. It also allows some air to be trapped in the lungs, which decreases the two-gas exchange and makes the act of breathing difficult. The alveoli also can become less elastic, making them loose and baggy. This also adds to the problem.

With air going in, certain toxins and harmful particles like pollution, smoke, germs, and dusts can enter as well. Healthy lungs have self-cleaning and filtering structures, like mucus—a source of unlimited fascination during elementary school—and small hairlike structures called cilia that move the sticky particle-laden mucus toward the throat, nose, and often eventually the playground. As we age, the function of those cilia can also decrease, allowing material to be retained all along the respiratory passage. This in turn decreases the diameter of all parts of the airway. They are also affected by a number of environmental factors (we'll get to that in the chapter on the physical environment) and by certain medications and behaviors.

The ability of the lungs to respond to greater metabolic demands like increased altitude and exercise also decreases. As with other systems, maintaining good health habits, like activity, diet, and regular exercise, preserves as much function as possible.

The Digestive System

You have probably figured out by now that I have the comedic sensibilities of your average ten-year-old, so it shouldn't come as a surprise that I find the gastrointestinal (GI) or digestive system, also known as the alimentary tract, a source of unlimited hilarity. I mean, I subscribe to the maxim that the holy triad of comedy is flatulence, testicular trauma, and anything where a cat makes that distressed sound out of frame. In short, I am an American.

Alternatively embarrassing and offensive, these emanations are part of the processes of the GI system, another veritable anatomical ballet of elegant function and beautiful synchronization.

Now, repeat after me, "Beans, beans, the magical fruit . . ."

Sorry.

The digestive system, like many others, can be considered by its structural composition and by function. Structurally, it starts at the lips and mouth where everything, depending on the age of the owner, from filet mignon to fingernails, goes in. It includes the oral cavity and the esophagus, which terminates in a smooth ringed muscle, the lower esophageal sphincter, which opens onto the stomach. The stomach, which is a curved structure, empties into the first part of the small intestine.

Now here is something interesting and to me pretty arbitrary about human anatomy. The "small intestine" is really misnamed in my opinion. Since there is a small intestine, there just has to be a large intestine, right? Yes, there is. But here's the thing: the small intestine is actually much longer than the large intestine. Much longer! The large intestine is bigger in diameter only. Now, I don't know who was in charge of this decision of nomenclature, but I have had an issue with him or her since the sixth grade.

I've gotten over that, sort of. Anyway, back to the digestive system. The small intestine is divided into the duodenum, where enzymes from the pancreas and the bile duct enter, the jejunum, and then the final segment, the ileum.

The small intestine ends at the beginning of the large intestine or ascending colon in a small outpouching called the cecum. By the way, this is where the appendix is located. The real name for this puzzling, troubling little structure is the vermiform appendix. It's more Latin, as if we hadn't had enough of that already, and means "wormlike." There are lots of opinions regarding the function of the appendix, and I won't belabor them here. Almost everyone, however, agrees that one function is to pay for a surgeon's lake house.

The large intestine includes the previously mentioned ascending colon, rising from the cecum to about the level of the base of the right rib cage, and becomes the transverse colon, which crosses the abdomen to about the level of the left rib cage, where it takes a southward turn to become the descending colon. From there it transitions to the sigmoid colon, then the rectum, and it ends at the anus. That's the end, literally. Poetic, isn't it?

That's the architecture. The function, which I will say, is the other way to appreciate the gut or digestive system and is far more interesting. So let's start with the lips. It's been said (I think by someone French) that the lips are the fingerprint of love and the last barrier against a harsh word. Its function is pretty obvious. At my house, we use it for kissing. From a digestive standpoint it's the voluntary sphincter that keeps food from spilling back out during a meal, elementary cafeterias aside.

From my caveman's perspective, it's the first step in my inevitable processing of a delicious mammoth burger. Alternatively, it is also where Wendell the saber-toothed cat takes in the first tasty morsel of me. The teeth and tongue process the burger, and the tongue manages additional separating and mechanical manipulation. It also provides a nifty, estheti-cally gratifying function of taste. Considering my lengthy dedication to kissing, it's also useful for that too, especially in France. I'll get into that more in the section on the pursuit of happiness, specifically the part about sex. No fair, skipping ahead!

While the structures of the mouth are busy dismantling the burger and the bun, the salivary glands in the cheeks discharge an enzyme called amylase. Amylase is also produced by the pancreas and acts to break down starch. So already in the mouth chemical action is taking place on the burger bun to prepare it for digestion and absorption down the road. When I am finished chewing, I swallow, and the burger or what is left of the burger moves into the esophagus, that long muscular tube that moves food along to the stomach. It does this by a coordinated series of rhythmic contractions called peristalsis. Now this is a really underestimated struc-ture and process. The esophagus has a unique combination of interactive sympathetic and parasympathetic innervation. The major nerve control-ling this process is called the vagus nerve.

Repeat after me: vagus, baby, vagus. Or, as I like to really say, what happens in the esophagus better not stay in the esophagus.

Now the esophagus has another function that is equally important. At the lower end is a ring of muscle called a sphincter, remember? It's the lower esophageal sphincter (LES), to be exact. Finally, something intui-tive. This sphincter prevents acid from washing back up from the stom-ach, a condition also known as reflux. If this condition is chronic, it's known as gastroesophageal reflux disease (GERD). This is a condition that is not only uncomfortable, but it can also potentially be deadly. If it is not addressed over time, the refluxing material can cause damage to the lining of the esophagus and can even lead to cancer.

Once the chewed-up mammoth burger gets into the stomach, the real processing begins to happen. At this point, the burger is now called a bolus. Certain cells in the lining of the stomach release digesting enzymes to break down the bolus so that it can be absorbed and put to work feed-ing our tissues so we can run away from Wendell. One such enzyme is called pepsin. It is a protease, meaning it breaks down proteins, like mam-moth meat. In order for it to work, it has to be activated by acid, which the stomach also produces. At the same time, the muscles of the stomach begin a vigorous peristalsis that mechanically aids in the breakdown of the enzyme-treated food. Now the bolus is called chyme.

My best childhood friend and I first learned about chyme in a junior high biology class. He instantly ruined the classic song "Scarborough Fair" by Simon and Garfunkel for me by inserting the word in the line "parsley, sage, rosemary, and thyme." Even now every time I hear that song I hear "parsley, sage, rosemary, and chyme." And now I have done that for you. Sorry.

The action in the stomach generally takes about an hour before the chyme moves into the next part of the digestive tract. If you think about it, kind of reminds you of what your mom told you about going swimming after eating, huh?

Thanks, Mom.

Now here is an interesting fact. The stomach can actually "sense" the nutritional makeup of food, such as carbohydrates, fats, and protein. This allows the brain to link tastes on the tongue to food content. Beyond the mechanical function, the stomach also has a small amount of absorptive activity. It's nothing like what occurs later in the intestine, but it is worth acknowledging. Water is absorbed, along with caffeine, some medications, and fortunately or unfortunately, depending on your perspective, alcohol. In fact, if you think about that, it explains why, when you are drinking with dinner, generally you feel the effects of alcohol before you get the nutritional benefits of the dinner.

Eventually the chyme moves across another sphincter at the lower end of the stomach, called the pyloric sphincter, into the first part of the intestine. This is where additional enzymes and chemicals that aid in digestion also occur. Three important enzymes are bile (or to use an old term, gall), lipase, and amylase, which I mentioned earlier.

The bile or gall is produced by the liver and collects in a small bag, the gallbladder, and connects to the small intestine by a small tube or duct. So the next time you hear the question, "Where does he get the gall?" you'll have the answer.

"From right under his liver."

These other enzymes I mentioned, lipase and amylase, are made in the pancreas, which also empties in the same area as the gallbladder. You've heard of a gallstone? A lot of people think these are not that big a deal.

Well, they can be. Sometimes if a stone forms in the gallbladder and gets stuck in the duct, it can damage both organs. This can even be life-threatening.

The enzyme lipase is important along with bile in order to break down fats. Amylase, which you may recall as also being produced by glands in the mouth, breaks down starches and carbohydrates. From there the food is considered to be digested. Now the intestine functions primarily to absorb nutrients. An additional function is bolstering the immune system. This is accomplished by the presence of probiotic flora, a fancy term for "good" bacteria, colonizing the small and large intestines.

The main functions of the large intestine are absorption of water and minerals and the formation and, eventually, elimination of feces. As mentioned, a substantial portion of the probiotic bacteria are located here. Two of those, *Bifidobacterium* and *Lactobacillus*, constitute the majority of healthy bacteria. These good bacteria provide important functions, such as the synthesis of folic acid and valuable nutrients from foods, including vitamins K and portions of the B complex.

The descending and sigmoid colon and the rectum are responsible for the last absorption of water and the final transformation of the chyme to solid waste or feces, also known as stool, poop, doody… the list goes on. I am pretty sure most people reading this book have the remainder of the elimination process down pat, so I won't bother with that. Suffice to say, if you've ever experienced the unfortunate coincidence of drinking an espresso after eating at a disreputable restaurant, well, you know how important the proper and timely execution of this function is. Remember the famous words of NASA, "Houston, we have lift-off," and you'll know what I mean.

HOW THE DIGESTIVE SYSTEM CHANGES AFTER 50

For the most part, the digestive system holds up pretty well throughout our later years. As with other systems dependent on smooth muscle integrity, your overall health and fitness will keep this running at near top form. Of course, medications, bad habits, and unfortunate biology will affect this, but in general, the major things to consider have to do with your actions.

Motility will slow. This often leads to constipation. The flora of the gut, those colonies of good bacteria, need care and maintenance; otherwise they can change, causing other problems like indigestion and bloating. In some cases lactose intolerance may also occur in later years.

The sphincter mechanisms throughout also tend to function less effectively, and GERD or reflux may cause issues. If it has been going on for a long time, scarring, called achalasia and stenosis, in the esophagus can cause restriction and discomfort.

In some cases, areas in the intestines can weaken and outpouchings called diverticula can form. This is especially prevalent in the colon and the sigmoid colon. The condition is known as diverticulosis. Sometimes they can become inflamed and infected. This is known as diverticulitis and can be extremely serious. Other conditions that tend to occur are the formations of polyps or little abnormal cell growths in the colon. They are not normal structures and have a potential to become cancerous, so generally they will have to be removed. Vigilance is key here. I will go into more depth about early detection and annual medical exams in the section on access to health care.

And now a word about hemorrhoids.

If ever there was a misunderstood part of the body, it has to be the hemorrhoid. Just the word makes some people cringe and others giggle. In that way it is as divisive and inflammatory a subject as discussing who gets what when crazy, rich Uncle Bob kicks the bucket. Still, it really does need for some justice to be applied, and I am going to do it now. Not to channel Gordon Gecko, but hemorrhoids, for lack of a better term, are good. They are little vascular cushions, batches of small blood vessels, in the anal area that help with a bowel movement. It is only when they weaken and become inflamed that they turn into a condition known as piles, even though some people, including clinicians, still just refer to them as hemorrhoids. Now piles can be painful and bad, and if they are serious enough, they can require medical treatment such as antibiotics and even surgery. When I was a kid, there was a joke to illustrate this, based on a popular television character. It went, "What makes you sit funny and yell Shazaam?"

Gomer's piles.

Yes, I know what you are thinking, but you won't forget the distinction between hemorrhoids and piles ever again now, will you?

The Endocrine System

This is another really fascinating system and one that, as we age, really has a huge impact as much on our "pursuits of happiness" as our overall health. Basically it's a communication system like the nervous system, only with a much different means of communicating. A bunch of glands in many different areas of the body release hormones, special chemical compounds, into the bloodstream. These hormones then swirl around until they encounter receptor sites on certain tissues. Think of a bunch of magnetic keys floating around in search of their matching locks. When they link up, voilà, a miracle happens.

Well, not exactly. But it is pretty magical.

In fact, it's a system that involves many of the systems and organs we have already talked about.

To give you an idea, here is a quick listing of the organs that secret hormone into the bloodstream. Three of the organs are in the brain: the pituitary gland, which secretes a whole bunch of hormones; the pineal, which secretes melatonin (thought to be important to sleep); and the hypothalamus, which secretes a bunch of regulating hormones for other organs. Two are in the neck: the thyroid, affecting metabolism, and the parathyroid, which influences how calcium is absorbed and retained in bone. In the chest we find the thymus, which disappears in adulthood, and the heart, which secretes hormones affecting everything from the kidney's function to blood vessels to fat tissue. In the abdomen, the kidneys secrete hormones affecting blood cell production in the bone marrow, the retention of salt, and blood pressure. Sitting on top of the kidneys are the adrenal glands, which secrete the anti-saber-toothed-cat-named-Wendell fight or flight hormone adrenalin—also called epinephrine—and stress-related hormones cortisol and some natural steroids and sexually related hormones called androgens. The digestive tract releases a number of hormones, many of which have already been covered, and the pancreas, which affects sugar uptake via insulin and another hormone called glucagon secretion.

The sexual organs or gonads are what most people associate with the endocrine system. These are located . . . well, you already know where they are located, though I might point out that individual results may vary.

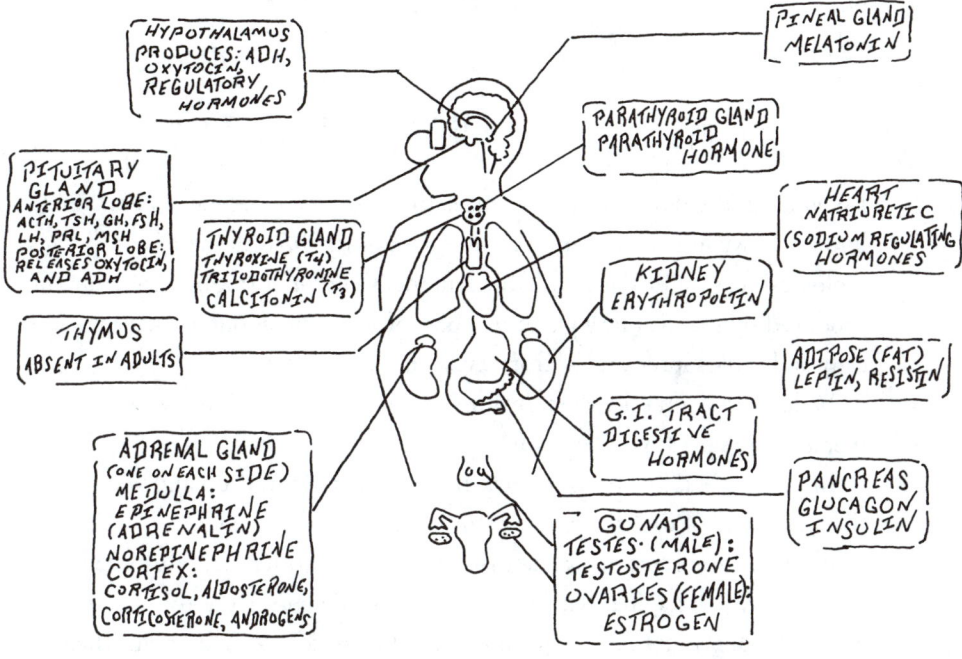

The testes, male organs, secrete testosterone and some other hormones. Ovaries, female organs, secrete estrogens—yes, there are more than one kind—and some other hormones as well.

Finally there is one tissue that is not in just one location of the body, but all over it. That tissue is adipose or, brace yourself, body fat. The hormones it secretes affect appetite and insulin function.

Now these are just the organs that secrete hormones into the blood stream. The organs that "feel" their effects and react to the magical keys entering their respective locks are all throughout the body.

So you see how complicated this system is, accounting for many of the regulatory functions of the body, ranging from thirst to the way calcium is stored or removed from our bones to the expression of male and female sexual characteristics. The latter is the function that most people equate with the endocrine system, and if you've ever had a hot flash, you understand why, but there really is a lot more to it than that.

The chart above lists some of the organs, the hormones they produce, and the function of the hormone. Take a look. You just might just realize that the endocrine system may be the most underestimated system in the body. You certainly will be reminded of how, as I like to say, it is all connected.

HOW THE ENDOCRINE SYSTEM CHANGES AFTER 50

If you recall the description of changes to the musculoskeletal system, you know that we lose muscle mass as we age beyond 50. Well, here is one biological reason for that: growth hormone. Growth hormone is actually produced by the pituitary gland in a part of the brain about as anatomically and philosophically far from musculature as it can get.

Well, unless you take the term "muscle head" literally. I know I have met a few people I wonder about.

In seriousness, the levels of growth hormone tend to drop and with them go some of the triggers that stimulate size and strength.

Another important hormone that decreases is aldosterone. For some reason I always imagine that word as the name of an over-the-top Italian action star anytime I hear it. I can just see the preview—"In a world where bad bacteria want to harm the colon, one man stands ready to dish out payback with yogurt AND bullets. He's Aldo Sterone in *The Pro Biotic*."

Or something like that . . .

Actually aldosterone has nothing to do with the gut. It acts on the kidneys to regulate salt absorption and thus water during the blood's filtration and production of urine. As the levels change, the tendency toward dehydration can increase. Finally there is insulin, maybe one of the most important hormones with regard to impact on all other systems in the body. Insulin is produced by the pancreas, as you already know. It allows sugar to be absorbed into our cells and used as fuel for energy production. Remember the three things a cell needs—water, oxygen, and fuel? Well, when the pancreas doesn't make enough insulin or the cell does not respond to the insulin we make, that is how the condition we know as diabetes occurs. If the pancreas stops making insulin, that is type I. If the cell and body's response to insulin is the problem, that is type II. Type II is the more likely variety to develop after 50. There is a lot an aging individual can do to enhance the function of insulin, and we'll get to that when we talk about behavior.

The Genitourinary System

Now for all you fans of aqueducts and indoor plumbing, get ready to be dazzled. This system is easily one of the most entertaining and frankly fluid systems within us. I know, it was a terrible pun.

The truth is you can look at the genitourinary or GU system and realize it is critical to our continued existence on both an individual level and as a species. Sounds lofty and complicated, huh?

Simply put, this is the system of structures and organs responsible for reproduction and the elimination of urinary waste. Probably the best way to describe it is by separating the urinary and the reproductive and then describing where they come together.

You may have noticed that I used the term reproductive instead of sexual. There is a good reason for that. Those things sexual and associated with sexuality are both structurally and functionally so multifactorial that I am saving that discussion for the section devoted to the pursuit of happiness. I feel pretty justified in doing so mostly because of an answer given by the famous psychiatrist and sexual obsessive, Sigmund Freud, who, when asked about the largest sexual organ in the body, replied, "The brain!"

So I am saving the subject of sex until the end of this book. That way, I know you'll keep reading!

And again, no skipping ahead.

Structurally, the urinary system is composed of the kidneys, the tubes connecting them to the bladder called the ureters, the expandable bladder, which is admittedly much less expandable in some, and finally the urethra, the tube the empties the bladder when you go to the bathroom. Now it goes without saying that the major urinary difference in men and women is the ureter, its length, and how it exits the body.

Which begs the question, "Why are you saying it, then?"

Good question. Because that difference accounts for a lot of problems and stating the obvious lays the groundwork for explanation. The urinary tract is actually a sterile environment. When bacteria or other infectious material enter it, an infection can occur. The most common way for bacteria to enter is via the external opening of the urethra. Since it is much shorter in women, the risk and prevalence of infection getting to the bladder and beyond is higher.

So that is why I said it.

The kidneys, as you have already learned, have many other functions, but their primary role is in the filtration of blood and removal of metabolic waste that is carried away as urine. The mechanism is pretty incredible, really. It all occurs due to a thing called the Bowman's capsule. That always sounded like a space vehicle to me, but there you go. The Bowman's capsule is a microscopic structure of a collecting tube shaped like a cup and it "holds" a ball of tangled blood vessels called a glomerulus. Try saying that ten times fast. I dare you.

When you go to your healthcare provider and they order blood tests, one of the things they look at is a value for the glomerular filtration rate (GFR). This is a really good indicator of how your kidneys are functioning.

After that, the urine then passes through the collecting tubules and tubes to the ureters that descend to the bladder, where urine collects. At some point, enough urine stretches the bladder signaling your central nervous system that you need to go to the bathroom and void. For me that is usually right about the time someone corners me in a hallway and says, "Hey Doc, I have a quick question about something my doctor told me . . ."

This statement is almost always a lie. Well, technically I guess it isn't a lie because the question *is* short. The answer, on the other hand will, for certain, never be.

Eventually, however, you will be in a situation in which you can relieve yourself and the bladder, via a small sphincter, evacuates into the urethra and then out to the world.

The reproductive organs or gonads are the ones responsible for reproduction and the generation of sexual hormones. "Gonads" sounds like a cheer for a really awful high school team, right? Can you imagine sitting in the stands yelling, "Goooo Nads"? I can't even imagine the team mascot. Even so, they are important.

The male gonads—known as the testicles—serve a dual use of sperm creation and creating the male hormones like testosterone, which promote male sexual characteristics. The root of the word is interesting. Some believe it comes from the Roman legal phrase *testis unus, testis nullus*, which meant that one witness's testimony means nothing without another. So it speaks to the pairings. Talk about the buddy system!

There is a lot of discussion in the news about the need for men to have a certain level of testosterone in order to function. While that is certainly true, there have been cases in which men have started this form of therapy only to find that their issues with fatigue, lethargy, etc. are really related to a cardiac or another chronic disease issue. So what does this mean? Make sure your healthcare provider addresses your overall health before blaming your poor old testicles.

The female version of the gonad is the ovary. This comes from the Latin root for "egg." Ovaries secrete the hormones estrogen, progesterone, and testosterone. How about that, guys! This is important for the expression of female sexual characteristics and for the maintenance and production of egg or oocyte formation. Now one little interesting but completely unfair thing in the differences of the sexes is that a man makes sperm throughout his life, but a woman is born with all the eggs she will ever have, so no new eggs are created. As a woman ages, the eggs deteriorate and eventually become relatively nonfunctional. The development of an egg from its primitive state in the ovary is due to a number of other hormones. At menopause these other hormones diminish, and the generation of a mature egg ceases. I'm suddenly reminded of the words of that immortal philosopher Tammy Wynette who sang, "Sometimes it's hard to be a woman."

I am not sure this was what she had in mind, but it sure seems to fit. In any case, if only considered in the hormonal context, women certainly are infinitely more complex than men.

HOW THE GENITOURINARY SYSTEM CHANGES AFTER 50

In general, the kidneys tend to lose cells and shrink as people age. Less blood flows through them, and they progressively process and remove waste products less effectively. The efficiency of salt and water balance and removal decreases, which can lead to dehydration. The bladder volume also decreases, increasing the frequency with which urination occurs. The predictability and strength of the bladder's contraction will decrease, thus causing urinary retention and increasing the potential for infection. The sphincter that controls release is less reliable, creating potential for accidental incontinence or leakage and in postponing urination.

Which reminds me, I'll be right back . . .

In women, the urethra gets even shorter, and its tissue becomes thinner with age. Talk about your rotten luck. This also increases the potential for trauma and infection. But it's not all whitewater rapids and cascading waterfalls for the men either. For men the prostate enlarges. This can impede urination and prevent complete emptying of the bladder. This condition can also decrease the force with which a man can urinate and can lead to prolonged dribbling at the end of the stream. (I am suddenly imagining the Harlem Globetrotters outside a men's room. I'm not sure why.) Another condition that can occur is urinary retention. This means that despite having a full bladder, a man may not be able to void. I don't have anything funny to say about that. In fact, if anyone experiences that, they should seek medical attention immediately.

The changes in the reproductive organs are much more obvious in women, but no less significant in men. For a long time, change of life or menopause was thought to be a female phenomenon by the medical profession. Now we know that is not entirely true. For women the changes are generally related to declines in estrogen levels. Menstrual periods end and pregnancy is no longer possible. The ovaries and uterus begin to shrink. The tissues in the vagina become thinner, drier, and less elastic. At its worst, this condition can lead to bleeding and pain during certain activities like intercourse and even a need to urinate urgently.

In men it's testosterone that is the culprit. The decline results in fewer sperm being produced and some decline in sex drive. Blood flow to the penis tends to decrease. To shed some light on another misconception, erectile dysfunction is not necessarily an age-related issue as much as it may be an indicator of an underlying health problem. If you or someone you know is experiencing this, see a physician.

The Immune System

I like the immune system. I certainly like mine. I like to think of it like my very own little department of defense, a veritable army of troops and command centers that react to any threat against me with a sense of duty and purpose. It doesn't matter the odds. It doesn't matter the threat. It can be a splinter in my finger or pandemic flu or a bad oyster I consumed in an ill-advised moment. My immune system doesn't ask questions or chastise me with a "what were you thinking?" message.

That's what the gastrointestinal system is for.

No, the immune system is pretty wonderful. So why don't I treat it better? I'll get to that soon enough.

So what is it, really? Well, it's a complex system of barriers and reactive cells and chemicals that attack, eat, eliminate, or neutralize offending agents like viruses, bacteria, and even parasites. Like most of the systems I have described, the immune system is dependent on different influences, organs, and other systems. Primarily, it is often described by the lymphatic system, white blood cells, surface agents, and inflammatory cascades of a bunch of chemical pathways.

Surface agents include things like tears, urine, or mucus that carry offending agents away. White blood cells or leukocytes include a bunch of different actors, like macrophages and neutrophils (think cellular Pac-Mans); eosinophils, which carry antiviral and some protein-destroying enzymes; lymphocytes, which produce enzymes that destroy infected and cancerous cells; and basophils, which are not well understood at all—kind of like the infield fly rule.

The chemical pathways include those enzymatic reactions generated by the white blood cells as well as inflammatory cascades in the bloodstream. These are reactions that yield a bunch of caustic and cell-destroying compounds like cytokines. These make it difficult for an infecting or offending item like a bacterium or virus-infected cell to stick around long.

If enough white blood cells and their dead targets pile up, they can often be seen by the naked eye as pus. Similarly, if the destruction takes place inside the body, the material is often carried away by the lymphatic system. This is a series of interconnected drainage vessels or tubes and nodes of collection. You've likely felt an enlarged lymph node under your arm or in your neck? Well, that is what it is, a part of the lymphatic drainage. In cases of cancer, the lymph node may be enlarged but not painful. This is one situation in which an absence of pain should spur you to see your healthcare provider even faster than if it hurts. Eventually the lymphatic system drains into the circulatory system, and the waste products are processed and eliminated via the liver and kidneys.

Generally, the immune system's cells act more slowly as we age. Since the flow of lymph and the reaction of the chemical pathways trigger more slowly, the reaction and efficiency of the system in fighting infection are also less effective. The ability of the immune system to react to abnormal or cancerous cells is also diminished. Vaccinations tend to result in less reliable immunity due to the reduced vigor of the antibody generation of the immune system as well. For the above reasons, older people are less effective at fending off and reacting to some infections like pneumonia or influenzas. In the most severe cases, the infection can even result in death. This is also the reason that in addition to influenza shots an older person's physician may suggest they get a pneumococcal vaccine for added protection.

The Skin

It's the birthday suit. Nature's shrink wrap. Your hide. And if you look like a guy I saw in the Speedo with the very hairy back, it's potentially your pelt! The skin is actually an organ, but I am including it in a discussion of systems because of its encompassing application and multitude of functions in the operation of the human body. It protects us, represents us, identifies us, and, if you are so inclined, at times even indicts us.

So who would want leave something like that out? Well, I wouldn't.

Like the rest of the descriptions, I will start off in consideration of the structure and then get into the function of skin.

Structurally, our skin is the three-layer-deep outer covering of a human being composed of an epidermis, a dermis, and a membrane. The epidermis is the outermost covering and differs slightly in its composition and thickness depending on the part of the body it covers. It makes sense if you really think about it. You would not want the same quality of skin on the soles of your feet that you have on your face, right? Similarly, reading Braille with your nose could present a challenge. So skin is really quite a diverse structure.

The outermost layer of cells exposed to the outside world is called squamous epithelium. The majority of the rest of the cells in the skin are called keratinocytes. These cells are really incredible. They have both structural qualities and yet when a foreign body like a splinter penetrates, an infection occurs, or a parasite invades, the cells can actually become a part of the body's defense. In the spirit of the Founding Fathers, keratinocytes are just like the Minutemen. They go from little skin citizens to skin citizen-soldiers cranking out weapons like inflammatory peptides, enzymes, and proteins. Subtle signals bring in white blood cells to join the fight and, well, you know the rest already.

The bottom layer of the epidermis is the basement membrane. This is the layer that acts as the nursery of the emerging keratinocytes and other cells. It is, as you can imagine, extremely delicate.

The dermis is the layer below the basement membrane and above the underlying fat and muscles. It is composed of connective tissue like collagen and elastic tissue. This is where the hair follicles and sweat glands are located. The lymphatic structures and the nerve endings and smooth muscle that tighten around the hair shafts, also called piloerectors, are found here as well.

So I have already started to talk a little about the function of the skin. It's an important line of defense. It's critical to sensation with special distinct nerve endings for heat, cold, touch, pressure, and vibration. It plays a huge role in regulating body temperature. If you have ever been to the gym and had to wipe off the equipment, you already understand this. It prevents dehydration and protects us when we are in the water, at least for a while. Anyone whose mom has warned them that they were getting pruny has seen evidence of that. It also provides additional protection from one of the greatest threats to our bodies, the effects of the sun's ultraviolet light. This is accomplished by the pigment melanin, which comes from cells called melanocytes. The amount of melanin produced varies with race and genetics and is the reason the sunscreen industry makes about a billion dollars a year, especially off pigment-challenged guys like me.

HOW THE SKIN CHANGES AFTER 50

As we age, the skin becomes thinner. It loses its elastic quality, which makes it become wrinkled and more likely to tear. Unprotected exposure to the sun increases this quality. There is also less collagen, which provides added strength, and elastin, the compound that makes skin stretchy. The fat layer beneath the dermis thins as well, and the nerve endings decrease, reducing a person's ability to detect potentially injurious sensation. The number of sweat glands and oil glands decreases, as does circulation. This affects the skin's ability to efficiently counter heat and cold stress. The risks of heatstroke and frostbite increase respectively. Finally, melanocytes decrease, making sun-related injury a greater possibility and reducing the ability of the skin to produce vitamin D.

Summary

Long before I became a doctor, I was fascinated by the human body. Later, when I was in school, I also became intrigued with the power and emotional impact of literature and language. The principal considerations of the dramatic struggle between tragedy and comedy seemed to somehow perfectly complement the study of human biology. Nowhere can you see a better example of ridiculous hilarity and drama, even at times succeeding to tragedy, than in the chronological progress and aging of our bodies. Usually we start off as pleasant-smelling, beautiful, innocent creatures. Then along comes something called puberty. If there was ever something simultaneously pitiful and laughable, it is the human being as a pubescent. For most of us, somehow, we get through it without being committed or chained up in the attic and emerge into young adulthood, where we enjoy—for lack of a better term—the physical state of Michelangelo's David or Venus on the half shell. Then by a combination of sheer luck and effort, we made it to middle age with our bodies and minds relatively intact.

Congratulations!

Now what? Well, since you can change your jeans, but you can't change your genes, you have to consider what you can change. In many ways it's also a Popeye thing. You are what you are. What you aren't is helpless, though. If you have an unusual family medical history, be sure to discuss it with your healthcare provider. You can't help your genetics, but you might be able to help how they affect you, which leads us to the next chapter. . .

Just remember, with any disease process or genetic condition a medical situation may be exacerbated as we age. To use a three-o'clock-in-the-morning-advertisement constant, your results may vary.

CHAPTER 2

BEHAVIOR

I AM A JELLY DONUT!

It was a beautiful day in June 1963 when President John F. Kennedy spoke to the eager crowd of German citizens in front of the Schöneberg Rathaus (town hall) in Berlin. What he said next would soon go down in political lore as the greatest gaffe in foreign policy. In an attempt at solidarity the president spoke the now famous line.

"Ich bin ein Berliner." I am a jelly donut.

At least that is what the *New York Times* reported that he said a few days later.

It wasn't true. Kennedy was a writer and a gifted speaker. The fact is that his interpreter had carefully translated the line into German and Kennedy had practiced it phonetically. He had really, correctly said "I am a Berliner," as he intended.

But the legend stuck. Frankly, I kind of like the legend. It makes him seem sweet and accessible and kind of delicious. It also makes me think of another famous line. You are what you eat. I can't say it with certainty, but I bet even if Kennedy had said he was a jelly donut, at some time in his life he *had* eaten a jelly donut and so he wouldn't have been incorrect. Of course, had he been into cannibalism, "I am a Berliner" might have been even more true and more of a reason for a *New York Times* editorial. Regardless, since this chapter is going to be all about how we are what we eat and do, then I have a confession to make.

I really am a jelly donut. Cherry, with powdered sugar.

The first chapter of this book was all about the things you can't really choose or control—your biology and genetics. This chapter is all about the things you can, and I would even go so far as to say that your health behaviors can optimize the hand nature dealt you. Certainly, good health behaviors can delay the onset of certain disease processes and sometimes even prevent them.

Of course, most people could come up with a couple of common behaviors that promote good health. They generally say with a kind of dour tone, "Well, I could exercise more or eat better," but there are a lot of other things that they don't immediately consider. Which is why I wrote this chapter.

Exercise

Given my affinity for the whole life, liberty, pursuit for happiness construct, it is only logical that I should go back to the Founding Fathers as we consider the subject of exercise.

Bear in mind that exercise is a complex consideration even as it is a fundamentally simple idea. So, what did the Founding Fathers, a group of wise and incredible if imperfect people, think of exercise? Well, because exercise has so many applications—as many applications as there are people who practice them—the very different members of the original Continental Congress approached it, just as you might expect, distinctly. They also had a lot to say about it, because as we know today, if there is one thing a member of Congress can do, it is talk. And yet, with exercise and exercise-related issues in mind, no one ever seems to sprain their tongue. Now there is irony for you.

In particular, I found that three very physically and emotionally different figures, Adams, Jefferson, and Franklin, had the most to say. As you read this, I think you'll find that they weren't so different from us.

First, there is John Adams, who from all accounts didn't look like he exercised a whole lot. Adams was short and somewhat pudgy, and yet he lived to the ripe old age of 90. I looked into it, and despite his body habitus or shape, John Adams had some very regimented health maintenance activities that he adhered to religiously, not the least of which was a daily walk. Such exercise, he believed, roused "the animal spirits" and "dispersed melancholy."

Must have been some walk, huh?

Thomas Jefferson, his close colleague and friend and a polar opposite in terms of physique, said, "Exercise and application produce order in our affairs, health of body, cheerfulness of mind, and these make us precious to our friends." He also said, "Not less than two hours a day should be devoted to exercise, and the weather should be little regarded. A person not sick will not be injured by getting wet. It is but taking a cold bath, which never gives a cold to any one. Brute animals are the most healthy, and they are exposed to all weather, and of men, those are healthiest who are the most exposed."

Now, I know some people are going to see this as an early American endorsement of nudism. Please don't quote this book if you do. I think it is fair to assume *that* is not what Jefferson meant, and I offer the remainder of his thoughts in support of a premise of "Simple diet, exercise and the open air, be its state what it will; and we may venture to say that this recipe will give health and vigor to every other description."

And finally, he advocated, "I repeat my advice to take a great deal of exercise, and on foot. Health is the first requisite after morality."

Now I'm not dumb enough to start in on the subject of morality, but it's pretty safe to say Jefferson was in favor of exercise and it was very important to him. It makes some sense considering the man lived to the age of 82 and died only five hours shy of his friend Adams.

Finally, there is the Founding Father that I never would have associated with exercise, but who had very strong feelings about it and, in fact, lived his ideals. When most people envision Ben Franklin, they think of an older fat man inclined toward the indulgences of diet and sensuality. While this was true in his later years—hey, the man was in France, for crying out loud—as a young man Franklin was very involved in physical fitness and fitness-related activity. In particular, Franklin liked to swim. He actually taught himself, which is a fairly nervy thing to do considering all he had access to was a river, not the neighborhood pool. According to his personal documents, he even seriously indulged the idea of pursuing a career as a full-time swim instructor. Forget the Declaration of Independence, forget bifocals, forget electrified keys; he wanted to swim! If he had gone that route, you can imagine how the world might have changed. Regardless, in typical Franklin fashion, he invented an early American set of swim fins and swimming paddles to increase his speed in the water. With all that in mind you might not be surprised to learn that Franklin is actually an inductee in the Swimming Hall of Fame. Hopefully, that is enough for him. I think the rest of us are grateful he chose the course in life that he did.

So what is the point? That a bunch of guys in uncomfortable shoes went for walks and a guy without a Speedo took a dip? No. They all were pretty clear that incorporating exercise had multiple benefits, not just the physical. They were also adamant about the overall benefit of this on the mind, body, and spirit.

They were right. Modern research on exercise's impact on the brain indicates—in addition to the obvious benefits of improved circulation, blood sugar management, and cardiovascular improvement—that the most immediate benefit is psychological. This is due to a couple of concepts: endorphin release and the idea of meditation in motion.

In an effort at fairness, another anonymous school of thought says that the advantage of exercising is that you die much healthier.

I don't agree, but in the spirit of fairness I had to include it. Plus, I think it's funny.

Now here is where I am going to say something that is just my opinion and may seem a little heretical on the surface.

I don't think most people should "exercise."

After going on and on about it, how can I say that? Well, it's because of what the word has come to mean, and I would remind that words *do* matter.

I think most people don't exercise for one reason. I think it is because we approach exercise as work. It's often no fun at all. That is where it breaks down for most people. It becomes one more unpleasant task in the day. I want people to be healthy, so if that requires a different perspective or a change of wording to get to that end result of improved health, then so be it.

Remember when you were a kid? Think waaay back. Did you exercise? No, you played, but you got all sweaty and you were breathing hard. You laughed and you had a blast!

Somewhere along the line—I am guessing gym class—that enjoyable pursuit changed to a task of exertion. The best way to maintain an "exercise" regimen is to not exercise at all but to play.

I mean, if you think about it. . . it makes sense. The concept of a lonely athlete toiling agonizingly away at ungodly hours in pursuit of a distant shot at a title or trophy is fairly awful. Admirable, but awful.

And as a friend of mine once said, "The trouble with jogging is that by the time you realize you are not in shape for it, it's too far to walk back."

On the other hand, a game of hide and seek can be a blast. Granted, playing hide and seek at my age could potentially lead to some activation of the neighborhood watch, but the principle of finding that thing that is kinetically fun for you is critical. For some of you, it may well be that a long distance run is the perfect Zen-like liberation. For others it's a sport, a game—and, no, canasta does not count as exercise. Still others may like dancing or a nature walk. For still others it is gossiping while you watch and accompany an old episode of *Sit and Be Fit*. The point is that there are no wrong answers for how someone improves their activity, outside of joining the beer-drinking team. You just need to do it.

All apologies to the good folks at Nike.

There are some tools that can help. For people who like spinning or a stationary bike, there are video game attachments that simulate the action you have to undertake, like competitors you overtake or obstacles you have to steer around. Of course you could always go for an actual bike ride, if you are able. Just saying…

There are machines that simulate cross-country skiing, jogging, climbing stairs, running in soft earth, on air, etc. There are computer and television/video programs that allow you to play a game of tennis against an electronic version of a friend or that allow you to simulate Pete Townsend's guitar gyrations. Then again, as I alluded earlier, if you are able and prefer, and, like Jefferson, see the value in outdoor escape, then you can actually do something in the real world. The point I'm making is that, in the words of the epicurean Julia Child, "You simply must find something to do!"

Want to know why?

Here's why. According to the National Institute on Aging at the US Department of Health and Human Services (HHS), as a person ages beyond 50, exercise and activity can help boost energy, maintain independence, and manage symptoms of illness or pain. Exercise and activity can even reverse some of the symptoms of aging. Not only is exercise good for your body, it's also good for your mind, mood, and memory. Whether you are generally healthy or are managing an illness, there are plenty of ways to become more active, improve your health, and boost your fitness.

Helping Older Adults Maintain and Lose Weight

As your metabolism slows with age, maintaining a healthy weight can become a challenge. I've already mentioned that exercise and activity help increase metabolism and build muscle mass, helping to burn even more calories. When your body reaches a healthy weight, your overall wellness naturally improves, too.

ACTIVITY AND EXERCISE

Again, I am not just using the word exercise, but the words exercise *and* activity. It is not by accident. Both terms refer to the voluntary movements you do that burn calories. "Activity" is defined, for the purposes of our discussion, as 150 minutes of physical activity per week. Those numbers apply whether you are trying to lose weight and are active or inactive. Physical activities are actions that increase bodily movement, such as gardening, walking the dog, raking leaves, and taking the stairs instead of the elevator. "Exercise" is a form of physical activity that is specifically planned, structured, and repetitive, such as weight training, tai chi, or an aerobics class. It can include everything from a walk to a run to some form of structured dance, like Zumba, ballet, tap, clogging, or exotic. Well, maybe not exotic, but then again, if that really works for you, who am I to judge?

Physical activity and exercise are both important and can help improve your ability to do the other everyday activities you enjoy. And now we are back to the concept of play again.

There are many ways to be active every day. The important thing is that you find something you enjoy doing, include it in your regular routine, and try to increase your level of activity safely over time.

The National Institute on Aging (NIA) at the National Institutes of Health (NIH) believes in this so strongly that the agency even has a program, G04Life, designed to help seniors fit exercise and physical activity (read *play* here) into their lives. G04Life is really pretty fantastic, and are you ready for the best part? It's free!

So it is well within your budget.

Just check out https://g04life.nia.nih.gov/. Once there, you'll find videos, self-determination tools, and a lot more.

Now I know what some of you may be thinking. "I exercised a lot when I was younger. I've earned the right to eat a gallon of ice cream and take a nap."

Actually, that is specious. As you pass the age of 50, activity is actually much more important than when you were young, and unfortunately it is not like you can build up a surplus of good health from your youth so you can coast later on.

Not yet sold? Well, try this on for size.

As I said earlier, *exercise and activity help increase metabolism.* Increased activity also *reduces the impact of illness and chronic disease.* According to HHS, the many benefits of exercise for adults over 50 include an improved immune function, better heart health and blood pressure, better bone density, and better digestive functioning. People who exercise also have a lowered risk of several chronic conditions, including Alzheimer's disease, diabetes, obesity, heart disease, osteoporosis, and colon cancer.

EXERCISE AND WELL-BEING

Exercise generally improves overall well-being. It does this by improving your mental health, strength, stamina, flexibility, and posture, which in turn will help with balance and coordination and reduce the risk of falls. It also helps alleviate the symptoms of chronic conditions such as arthritis, but the benefits are not just physical.

EXERCISE AND SLEEP

Exercise and activity, especially vigorous activity, often improves sleep, helping you fall asleep more quickly and continue to sleep more deeply. I'll go into sleep in more depth later, no pun intended. Additionally, endorphins, our body's naturally produced molecules that cause euphoria and blunt pain input, are produced by exercise and can actually help you feel better and make rest easier to obtain. Studies have also suggested that naturally produced endorphins, especially from chronic activity and exercise, can reduce the need for pharmaceutically provided pain medications and enhance recovery from illness and injury.

Exercise improves blood flow to the brain. That improves function and performance. Some research has suggested that exercise may help slow the progression of brain disorders such as Alzheimer's disease.

So there is no reason not to do this. No matter how old, restricted, ill, or even partially disabled, there is something you can do to increase your activity and exercise.

So, you may ask, how do we start?

A Word about Safety

Well, first, you do it with an eye toward safety. There is nothing more demoralizing than starting out strong, only to be stopped by an injury. So, first, I want you to see a healthcare provider and make sure you are healthy enough to begin some kind of program. Your current state of health may not define what you ultimately can do, but it is important in defining where you start. Specifically, ask if there are any activities you should avoid.

Certain health problems will affect your workouts and conversely are affected by increased physical activity and workouts. For example, diabetics may need to adjust the timing or amounts of medications and meal plans as they set up an exercise schedule; then as their body changes, those adjustments may need to be made again at intervals. Similarly, conditions that come and go or that are cyclic, such as myasthenia gravis, may require an alteration of schedule. This requires that you maintain a constant and open line of communication with your healthcare provider.

Above all, if something feels wrong, such as sharp pain or unusual shortness of breath or any other distress, simply stop and get help. Consult your healthcare provider. In the long run, you may need to scale back or try another activity.

Getting Started

Remember the hypothetical "If you were going to be stranded on a desert island for the rest of your life and could only have one kind of food, what would it be?" That always bothered me. It led to too many questions.

Why did I plan so poorly as to wind up stranded? How is it possible that the "island" has a menu so I can order ahead? Why is the menu à la carte?

You get the idea. Well, with exercise you are not just choosing one thing. In fact, most exercise experts feel that variation keeps things fresh and allows adequate recovery. Even if you are doing something you enjoy to begin with, you will still eventually want to supplement or try some other activity. The key is finding activities that you enjoy. Here is an overview of the four building blocks of senior fitness and why your body needs all of them.

According to the Committee on Accreditation for the Exercise Sciences and the National Coalition for Promoting Physical Activity, mixing different types of exercise helps both reduce monotony and improve your overall health. Regardless of the activity or exercise program you choose, according to the NIA, it should include elements that improve cardiovascular or aerobic fitness, strength training, flexibility, and balance.

Cardiovascular endurance uses large muscle groups in submaximal, rhythmic motions over a period of time. "Cardio" workouts get your heart pumping and may even make you feel a little short of breath. Cardio includes walking, stair climbing, swimming, hiking, cycling, rowing, tennis, and dancing. Basically, it's anything that increases your heart rate and metabolism. One additional benefit: it also promotes independence by improving endurance and capacity for all daily activities. Unfortunately, this is what most people think of when they use the term exercise, even though the word includes much more. Cardio should be a part but doesn't have to be the entirety of exercise, and in fact, I'd recommend it not be.

Strength training builds up muscle with repetitive motion using weight or external resistance from body weight, machines, free weights, or elastic bands. Generally it allows brief intervals for recovery before resuming the action. It also focuses more on a specific muscle group, such as the back, legs, or arms, and less on the overall increase in metabolism or cardiovascular system. "Power training" is often strength training done with more resistance or with heavier weights to increase power and reaction times.

The benefits? Strength training helps prevent loss of bone mass (density). It builds muscle, and it improves balance—all important in staying active and avoiding falls. Most people don't think about it, but strength training can also improve your speed. This factors in to things like crossing the street or preventing falls by enabling you to react quickly if you start to trip or lose balance. Building strength and power will also help you stay independent as it makes day-to-day activities easier—anything from opening a jar to getting in and out of a car to lifting objects... like, say, grandchildren.

Flexibility activities challenge the ability of your body's muscles and joints to move freely through a full range of motion. Flexibility can be improved through stationary stretches and stretches that involve movement to keep your muscles and joints supple so they are less prone to injury. It also increases blood flow to muscles, tendons, and ligaments, which allow safer initiation of other activities. Yoga is an excellent means of improving flexibility. It helps your body stay limber and increases your range of movement for ordinary physical activities such as tying your shoes, shampooing your hair, or looking over your shoulder for the odd saber-toothed cat.

The last of the building blocks is, ironically enough, *balance*. I think it is ironic because everything I have said so far has to do with building balance and joy into increased activity and exercise. Balance depends on proprioception—or the inherent perception of your body's position and its orientation in space—and the ability to maintain that position. Balance helps to maintain standing and stability, whether you're stationary or moving around. Activities that improve this include yoga, tai chi, and posture exercises.

Balance improvement also improves posture and the stability of your gait as you walk. It also reduces the risk of falling and the fear of falling, which often leads to hesitation and, ironically enough, increased falls.

So how do you prepare for all that? After visiting with your healthcare provider, seek out good advice. If you have the financial resources, you should consider consulting a qualified trainer or certified physical fitness expert. Just make sure you check their qualifications. This is often tricky. There are many organizations that offer certifications. Some are reputable, others are not. A good starting point is to begin with your local university's sports training or kinesiology department.

You can also contact your local senior center for recommendations. Once you have chosen someone, make sure you clearly explain your level of fitness, your goals, your experience, and any recommendations or restrictions from your healthcare provider. Better yet, link up the two. Both are providing a service for you. It's a business relationship with potential life-improving or life-threatening effect. Treat it like that. Research the prospective trainer. Ask for the trainer's credentials and references and review it with your healthcare provider. You can also get more information from a number of agencies at this website: http://www.nia.nih.gov/health/publication/exercise-physical-activity/resources. Once you have reviewed a candidate on paper, interview him or her.

Here are some things you should definitely consider. Make sure he or she has had experience with senior fitness, at least two years' worth. Make sure he or she has had experience with designing and implementing a senior fitness program. Ask if he or she has dealt with people who have your kind of medical issues, restrictions, and illness. Additionally, the website www.Shapeup.org has some more great tools for a starting self-assessment.

Again, when you have finally chosen a trainer and a regimen, discuss the exercise plan with your healthcare provider. Get your provider's opinion on the recommendations offered by the fitness consultant.

Regardless of the activity, with a consultant or without, you will want to do everything you can to make it fun. As I wrote earlier, increased activity and enjoyment are the goals. So ask yourself, what do I want to do? What will be fun?

Think about activities that you enjoy and how you can incorporate them into an exercise routine. Take music, for example. All you have to do is look around and you'll see that almost everyone is listening to music while they work out. There is a good reason for that. It enhances the experience, gives pleasure, and with a personal device and earphone or earbuds, it allows personalized volume and selection of your very own soundtrack. Suddenly, you're Rocky with Bill Conti's rousing number as you run up those steps in Philadelphia.

Yo, Adrian!

Since I mentioned Rocky, competition is another component of some workouts that many people find a great enhancement, while others would rather do without. If this is something that interests you—I'm envisioning some heavily wagered outcomes on a mall walk—just make sure that your opponent is on the same wavelength. Another consideration that is very individualized is how focused you need to be.

If you have decided on the Flying Wallendas workout and are going to undertake a high-wire component, then focus is likely to be a big factor. If you are walking laps at the mall, then enjoying less focus as you simultaneously window shop is probably a part of the fun.

If your preference is something that allows a more social venue, look into the offerings at senior centers or senior social groups that incorporate an interactive element to their activities. I'm talking about things like a yoga class (those are offered at different levels so you will be challenged without being overwhelmed), aerobics classes, or hiking and walking groups. On that same note you can often find a similarly inclined friend to work out with, and the interaction as you stretch, work out, and cool down can be even more enriching. Just remember, figure out what works for you. Find out what is *fun* and prepare appropriately.

If you do decide to work out alone, you can enhance the experience by watching a favorite movie while on the treadmill. Just make sure it doesn't increase your risk for a fall.

A Word About Safety

Once you have been "cleared" to start, decide what form of activity or exercise you are going to undertake. Also be prepared to change. As you get in better shape, you will probably want to try different things. That is perfectly normal. It is also smart.

I don't necessarily recommend the Pamplona Fun Run.

In any case, in the interest of physical safety you also really have to assess *where* you will be working out, walking, biking, doing yoga, or whatever your chosen pursuit will be. I mean, think about it. If you are planning a nature walk, taking it through an all-carnivore wildlife preserve may not be the best idea, right? Do some homework about the area. Find designated exercise trails if you are planning to walk.

If that is not an option and you are walking alongside roads, always walk facing oncoming traffic. Look for a good, flat, stable surface. If there are guardrails, see if there's a smooth, flat surface behind the barrier where you can walk. If you need to walk on a paved shoulder, stay as far away from traffic as possible. Watch for bridges and narrow shoulders. Be sure

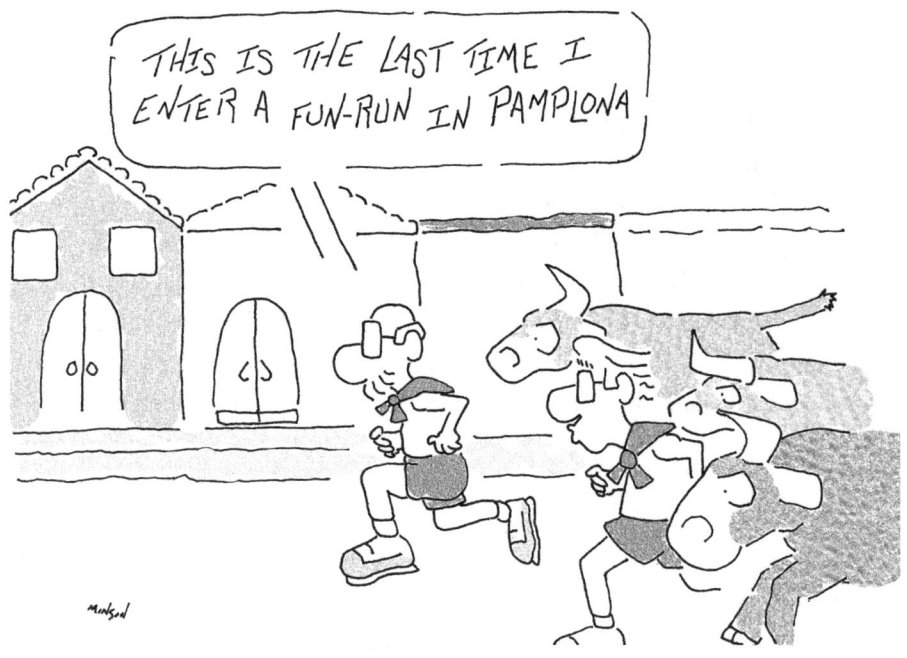

drivers or bike riders can see you. Always wear brightly colored clothing, and if you walk during low-light hours—dusk or dawn—be sure you have reflective material on your jacket or walking shoes and carry a flashlight. Consider wearable flashing lights. Rescue research has shown that a flashing light catches the eye better than a sustained beam of light. Of course, when you are out for a walk, *that* is the only flashing you should be doing. Sorry, I'm still obsessing about Jefferson's comments on exposure.

You might also want to take along a whistle, a charged cell phone, and an ID, especially if walking alone.

If biking is more to your liking, you should probably stay off the Interstate. With respect to the movie "Breaking Away" look for areas that have biking lanes or specific trails. If you are a swimmer, see if municipal pools have actual swimming times for adults and stay out from under the diving board. You know, stuff like that.

In the greater interest of safety, also check to see if a rash of crime has occurred in the area and stay aware of your physical environment. Oh, and if you see a saber-toothed cat named Wendell, take the following steps: (1) call animal control and (2) seek out a psychiatrist.

Breathing

I'm a big fan of breathing. Just ask anyone that knows me. As goofy as this may sound, you need to make sure you breathe regularly as you exercise. Honestly, a lot of people don't focus on their breathing. Breathe in slowly through your nose and breathe out slowly through your mouth. When lifting weights, breathe out as you lift or push, and breathe in as you relax. This may not feel natural at first, and you probably will have to think about it for a while as you do it. Whatever you do, don't hold your breath. It increases strain and can reduce blood flow to the brain and heart.

PROPER FORM

On that note, proper form and safety also go hand-in-hand. For lifting exercises, you may want to start alternating arms and work your way up to using both arms at the same time. If it is difficult for you to hold hand weights, try using wrist weights. To prevent injury, don't jerk or thrust weights into position. Use smooth, steady movements and focus on maintaining good form.

Avoid "locking" your arm and leg joints in a tightly straightened position. To straighten your knees, tighten your thigh muscles. This will lift your kneecaps and protect them.

For many of these exercises, you may need to use a chair to start out, even if you are not chair-bound. Just choose a sturdy one or a support structure that is stable enough to support your weight when seated or when holding onto it during the exercise.

Muscle Soreness

Muscle soreness lasting a few days and slight fatigue are normal after muscle-building exercises, at least at first. After doing these exercises for a few weeks, you will probably not be as sore after your first workout. If it persists or worsens, talk to your healthcare provider.

So you may be thinking what about those of us that are chair-bound or are already restricted? You want we should just prop a chair out by the highway with our whistle and cell phone?

Of course not.

The NIH actually has some great recommendations for seniors who have restrictions. It advocates that even if you are frail or chair-bound, you can still experience the physical benefits and mood-boosting effects of exercise and increased activity. Chair-bound adults can improve fitness with strength training, flexibility, and even some cardio activities. If being chair-bound has prevented you from trying exercise in the past, take heart knowing that when you become more physically active your potential future activities will expand. The results will amaze you. Like any exercise program, a chair-bound fitness routine takes a little creativity and personalization to stay fun and to remain effective. With reference to the building blocks of strength, balance, flexibility, and cardio, here are some activities that you might consider:

- *Strength*: Use free weights ("dumbbells") to do repetitive sets of lifting. Don't have weights? Use anything that is weighted and fits in your hand, like soup cans. Personally, I like pork and beans cans. There is something magically metaphoric about pushing the pork away that really speaks to me on so many levels.

- *Resistance*: Resistance bands are like giant rubber bands designed to give your muscles a good workout when stretched and pulled. Resistance bands can be attached to furniture, a doorknob, or even your chair. Use these for pull-downs, shoulder rotations, and arm and leg extensions. Giant rubber bands always makes me think of every Wile E. Coyote cartoon I ever saw, and if there is a pesky roadrunner about, you can consider launching yourself on a pair of roller skates too. That's a joke. Don't do that.

- *Flexibility*: By practicing mindful breathing and slowly stretching, bending, and twisting, you can limber up and improve your range of motion. Some of these exercises can also be done lying down. Ask your doctor or search online for chair-yoga possibilities. Another option is to use the exercises that are on that ubiquitous flyer in the seatback pocket on airplanes. It includes stuff like rolling your neck, shrugging your shoulders, rolling your ankles, pointing and flexing your toes, and more.

- *Cardio/Endurance*: Check out pool-therapy programs designed for wheelchair-bound seniors or those with limited range of motion. Also, wheelchair-training machines make arm-bicycling and rowing possible. If you lack access to special machines or pools, repetitive movements (like rapid leg lifts or modified pushups) work just as well to raise your heart rate.

Now what I have described so far falls definitely in the exercise category, that is, organized intentional pursuit, but there are a lot of other ways to increase *activity* without being in a class, biking group, or organized cohort. For example, as you indulge in your daily activities you can choose stairs over the elevator, park at the far end of the parking lot when arriving at appointments and meetings, walk down every aisle of the grocery store while shopping, practice balancing skills while standing in line, or do neck rolls while waiting at a stoplight. Those last two, of course, you can do if you don't care what other people think. At home you can do a set of wall pushups while waiting for water to boil, vigorously vacuum (personally, I am putting this up for an Olympic event at the next Summer Games), tend to the garden, sweep the sidewalk, rake leaves, lift weights while watching the news, try toe raises while talking on the phone, or do knee bends after sitting for a long period of time.

In general, the amount of effort you need to do any activity will depend on your starting point, your fitness level, how strong you are, and how active you've been. Walking a mile in 15 minutes will be a lot easier for someone who does it every day compared with someone who has never done it. You can use the following informal guidelines from the NIA to estimate how much effort you are putting into your endurance activities when you first begin:

- Brisk walking is an example of moderate activity, while jogging is a vigorous activity.
- Talking is easy during moderate activity. During vigorous activity, talking is difficult.
- If you tend to sweat, you probably won't sweat during light activity (except on hot days).
- You will sweat more during vigorous or sustained moderate activity. (Just remember to drink fluids even if you don't sweat.)

As you become more active, you'll probably notice signs that you're getting more fit:

- You'll have more energy.
- Your overall mood and outlook on life may improve.
- It's easier to do your usual daily activities.
- Climbing a flight of stairs is easier.
- It's easier to get in and out of the car.
- You can get down on the floor and play a game with your grandchildren or other peoples' grandchildren… or even a dachshund, and get back up again more easily when the game is over.
- You're sleeping better at night.
- You have less pain when you move around.
- Symptoms of an ongoing health condition may improve.

Injuries

The most important thing to remember when it comes to the subject of injury is this: don't get one. It's discouraging, painful, and potentially very unhealthy. Here are some ways to avoid becoming injured.

When starting to exercise, begin slowly. That means warming up. Most people think of warming up and stretching before they run, but even if you do something like swimming, like old Ben Franklin, you need to do this. And, of course, my mom would kill me if I didn't tell you to wait an appropriate amount of time after eating before you go in the water.

Seriously though, it is actually a good idea to wait at least an hour or two after eating a large meal before doing any strenuous exercise.

Who knows, what I am about to offer next may be the best advice in the whole book, aside from "Don't forget to floss" or "Wear sunscreen" or the diet advice. Well, there's a lot of good advice in this book, but this one *is* really important. If you feel pain, back off.

Pain is nature's stop sign. I am pretty sure Louis Pasteur said that, or maybe it was my high school track coach. Anyway, this is where I again endorse activities with low injury potential, like yoga or tai chi.

You should also stop what you're doing if you experience pain or pressure in your chest, neck, shoulder, or arm. These are potentially major warnings. You should also stop if you start to feel dizzy or sick to your stomach or break out in a cold sweat. If you start to experience muscle cramps or feel severe pain in joints, feet, ankles, or legs, you should stop immediately and seek medical care.

Warming Up

I said it before, I'll say it again. You must warm up. I have actually come to believe that we should really start out each day with some light stretching and gradually accelerated movement to get the blood flowing and to increase our flexibility. I mean, think about it. What do they tell you about starting a car on a cold morning? They tell you to let it warm up. Your own soft machine, your body, needs the same thing.

By the way, in case you didn't notice, I just moved us from the horse-drawn era to the industrial, mechanical era metaphorically. Now, no one can accuse this book of not being progressive.

So what is a good way to warm up? Well, this is where I get back on the yoga kick. When you consider the progressive vigor of any yoga workout and the specific need for this among people over 50, it really makes sense that yoga is a perfect way to start any workout or activity session.

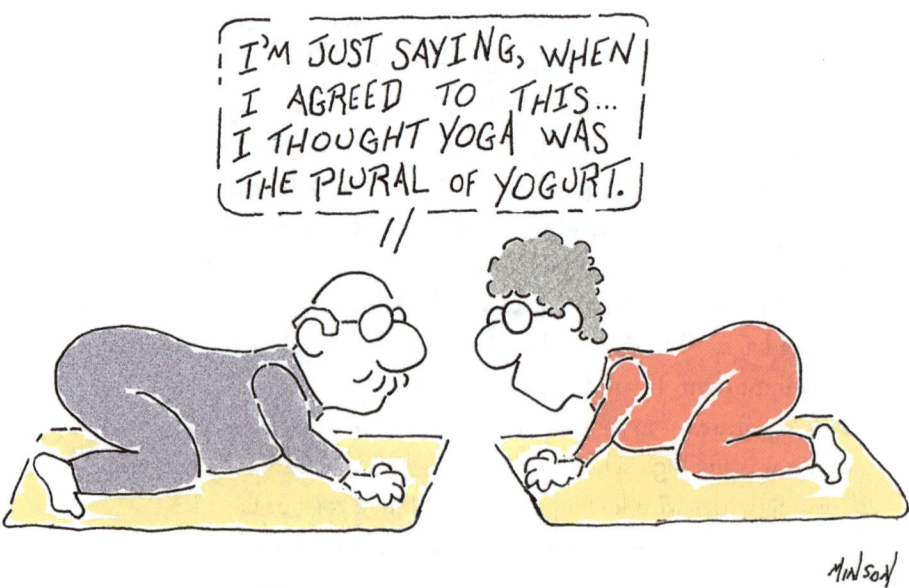

Even if it seems like a foreign concept, even if you thought yoga was the southern pronunciation of a cartoon bear's name or the plural of yogurt, now is the time to look into it. It is low-impact and can be tailored to any fitness level. The benefits are many. The actions of yoga help increase and improve balance and flexibility. The changes in the brain help lower blood pressure and improve cardiovascular function, and, as I referenced earlier, it makes you look better naked. So what's not to love?

Clothes Make the Athlete

Another thing you can do to prevent injury is to wear proper clothing. Now I know your bell bottoms and platform soles may still look really good on you, but for a safe and effective workout, you need to think about function over form. It starts with the shoes.

Rule number one, don't throw one. It is impolite and you know what they do to lame horses in old cowboy movies, don't you?

Choose shoes that are made for the type of physical activity you want to do (walking, running, dancing, bowling, tennis). Look for shoes with flat, nonskid soles, good heel support, enough room for your toes, and a cushioned arch that's not too high or too thick. Make sure your shoes fit well and provide proper support for your feet. This is especially important if you have diabetes or arthritis. Shoes should feel comfortable right from the start. Think of your shoes as safety equipment for your feet. Check them regularly and replace them when they're worn out. You can tell you need new shoes when the tread on the bottom is worn down, your feet (especially your arches) feel tired after activity, or your shins, knees, or hips hurt after activity.

You should also make sure that your clothing is appropriate for the weather. Moisture-wicking materials like silk or some synthetic blends worn next to the skin are best, as they help keep you from overheating and reduce issues of skin irritation. Protective garments may also be worn as layers, farther away from the skin. If you anticipate activity as the temperature changes during the day, definitely consider appropriately layered clothing. Finally, make certain that the garments fit well and don't increase your chances of tripping or getting caught in exercise machinery.

I'm suddenly envisioning the ball-gown-hundred-yard-dash as a very

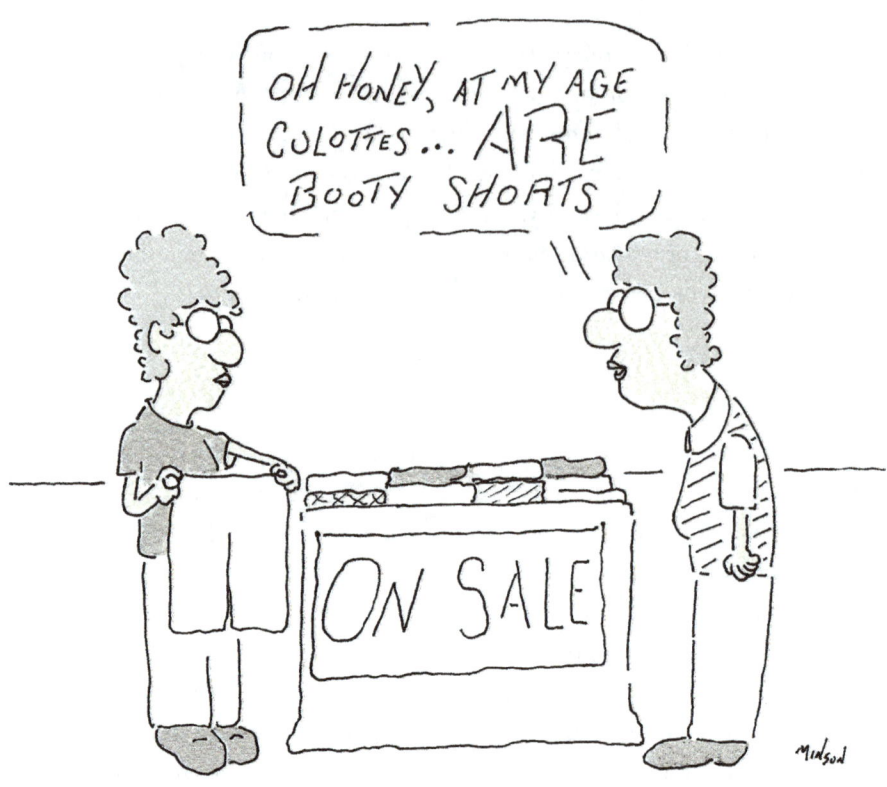

bad idea for a competition. Clothes may make the athlete, as they say; just make sure they don't make the athlete injured.

Cooling Down

Of equal importance is the act of warming down or cooling off after a workout. In any vigorous activity or exercise, the muscles heat up and create more metabolic waste from all that cellular consumption of oxygen, water, and fuel. There needs to be adequate time to mobilize those metabolic wastes for elimination. If you don't, you are likely to be much more stiff and sore the next day, and you run a greater future risk of injury. A rule of thumb is to gradually slow down until your heart rate returns to normal before stopping completely. This is not particularly scientific, but I use it as it is a simple and medically valid way to assure that I am back to normal, metabolically—or at least as normal as I am ever going to get. Notice that I did say "metabolically."

And finally, with the oxygen, fuel, and water recipe in mind, make sure to drink plenty of water before, during, and after your exercise session. This is said all the time by exercise professionals, sports trainers, and healthcare experts, but it's the most commonly neglected preventive activity.

Hydration

So since I brought up hydration, let's really consider the subject of *proper* hydration. It is really important—way beyond just the consideration of exercise.

According to the Agency for Healthcare Research and Quality, 7.3 percent of hospital admissions for senior and elderly patients are related to, or aggravated by, dehydration. It generally can be avoided or corrected in the outpatient setting, but can be extremely deadly if it occurs in a patient with a comorbidity (a medical condition that increases in severity with other factors like dehydration).

I spoke with a patient the other day who was understandably concerned that her mother had been admitted to the hospital twice in the last six months for dehydration. In both cases the first sign that something was wrong was that the woman was slurring her words and appeared terribly confused. In both cases she was initially assessed to rule out a possible stroke. Eventually, after a laborious and expensive workup, she was found on one occasion to be severely dehydrated and on the other to have a urinary tract infection aggravated by dehydration.

I asked my patient if her mother had any other signs or symptoms. As I expected, she affirmed that in addition to the change in her mental state she also was not sweating and seemed pale. I took the opportunity to share some of the common presentations of dehydration in order to catch it, or hopefully to prevent it, in the future. The first thing is remarkably simple, but always the first thing overlooked. Had anyone observed that she wasn't actually drinking water? Of course, the answer was no. I went on down the list, which included these signs of dehydration:

- Being thirsty
- Urinating less often than usual (though this can be offset by certain medications or diabetes)

- Dark-colored urine (though this also can be affected by diet and certain medications or supplements)
- Dry skin or skin that *suddenly* loses elasticity or that tents up when pinched and doesn't snap back as fast as normal
- Fatigue or feeling tired
- Dizziness, irritability, and fainting

I will offer that that irritability thing should be included with other signs, not as a stand-alone sign of dehydration, otherwise I might be accused of having been dehydrated my entire life.

As it turned out all of those were present in my patient's mother.

In truth, dehydration is one of the most preventable problems and it's all too common.

If you don't think this important, consider the following. According to the US Geological Survey, water makes up approximately 60 percent of the human body, 70 percent of the brain, 90 percent of the lungs, 75 percent of lean muscle mass, 10 percent of body fat, 22 percent of your bones, and 83 percent of your blood. Just call me Aquaman!

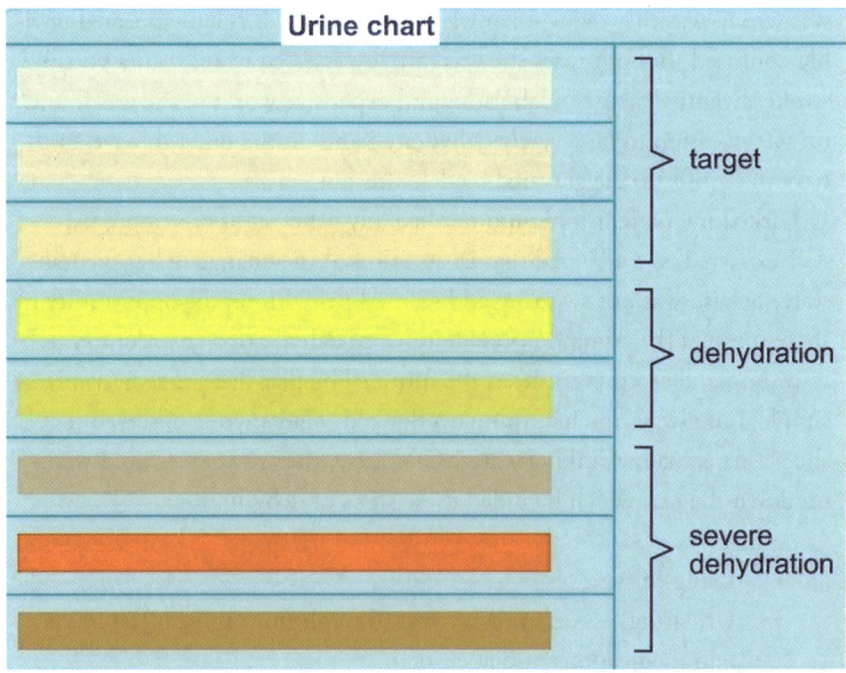

Urine chart

Proper hydration depends on a number of things: the heat, the heat index, medical conditions, medications, the sort of activity being attempted, overall fitness, and the health of the individual. All of those affect what is proper hydration. A 2004 report by the Institute of Medicine (IOM) at the National Academies provided guidelines for daily normal hydration, meaning water consumption. For male adults 19–70 years of age it was 3.7 liters (approximately 125 ounces… but let's stay with liters). For adult females the amount was 2.7 liters. Understand that these are general recommendations, not absolutes. Now, the water we consume is not just the water we drink. Some is in the foods you consume. So this is the cumulative number related to hydration. This number may also vary, as you might imagine, with a person's size and the other conditions mentioned earlier.

This also concludes my introductory lecture on the metric system.

Now, if you factor in additional requirements of exercise or increased activity, temperature, and humidity, for yourself you might find you get some very different numbers.

If you really want to be more exact, you can calculate your basic daily drinking water requirement by taking your weight in pounds, dividing it by half (or multiplying it by .5—it's the same thing!), and then dividing that number by 8 (the number of ounces in a cup).

For example, if you weigh 140 pounds:

140 / 2 (or 140 × .5) = 70

70 / 8 = 8.75, or approximately 9 cups of water per day!

Or if you're a metric type:

Weight in kilograms multiplied by 30 = milliliters per day.

If you are a stickler for math, you will realize that equation doesn't amount to the IOM numbers. That said, these are very broasd estimates and they vary. Suffice it to say you should *consult with your healthcare provider* for your individualized personal intake recommendation and then make sure you consume enough.

Of course, this all depends on being healthy, the weather or climate you are in, your medications, and more, so again, talk to your healthcare provider to get specific advice.

Suddenly, I see a *Schoolhouse Rock* entry in my future!

If you have any ideas about how I can create a really catchy song about hydration, let me know. I'm thinking of something like, "*hydration station, helps constipationnnn . . .*"

Maybe not.

Nutrition

Call it whatever you like: nutrition, food, intake, mangia, comida, the reason for being . . . we all have to do it. If you recall the Kennedy story, you *are* it. That is truer even than it initially seems. Food is the substrate of the building blocks of our body, so it makes sense that you would want it to be of the highest quality, right? And yet this may be the area where we have the least effective knowledge and often feel least in control to do what is in our own best interest. I have an anecdote that sums this up perfectly.

I was watching the news on television, and the featured story was a series dedicated to the American obesity epidemic. The on-air personalities interviewed a whole gaggle of experts who offered their theories on why Americans were becoming more obese (and at the same time less healthy from what we eat) and what we could do about it. It was a fascinating, pertinent, and disturbing discussion. I was just getting into it when the show broke for a commercial. The screen suddenly filled with a gigantic, gorgeous, perfectly grilled hamburger. It looked, in fact, like a hamburger version of a movie star, absolutely perfect for the big screen. Its pickles were just the right size, voluptuous without being tackily displayed. The mustard and ketchup were applied skillfully without being overdone and tarty, and the bun showed just enough burger to be attractive and striking without violating the standards of censorship and good taste. The lettuce was fresh and perky, and don't even get me started on the tomatoes.

In fact, I kind of need a moment alone right now.

It was the kind of hamburger that made the pathetic versions I have seen and eaten look like completely mortal fare. This was the hamburger of the gods. The kind of burger they sold at a greasy spoon on Mount Olympus. And guess what? According the commercial's narration, and even more alarming, I could have it extra-sized. That commercial was followed immediately by an advertisement for a children's cereal that was, according to a happy cartoon bird that seemed intent on whipping America's children into a feeding frenzy, chock-full of flavor and was also fun, Fun, FUNNN to eat . . . and it came with a toy!

Right after that there was an ad for a heartburn medication, followed by a commercial advertising a local weight loss center. Then finally there followed an ad requesting assistance to end world hunger. All I could determine after that was that we may just be at our craziest and conflicting when it comes to nutrition. You notice I used the word *nutrition*, not *food*, and not *eating*.

After seeing all that, I just had to wonder if it wasn't true that some— if not a substantial part—of our health issues didn't result from what we are shoving into our mouths. Food is so tightly connected to our social enterprise: how we relate to and interact with our world and how we gratify, feed, and fortify ourselves and others that we somehow lose track of the very idea of getting actual nutrition. I really think we are, in some instances, actually poisoning ourselves, either by the quantity or the quality of the stuff we consume, and I am not alone in that thought. And in the spirit of complete honesty, as in the Kennedy anecdote earlier, I am a jelly donut, and in the interest of full disclosure, I am also a sunflower seed, an eggplant, a broccoli, a black bean, a chickpea . . . the list goes on and on. So, let's look at this.

Processed Food Products

Rule number one: if it's in a package, it's processed. How much it is processed is what matters.

Processed food products—you notice I don't call them foods—start out as real food. Real food grows in fields or ideally frolics about in pastures until harvest time, when it is subjected to certain processes. Those processes can include harvesting, heating, milling, pressure treatment, irradiation, and chemical treatments.

Heat processing is often employed with canned and dried foods. Think about all that stuff on the shelf and those deceptive little packets of "all natural dried fruit snacks" that make you think you are getting a healthy choice. You may not be, actually.

Milling sounds like a natural process. When I first heard the word, I imagined a rustic structure next to a happy little burbling stream with a waterwheel turning a grist stone. It's actually a little less pastoral in reality. Let's take flour for example. In reality whole-grain wheat berries, including the most nutritionally important parts, the germ and endosperm, are delivered from the field as technically living things. What I mean by that is if you took a wheat berry and planted it, it would germinate and grow as long as soil and adequate amounts of water were available.

En route to becoming flour, it often enters a factory where it is pulverized and the germ is generally removed. It is then subjected to chemical bleaching, mixed with preservatives to prevent mold and extend the "shelf life," a term that is terrifically ironic as what started as a living nutrient-dense product, a wheat berry, is now completely devoid of life. Its new "life" as a cracker or noodle or slice of bread is usually substantially nutritionally depleted and as lifeless as the plastic material housing it. Some estimate that as much as 60 percent of the nutritional value of the natural wheat berry can be lost in milling, bleaching, and processing.

Once on the shelf, its new definition of life is now a marketing and manufacturing term for how long it can sit and still not damage future sales potential or acutely poison the consumer.

In fact, there are often a lot of assumptions about those terms and dates stamped on the outside of the package. Didn't realize there was information like that on the outside of the package? If you didn't, you should check, and when you do, you'll discover that there is a subtle but wide variety of phrasing associated with the date. This language is very important because, after all, you are what you eat and you don't want to be an expired, old, lifeless commodity shrouded in plastic, or polyester, or cotton for that matter.

"Sell by" language can be really confusing. It tells how long the store can sell foods like meat, poultry, eggs, or milk products. It's a governmental determination based on studies and averages of the material's integrity if stored at proper temperature and in proper conditions. Basically, it is telling the store that it has to sell the product before the date. If you notice, it doesn't stipulate how long you have to consume it before it goes bad.

"Use by" does. It describes how long the food will be at peak quality. If you buy or use it after that date, some foods might not be safe any longer. If you see this language, make certain you are giving yourself enough time between purchase and consumption or you could harm yourself.

"Best if used by" (or "best if used before") tells how long the food has the best flavor or quality. It is a purely qualitative or product satisfaction term. It is not really a purchase or safety date.

So now that you know what it means, milling doesn't sound so good, does it? Sounds harsh even? Well, consider this. After going through the entirety of food product processing, in general, anywhere from 50 percent to 80 percent of the nutritional value—whether as vitamins or the actual *quality* calories—may be removed.

Now that *is* harsh. Ready for more?

Many foods are pressure-treated. In general, it is pressure combined with heat. If you are acquainted with the concept of pasteurization— quickly heating a liquid food material like milk or juice to kill contaminants and germs—then you have a rough idea, and while pasteurization is a life-saving and good concept, the application of pressure and heat also inherently depletes some of the vitality of the liquid food. It can also rob it of some of the nutritional value. Pressure treatment to further reduce the water content and preserve the material can take even more important nutritional material out of it.

Recently there has been considerable media discussion about irradiated and genetically engineered food. When I hear that, I immediately imagine some great Midwestern, 50s-era, sci-fi flick about giant vegetables running amuck, like *The Corn That Ate Omaha* or *The Adventures of Broccoli Man*. Unfortunately, it's not nearly that whimsical. As far as radiation goes, it has been used for years to sterilize food products that otherwise would not tolerate pressure and heat without becoming unmarketable. You generally see this used with herbs, spices, and some herbal infusions.

Genetic modification speaks to the actual manipulation of some aspect or sequence of an organism's genetic material. It is not like the artificial selection you know from selective breeding of, say, cattle, but it is more focused on the manipulation of a specific gene or trait of an animal. This is an area where a lot of people and some food advocacy groups have concerns. So as they say in the Saturday serial adventures, "Stay tuned."

Food additives are everywhere. They are in everything from bread to dairy products to commercially prepared sauces to baby food. About the only place you won't find them in your food is out in the orchard or in the garden.

So, you might be thinking, if it's not packaged, it is probably okay, right? Unfortunately, no. When I was boy, back in the Pleistocene era, there were certain times of the year when we could not get certain fresh fruits and vegetables. The grocer would shake his head and say, "It's out of season." So we had to get something else, like a processed fruit in heavy corn syrup (insert sarcastic tone here), and we made do. If you notice nowadays, there is never any shortage of fresh fruits and vegetables. Fantastic, isn't it? Well, maybe and maybe not.

If you see fruits and vegetables in your local grocery store's produce bin, especially if they are not in season in your area, they may be from a place that does not have the same regulatory requirements as we are used to in the United States. This really means that you should ask your grocer about the source of the produce and be sure to read the small print (you will want extra powerful readers) to determine if the produce is from another country. If so, then check the websites of the Food and Drug Administration (FDA) and US Department of Agriculture (USDA) for any warnings, and please use extra caution in washing your fruits or vegetables before you prepare or eat them.

Additives and Food Labeling

If there is only one thing you take away from this discussion of food, I hope it is the recommendation to *read* the label of any processed food package. And I am not just talking about the front of the package. In fact, I sort of look at the front of the package as nothing more than a last-ditch commercial effort. The back of the package, however, is where you'll find the required disclosure of the real ingredients of the package's contents. In particular, you should look for two things: the ingredients list and the nutrition facts label. What's the difference?

THE INGREDIENTS LIST

This is a required list of the ingredients of a processed food. The ingredients are listed in descending order—from greatest amount to least so. For example, if the first thing listed is processed flour, then that is what it contains the most. Oddly enough, the ingredients list does not tell you

> **Ingredients: Whole Grain Oats, Sugar, Oat Flour, Corn Syrup, Modified Corn Starch, Corn Starch, Dextrose, Salt, Gelatin, Trisodium Phosphate, Yellows 5 & 6, Red 40, Blue 1 and Other Color Added, Natural and Artificial Flavor. Vitamin E** (mixed tocopherols) **Added to Preserve Freshness.**
>
> **Vitamins and Minerals: Calcium Carbonate, Zinc and Iron** (mineral nutrients), **Vitamin C** (sodium ascorbate), **A B Vitamin** (niacinamide), **Vitamin B$_6$** (pyridoxine hydrochloride), **Vitamin B$_2$** (riboflavin), **Vitamin B$_1$** (thiamin mononitrate), **Vitamin A** (palmitate), **A B Vitamin** (folic acid), **Vitamin B$_{12}$, Vitamin D$_3$.**

the percentage of processed flour there is, so it could be 20 percent or 99 percent. Tricky, huh? Don't feel completely informed? We aren't.

Here's an example from a popular product.

It starts out pretty nicely. Whole-grain oats. Okay. Then the second most common ingredient is sugar. Uhhhhh, okay. Then beyond sugar the next most common ingredient is oat flour, which would normally make me feel a little more reassured, but remembering what I do about the processing of milling, I am not so sure. Next up is corn syrup. Know what that is? A whole lot of sugar! So, yeah, there is a lot of sugar. I mean this is a pretty good start to the day—if you are a hummingbird! My hands are starting to shake already.

NUTRITIONAL FACTS LABEL

The nutrition facts label is the breakdown of material in the processed food that contributes to the daily estimated nutritional requirements for an adult, based on a 1,200-, 2,000-, or 2,500-calorie diet. The nutritional facts label should always be read carefully in conjunction with the ingredients list. So for the same product let's consider this. At the time of printing the FDA was proposing the following label changes.

Nutrition Facts

Serving Size 2/3 cup (55g)
Servings Per Container About 8

Amount Per Serving

Calories 230 | Calories from Fat 72

	% Daily Value*
Total Fat 8g	**12%**
Saturated Fat 1g	**5%**
Trans Fat 0g	
Cholesterol 0mg	**0%**
Sodium 160mg	**7%**
Total Carbohydrate 37g	**12%**
Dietary Fiber 4g	**16%**
Sugars 1g	
Protein 3g	

Vitamin A	10%
Vitamin C	8%
Calcium	20%
Iron	45%

* Percent Daily Values are based on a 2,000 calorie diet. Your daily value may be higher or lower depending on your calorie needs.

	Calories:	2,000	2,500
Total Fat	Less than	65g	80g
Sat Fat	Less than	20g	25g
Cholesterol	Less than	300mg	300mg
Sodium	Less than	2,400mg	2,400mg
Total Carbohydrate		300g	375g
Dietary Fiber		25g	30g

Original nutrition facts label

Starting at the top, we see the serving size and the number of servings in the package. This is extremely important information, especially with some packages, as the assumption is that a package *is* a serving. Next up is the breakdown of calories per serving. Now, in this product's case, there are maybe two entries. The product in the box and the product with milk added, which is how most people would consume it.

Alternate Format

Nutrition Facts

8 servings per container

Serving size   2/3 cup (55g)

Amount per 2/3 cup

Calories   **230**

% Daily Value*

QUICK FACTS:

12%	**Total Fat** 8g
12%	**Total Carbs** 37g
	Sugars 1g
	Protein 3g

AVOID TOO MUCH:

5%	Saturated Fat 1g
	Trans Fat 0g
0%	**Cholesterol** 0mg
7%	**Sodium** 160mg
	Added Sugars 0g

GET ENOUGH:

14%	Fiber 4g
10%	Vitamin D 2mcg
20%	Calcium 260mg
45%	Iron 8mg
5%	Potassium 235mg

* Footnote on Daily Values (DV) and calorie reference to be inserted here.

Proposed nutrition facts label

Seems kind of vague and potentially misleading? Maybe. Seems like you need to read the fine print? Well, you do. So why are food producers doing this? What do they have to gain? In a word, money. A lot of it. Consider the following.

According to Michael Moss, the Pulitzer Prize–winning author of *Salt Sugar Fat: How the Food Giants Hooked Us*, "Grocery sales now top $1 trillion a year in the US, with more than 300 manufacturers employing 1.4 million workers, or 12 percent of all American manufacturing jobs. Global sales exceed $3 trillion."

That is pretty good motivation, huh?

In order to achieve that end, he found that

". . . according to high level industry officials and a trove of sensitive, internal records—a window opened on how aggressive the industry was wielding not only salt, but sugar and fat, too. These are the pillars of processed foods, the three ingredients without which there would be no processed foods. Salt, sugar and fat drive consumption by adding flavor and allure. But surprisingly, they also mask bitter flavors that develop in the manufacturing process. They enable these foods to sit in warehouses or on the grocery shelf for months. And, most critically to the industry's financial success, they are very inexpensive."

Now, consider that they literally control the market, that most Big Food industry products command the optimal shelf space in grocery stores, and that healthier and less refined products are relegated to the bottom or top of the shelf. These food companies control access to prime advertisement spots, and they know exactly what we like. In many cases they have even helped shape our palate so we do like what we like. Sometimes it seems we stand almost no chance at all in eating healthy.

Almost, but not quite.

By virtue of the fact that you are reading this book, you have one factor in your favor. You can read! So keep going.

In table 1 you will find a list of some of the prime offenders, a Minson's Most Wanted list of foods that can have significant health impacts. Bon Appétit.

Table 1. Dietary Offenders or . . . Hit Foods

Ramen Noodles: Offender=SALT

Ramen noodles are popular among college students, but they are not a healthy meal. One package of Ramen noodles adds 14 grams of fat to your day and 1,580 mg of sodium! Interestingly, it is actually the flavor packet that contains most of that sodium.

Pickles: Offender=SALT

Pickles are low-calorie, which is good, but they are loaded with sodium. One medium pickle (about 5 inches long) can have around 570 mg of sodium. That's over one-third of your sodium limit (2,300 mg) for the day.

Sauerkraut: Offender=SALT

Sauerkraut is great low-calorie way to add vegetables to a bratwurst, right? Not really. A half cup may only have 13 calories, but it also has over 460 mg of sodium.

Chicken Soup: Offender=SALT

Chicken noodle soup is often considered a comfort food, but it is not so comforting to know that there can be up to 880 mg of sodium in a one-cup serving. If you think about it, when you are potentially salt/electrolyte depleted or dehydrated when sick with a respiratory infection, you crave salt and this may be how and why it got its reputation as a remedy. Otherwise, be careful.

Processed Pot Pies: Offender=SALT+FAT

A single pot pie can contain about 1,300–1,400 mg of sodium plus about 35 grams of fat! Keep in mind that this is over 50% of your daily recommended values for both. The fat also includes trans fat, which you want to eliminate from your diet completely, and it also can have an unhealthy dose of saturated fat.

Alcohol: Offender=Blood Vessel Damage+Hypertension

This one is tricky and a matter of excess exclusively. Alcohol consumption can actively cause blood pressure to elevate. It can also damage the walls of the blood vessels while simultaneously increasing risks of further complications for diabetics.

French Fries: Offender=FAT+SALT

While many fast food chains are now frying their fries in trans-fat-free oil, not all of them are. Regardless, French fries still provide a large dose of fat and sodium. A medium serving of fries has about 19 grams of fat and 270 mg of sodium.

Bacon: Offender=FAT+SALT

Bacon is mostly fat. Three slices have 4.5 grams of fat and about 270 mg of sodium. Opt for lower-sodium varieties and try turkey bacon instead of pork. Even with these switches bacon should remain a "special treat," not an everyday indulgence.

Donuts: Offender=FAT

Donuts are the siren song of processed foods. Almost irresistible, they sure aren't very good for your health and body. Just one donut packs in 200 calories with 12 grams of fat.

Sadly, I like a lot of the stuff on that list, but every time I am tempted, I just envision myself standing on the railing of the Brooklyn Bridge, eating a nitrate-laced hotdog, on a processed bun, covered in kraut and pickles . . . right before I jump off? Sometimes it helps.

Food and Aging

Admittedly as we age, the issues of nutrition, food buying, and hydration often are an ever greater challenge. Many seniors find just considering the subject of nutrition difficult, even without the distractions, and not worth the trouble, as food itself may have lost some of its appeal. We often feel that food doesn't taste the same way it once did or as good, or that getting out to the store to shop is too difficult, or that we have no appetite at all, or that it costs too much. These are just a few of the many reasons that seniors don't eat healthily.

The National Institute on Aging has put together a number of free publications with guidelines and helpful nutritional strategies for people over the age of 50. They address issues like food safety, getting additional financial support, understanding your daily caloric requirements, and how to eat nutritionally on a budget.

In 2010 the USDA and Health and Human Services came out with *Dietary Guidelines for Americans*, which described healthy eating plans. The USDA "food patterns" suggest that people who are 50 and older should choose a selection of the following daily:

Fruit. Try to consume from *one and a half to two cups* of fruit every day. For the best results, I'd look to unprocessed fruit to make sure you are not consuming unnecessary calories from sweeteners and corn syrup. Not that I should have to describe a cup, but given what I have seen and the American propensity for supersized portions, a half cup as described here is roughly the same amount as a cut-up, two-inch peach.

Vegetables. Try to consume *two to three and a half cups* of vegetables. Again, I am going to make a plea for fresh vegetables—not canned or processed materials—if you can get them. With fresh vegetables, you control the amount of cooking and depletion that a vegetable undergoes before you eat it.

Grains. Try to consume *5 to 10 ounces of grains* each day. A small whole-grain (including the germ and endosperm) muffin, a slice of whole-grain bread, a cup of whole-grain cereal, or a half cup of grain or pasta should amount to roughly that amount. Now, I am aware that "small" is a relative term. For purposes of clarity and at the risk of angering well over half of the world, I will offer that "small" is roughly three by three inches. If it makes you feel like you are getting more, you can use the metric system and luxuriate in seven centimeters by seven centimeters of muffiny goodness.

Proteins. Try to consume *five to seven ounces* of protein. Most people immediately think of protein as a meat product, like, say, SPAM.

Actually, this is neither an endorsement nor a condemnation of SPAM, though it certainly made for a catchy Monty Python tune.

The truth is that you can get all the protein you need without the additional "bad" fats such as transfats or saturated fats by consuming other protein sources such as legumes. Legumes are things like chickpeas, beans, and lentils. They are low in fat and generally cheaper, in case you are considering budgetary issues.

Five to seven ounces is the same as one egg, a quarter cup of cooked beans, tofu, or lentils, nuts or seeds, or a little over a tablespoon of peanut butter.

Dairy foods. Try to consume *three cups* of fat-free or low-fat milk. Obviously for some individuals with lactose intolerance or other digestive problems, you should speak with a nutritionist and your doctor about alternatives. Professional consultation is the advice I have given for everything else, but I wanted to include it here as well. Dairy, of course, includes milk, which most of us think of as cow's milk. It can also include cheese, cottage cheese, and yogurt.

Now, when I was a boy, I encountered one of the greatest products, I then thought, in the history of food: spray-on cheese spread. It came in a can, and with the push of a button, expressed at high velocity, something that tasted exactly like cheese. It was simultaneously a food product, source of practical jokes, literary expression (you could write with the stuff), and, at times, even a weapon. What it wasn't . . . was cheese. I read the label, I think I was eleven maybe, and it was like a lesson in organic and inorganic chemistry. Most of it was preservatives and manufactured edible oils. Following the ingredients list, I finally found—at about entry number thirty—"cheese flavorings." Years later, I still can't figure what cheese products actually are. I just know that the stuff I used to spray paint everything from a backyard fence to a saltine was definitely not cheese. Which leads to. . .

Oils. I have already talked about fats, I know, but this use of the term "oils" is a little different. This is oil added during the process of cooking as opposed to oils inherently included in a foodstuff. Again, in general, a healthy diet should include about *five to eight teaspoons* of healthy oil a day.

What's on the Plate

There is another way of thinking about this is a little more user-friendly. The National Institute on Aging's *What's on Your Plate?* program, https://www.nia.nih.gov/health/publication/whats-your-plate recommends using common items for measures of what should be included and the limits of what should be on a plate for a meal. For example, a deck of cards amounts to about three ounces of meat or poultry protein. Half a baseball amounts to a half cup. And, if you are doing the math, a whole baseball is roughly a cup. So is a balled up fist, roughly. Four dice together amount to one and a half ounces of cheese, not the spray-can kind. The tip of your first finger is roughly a teaspoon of butter or margarine. A compact disc or DVD is the size of a standard tortilla or pancake. And, finally, a Ping Pong ball is equal to two tablespoons. Frankly, all this discussion is making me hungry and oddly interested in a parlor game.

Fiber

To quote my grandmother, you can't swing a dead cat without hitting somebody that is talking about fiber. Now, I never understood that concept of swinging a dead cat. I assumed it was part of her ongoing, constant theme of how hard and impoverished an upbringing she'd had. I know for fact she walked to school in the snow and didn't have shoes and had to eat all sorts of unprocessed stuff, so I am just guessing that she was hard up for playthings (and apparently pets, too), not to mention adequate personal space. For the record, as a person interested in promoting good health, I don't recommend doing that with a dead cat. In fact, I wouldn't handle a dead cat. I would recommend just respectfully disposing of it. I'd also recommend taking better care of your cat so it doesn't end up that way in the first place.

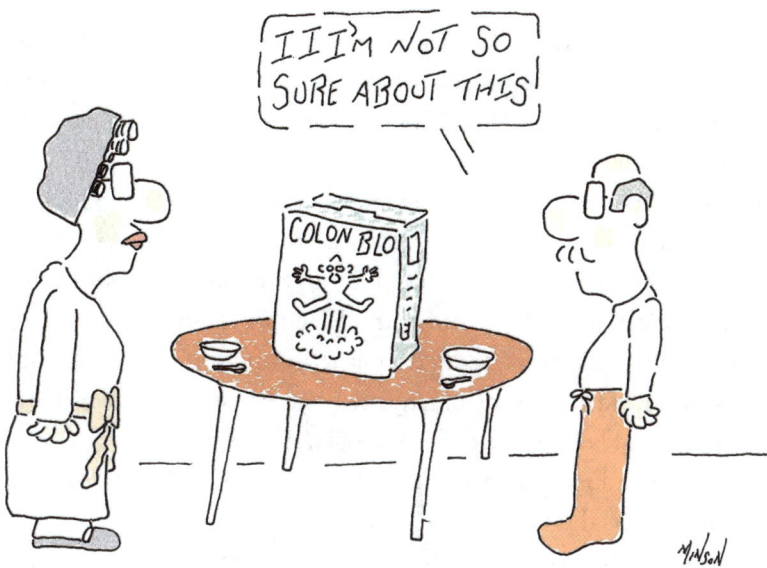

So, on to fiber!

In a word, fiber is good. It has been shown to aid in digestion and in promoting digestive health by reducing constipation, reducing diverticula formation, lowering cholesterol, and helping to normalize blood sugar. So it's good. There are a number of ways that you can get a proper amount of fiber. The best way is from natural sources. Tactics for increasing the fiber content of food can include eating cooked lentils, beans, and peas often, leaving the skins and peelings on fruits and vegetables, increasing the amount of fruits and vegetables in your diet, and using whole grains.

If additional fiber is needed, there are dietary cellulose supplements. One of the least expensive and natural sources is miller's bran. This is basically the outer seed covering of grain and is available in many health food stores or online. It is tasteless and odorless and can be added to almost anything from salads to prepared food. It is also extremely inexpensive.

Salt

Most people see the word salt and they think sodium chloride, as represented by its chemical symbology NaCl. Technically "salt" is anything that precipitates from an acid and a base encountering each other. Forgive me. I am in a *chemistry* kind of mood obviously. It's important, though.

A chemist, nutritionist, or physician may use the term salt, but they can also mean other things, especially when talking about medications and chemicals. For the purposes of this book, I'll stay with the popular term, meaning NaCl.

In general, the more processed a food is, the more likely a food has accumulated added salt, either in the process of milling and bleaching or as a flavor enhancement or preservative. It is not bad, but if all you are consuming is processed food, you are probably getting multiple doses of salt and sugar, which also osmotically is a salt. Need more of an explanation?

Back in the olden days, before my grandmother started playing with her dead cat and before proper food refrigeration resources, the preservation of certain food products was with sugar and salt. This is how the Founding Fathers did it.

Sugar and salt dehydrated the food and made the foodstuff inhospitable to bacterial growth. As a result, the salt content increased and our palates adjusted. Even today salt is added to food to increase its palatability and marketability. If you see a food product that is "cured" or "brined," be careful and be sure to read the back of the package. You'll be impressed, and maybe alarmed, by the amount of sodium it contains. Some raw or unprocessed foods also have inherently higher salt content. Meat, for example, that is high in protein often has higher salt amounts. Canned and preserved foods like beef jerky and canned goods often are quite high as well.

The simple fact is that our bodies need salt. Too much salt, however, can lead to a number of problems, including increased blood pressure and aggravation of certain diseases, especially cardiac conditions. Most people consume way too much. This may be due, in part, to their adding salt to their food at the table. More likely, they are consuming salt that is already in the food to excess. Don't believe me? Check out the nutritional facts entry on the package and look at the sodium content.

According to USDA and HHS, for people over the age of 50 the daily limit of the amount of salt or sodium chloride is 1,500 milligrams, or about two-thirds of a teaspoon. For younger adults it is 2,300 milligrams. This is not just what you shake on your dinner. It includes all the NaCl that is in your foods from processing *and* what you decide to add during preparation *and* what you add at the table. Want to do something about this? Read! Not the front of the package, the back!

You might also consider using salt substitutes. A good idea, but be careful. Many salt substitutes still contain sodium chloride. They may also contain potassium, which also has a daily limit and amount. In doubt? Talk with your healthcare provider and probably also a credentialed dietician. If you ask your healthcare provider for a consultation with a dietician or credentialed nutritionist, your insurance policy may cover the cost. There are additional risks of overdosing on salt for older people. Remember what I wrote in the last chapter about how the ability to detect taste changes, and how we tend to over season, most usually with salt? A safe alternative to this is to increase the amount of spice or citrus rather than salt. Doing this tends to satisfy the palate and reduces the amount of NaCl ingested.

Fats

I've already talked a little about fats, especially those inherent fats in foodstuffs, but I do want to add one additional thought in terms of "solid" fats like animal fat or tallow and certain manufactured fats like shortening. Generally, these are unhealthy fats. There are also healthier fats, such as vegetable oils or some nut-based oils (see table 2).

There are some other things you can do to reduce the amount of fat you consume.

Table 2. Bad Fat, Good Fat

Solid Fats and Oils	Vegetable Oil Alternatives
Beef, pork, and chicken fat	Canola oil
Butter, cream, and milk fat	Corn oil
Coconut, palm, and palm kernel oils	Cottonseed oil
Hydrogenated oil	Olive oil
Partially hydrogenated oil	Peanut oil
Shortening	Safflower oil
Stick margarine	Sunflower oil

- Trim fatty tissue from cuts of meat.
- Remove the skin before cooking.
- Choose unsaturated oils for cooking.
- Boil, broil, and steam your foods.

Can I Eat Healthy on the Cheap?

Now you may be thinking, thanks for all the advice, but I can barely afford one can of SPAM. What is all this fancy food selection going to cost me? Surprisingly, not necessarily a lot. In fact, it may save you money. I'll cover food assistance and resources for seniors in the next section, "Liberty." For now, you might want to look at the really great work done by Iowa State University. It has a website (http://www.extension.iastate.edu/foodsavings) that offers a calculator, tactics, recommendations, and recipes, which also break down nutrient-dense dishes for pennies a serving.

Alcohol

So this subject is tricky—mainly because people hear and read exactly what they want to when you start talking about the health benefits of moderate consumption. So with that risk in mind, I'm going to offer the following disclaimer. Please talk to your healthcare provider and get specific advice. What I am going to suggest is based on a very broad generality! I'll start off with saying that too much of a good thing is bad! So if every evening or weekend at your house is like an outtake of *Angela's Ashes*, then, yeah, you need to rethink your intake. That said, there are some reported benefits associated with modest imbibing.

You know I like the Founding Fathers. Well, they used to raise a glass and drink to health, and there is actually something to that. The beneficial effects, generally, of moderate or modest alcohol consumption and certain beverages have specific effects. Now, most people instantly say, "Oh yeah, I heard red wine is okay." Then they open the sluice gate and begin swilling away. There actually *are* many benefits to red wine. It has polyphenols, which act as antioxidants, and there is an antibacterial compound known as reservetrol, which helps prevent blood clots and reduce bad cholesterol, but before you sign up for the Robert Mondavi liquid health plan, remember, it is all about moderation. Similarly, white wine has benefits, though the concentration of its compounds compared with those in the darker grapes are reduced.

According to the CDC, a standard drink in the United States is 14.0 grams or 0.6 ounces of pure alcohol. This generally equates to 12 ounces of beer (5 percent alcohol content) or 8 ounces of malt liquor (7 percent; you know who you are!) or 5 ounces of wine (12 percent) or 1.5 ounces or a "shot" of 80-proof (40 percent alcohol content). If you are from Kentucky or West Virginia and you make "hooch" up in a "holler," then all bets are off. I watch reality TV, too, as you can tell.

According to the *Dietary Guidelines for Americans*, moderate consumption is one drink per day for women and two drinks per day for men. Sorry, ladies.

Now one thing I want to make really clear is that I am not suggesting anyone start drinking if they don't drink already. In fact, the initiation of drinking in a search for health benefits is not recommended. More like an excuse, really.

Also please understand that alcohol consumption is extremely biologically specific to the individual. There are a bunch of factors that influence why people differ. They are: age, gender, race and ethnicity, physical condition or health, concurrent food consumption, the period of time during which the alcohol was consumed, family history of alcohol issues or abuse, and the medication you might be on.

Some people should never consume alcohol. They include children, alcoholics, pregnant women, individuals who are about to drive an automobile or boat or who will operate heavy equipment, people who have a medical condition, including medications that prohibit it, and those whose healthcare providers have recommended against it.

Sleep
RESTFUL SLEEP

No matter how well we nourish ourselves, no matter how in shape we are, no matter how well hydrated, there is one additional factor in the healthy behavior category that can make or break how healthy we truly are. That is how well and how restfully we sleep. Of course, considering rest and hydration, when you hydrate is just as important, as any six-year-old boy caught between the urgings of his full bladder and the fear of the monster under the bed will tell you . . . but enough about me and my childhood traumas.

WHY WE SLEEP

Nobody seems completely, definitively sure why we have to sleep. There are a lot of theories, but one thing that is certain is that sleep is essential for survival. Animal studies involving rats show that if an animal, humans included, is not allowed to sleep, within two weeks it will die.

Experts have theorized that sleeping might be an evolutionary instrument to conserve energy. Others suggest that sleep offers the brain a chance to process experiences or exercise neurological pathways that are subverted to conscious thought while we are awake. Regardless, sleep has a therapeutic benefit in that it offers the body and mind the opportunity to revitalize, reenergize, and restore. We use it to organize long-term memory, integrate knowledge and experiences to our psyche, and repair and restore nervous-system tissue.

If you recall, earlier in the book I described the way the brain and nervous system send signals via electrical and certain hormonal and chemical mechanisms. These neurotransmitters and their receptors impact various functions. For example, serotonin affects mood, acetylcholine affects memory, learning, and concentration, and dopamine plays a role in movement, motivation, and learning. Now this is way oversimplified, but here's how it works. Over time, each day, as we are awake and thinking—or writing a book—the balance of these neurotransmitters get out of equilibrium and metabolic waste accumulates. These chemicals, a part of the neuroendocrine system, eventually need to be restored to balance after such prolonged neurological activity.

SLEEP THEORIES
Inactivity Theory
One of the earliest theories of sleep, sometimes called the adaptive or evolutionary theory, suggests that inactivity at night is an adaptation that

served a survival function by keeping organisms out of harm's way at times when they would be particularly vulnerable. Take, for example, our good friend, the cave-dwelling brother of Og Mammothtail, and Wendell the saber-toothed cat. It was much easier for them both to find food in the daytime and, for Og and his relatives, at least, to hide during the night. This theory suggests that animals that were able to stay still and quiet during these periods of vulnerability had an advantage over other animals that remained active. This is also known at my house as "the squeaky wheel gets removed." These animals did not have accidents during activities in the dark, for example, and were not killed by predators. Through natural selection, this behavioral strategy presumably evolved to become what we now recognize as sleep.

A simple counterargument to this theory is that it is always safer to remain conscious in order to be able to react to an emergency (even if lying still in the dark at night). Thus, there does not seem to be any advantage to being unconscious and asleep if safety is paramount.

Brain Plasticity Theory

One of the most recent and compelling explanations for why we sleep is based on findings that sleep is correlated to changes in the structure and organization of the brain. This phenomenon, known as brain plasticity, is not entirely understood, but its connection to sleep has several critical implications. It is becoming clear, for example, that sleep plays a critical role in brain development in infants and young children. Infants spend about 13 to 14 hours per day sleeping, and about half of that time is spent in rapid eye movement (REM) sleep, the stage in which most dreams occur. A link between sleep and preserving brain plasticity is becoming clear in adults as well. This is seen in the effect that sleep and sleep deprivation have on people's ability to learn and perform a variety of tasks.

The Restorative Theory

Another explanation for why we sleep is based on the long-held belief that sleep in some way serves to "restore" what is lost in the body while we are awake. Sleep provides an opportunity for the body to repair and rejuvenate itself. In recent years, these ideas have gained support from empirical evidence collected in human and animal studies. The most striking of these is that animals deprived entirely of sleep lose all immune function and die in just a matter of weeks. This is further supported by findings that many of the major restorative functions in the body, like muscle growth, tissue repair, protein synthesis, and growth hormone release, occur mostly or, in some cases, only during sleep.

Other rejuvenating aspects of sleep are specific to the brain and cognitive function. For example, while we are awake, neurons in the brain produce adenosine, a by-product of the cells' activities. The buildup of adenosine in the brain is thought to be one factor that leads to our perception of being tired. (Incidentally, this feeling is supposedly counteracted by the use of caffeine, which blocks the actions of adenosine in the brain and keeps us alert.) Scientists think that this buildup of adenosine during wakefulness may promote the "drive to sleep." As long as we are awake, adenosine accumulates and remains high. During sleep, the body has a chance to clear adenosine from the system; as a result, we feel more alert when we awaken.

Energy Conservation Theory

Although it may be less apparent to people living in societies in which food sources are plentiful, one of the strongest factors in natural selection is competition for and effective utilization of energy resources. The energy conservation theory suggests that the primary function of sleep is to reduce an individual's energy demand and expenditure during part of the day or night, especially at times when it is least efficient to search for food.

Research has shown that energy metabolism is significantly reduced during sleep (by as much as 10 percent in humans and even more in other species). For example, both body temperature and caloric demand decrease during sleep, as compared with wakefulness. Such evidence supports the proposition that one of the primary functions of sleep is to help organisms conserve their energy resources. This would apply to both Og and Wendell. Many scientists consider this theory to be related to and part of the inactivity theory.

Regardless of why we need it, getting adequate rest accomplishes a number of things. It allows our bodies to recharge and repair themselves. It also is necessary for proper neurological or brain function. This is not just true of people over the age of 50, but of everyone.

At a certain point we become sleepy, which is the result of the brain's signaling that it needs to cease conscious activity. And then, according to Shakespeare, we "sleep, perchance to dream," we hope. For many of us, achieving a restful night's sleep is not as easy as closing our eyes and drifting off. Illness, chronic medical problems, stress, medications, and other things can impede the ability to fall asleep or stay asleep for a sufficient period of time.

STAGES OF SLEEP

Sleep can be divided into two main categories: rapid eye movement (REM) sleep and non-REM sleep.

Non-REM sleep is further divided into four stages. Stage 1 is the "lightest" stage. You can be awakened without difficulty; however, if aroused from this stage of sleep, you may feel as if you have not slept at all. Stage 1 may last for 5 to 10 minutes. Many may notice the feeling of falling during this stage of sleep (hence "falling asleep"), which may cause a sudden muscle contraction called hypnic myoclonia. Personally, I like that term. I think that sounds like a really cool name for a jazz musician whose favorite head covering is a beret. As in "Appearing one night only, the Hypnic Myoclonia Five or Hypnic Myoclonia and Thelonious Monk present, 'Christmas Is a Real Gas.'"

Stage 2 is a period of light sleep during which polysomnographic (electrical sleep) readings show intermittent peaks and valleys, or positive and negative waves. These waves indicate spontaneous periods of increased muscle tone mixed with periods of muscle relaxation. The heart rate slows, and the body temperature decreases. At this point, the body prepares to enter deep sleep.

Stages 3 and 4 are the deep stages. They are also known as Delta (wave) sleep. This is the depth from which your being awakened makes you somewhat disoriented for several minutes. Think of brushing your teeth with Ben Gay liniment by mistake. These deep stages have been shown to be periods during which your body regenerates some tissues and strengthens its immune system.

REM sleep generally occurs about 90 minutes after you fall asleep. The first period of REM typically lasts 10 minutes, with each recurring

REM stage lengthening, and the final one lasting up to an hour. In people without sleep disorders, heart rate and respiration speed up and become erratic during REM sleep. During this stage the eyes move rapidly in different directions. Intense dreaming occurs during REM sleep as a result of heightened brain activity, but a relative paralysis occurs simultaneously in the major voluntary muscle groups. REM is a mixture of encephalic (brain) states of excitement and muscular immobility. Doesn't that sound exciting? It almost makes me wish I were awake so I wouldn't miss it.

During sleep the body cycles between non-REM and REM sleep. Typically, people begin the sleep cycle with a period of non-REM sleep followed by a very short period of REM sleep.

How much sleep do you need?

This really varies with each one of us. On average, and I stress this is really general, adults need from seven to nine hours of sleep each day.

SLEEP DISORDERS

One of the great fallacies about aging is that poor sleep is inevitable. It's not, even though according to the National Sleep Foundation, 74 percent of *all* adults experience difficulty sleeping once or twice a week. According to a report issued by the National Commission on Sleep Disorders Research, 30 percent to 40 percent of people in the United States have insomnia within any given year. Insomnia is defined by the National Institutes of Health as "an experience of inadequate or poor-quality sleep." Characteristics of insomnia include difficulty falling asleep, difficulty maintaining sleep, waking up too early in the morning, experiencing nonrefreshing sleep followed by daytime tiredness or a lack of energy and difficulty concentrating, and irritability.

Lack of sleep or poor rest can lead to a number of cognitive and behavioral issues, such as concentrating, making decisions, working with and getting along with other people, and unsafe actions.

It is such a prevalent problem that there are medical professionals who specialize in the treatment of sleep disorders exclusively. There are a lot of medical reasons that people fail to achieve restful sleep. One of the most common is soft tissue apnea, a narrowing or blockage of the upper airway, usually when the soft tissue in the rear of the throat collapses during sleep. If you have heard someone with this condition, you know it sounds like a broken buzz saw is being started in the next room or like an active murder by strangulation is taking place. It's no laughing matter, though. Obstructive sleep apnea is more common among older adults and among people who are significantly overweight. Obstructive sleep apnea can increase a person's risk for high blood pressure, strokes, heart disease, and cognitive problems.

Risk factors for sleep apnea include being overweight, male, and over age 40 as well as having a large neck size, enlarged tonsils and tongue, a family history of sleep apnea, gastroesophageal reflux disease (GERD), nasal obstructions due to a deviated septum, and allergies or sinus problems.

In some cases the airway is not blocked, but the brain fails to signal the muscles that control breathing. This is known as central sleep apnea.

Regardless, if you experience daytime sleepiness, no matter how much time you spend in bed, seek medical attention.

WHAT YOU CAN DO

- First, get help. Not by drinking or taking a pill on your own. Get a medical evaluation from your healthcare provider. This is critical. The cause could be something life threatening and you don't want to overlook that.
- If your healthcare provider determines that you need a Continuous Positive Airway Pressure (CPAP) device, dental devices, or surgery, follow through.
- Limit excessive noise and/or light in your sleep environment.
- Limit the time spent in bed while not sleeping, and use brighter lighting to help with circadian rhythm problems. Your circadian rhythm is your 24-hour internal body clock and is affected by sunlight.
- Utilize relaxation techniques like meditation.
- Keep a regular sleep schedule. Go to sleep and wake up at the same time, even on weekends. Indulge in ritual that is the same every time you are about to go to bed. By ritual, I'm talking about turning off the TV and letting things get quiet—not sacrificing virgins, then again . . .

- Try not to nap too much during the day. This one varies with different people and the length of the nap.
- Don't drink alcohol to try to help you sleep. Even small amounts of alcohol can make it harder to stay asleep.
- Create a safe and comfortable place to sleep.
- Use your bedroom only for sleeping. After turning off the light, give yourself about 15 minutes to fall asleep. If you are still awake and not drowsy, get out of bed. When you get sleepy, go back to bed.

Oh, and then there is the benefit of exercise. I can't say enough about this one, but I am about to try…

Exercise and Rest

If you recall, when we last left the mammoth-burger-eating caveman, he was all keyed up and balancing the desire to eat his lunch with the survival reflex to flee from Wendell. In addressing the relationship between exercise or physical activity and rest, think about the sympathetic and parasympathetic nervous systems. One controls fight or flight, the other controls rest and relaxation. So, in the caveman's case, when he is worried about running away from Wendell and less consumed with enjoying his burger, he is in sympathetic mode. His heart is beating faster, blood is shunted to the muscles, and the last thing biologically that his body wants to do is "take a little nap." So he runs from the big cat. His muscles heat up as they go into overdrive, his breathing rate increases, and his heart rate speeds up as he tries to escape with his burger in hand. Now if he is successful in his escape, after an interval of time, he starts to realize that he is in the clear, and so does his body. Eventually the muscles cool down, and his neglected stomach reminds him it is time to eat. So he gobbles the rest of his lunch, and as the muscles start to cool more, something happens. He gets sleepy.

Or, if you were rooting for Wendell, he charges after his burger-eating prey, and after running and tracking relentlessly, he manages to score both a caveman *and* a burger. Talk about supersizing a meal! As he settles down to a prehistoric surf-and-turf, or actually, turf-and-turf dinner, his muscles start to cool down and, eventually, guess what. He starts to get sleepy.

What's the point? There is a scientifically supported relationship between exercise and improved sleep. How does it work? Glad you asked.

During a twenty-four-hour day our body temperatures naturally go up slightly in the daytime and back down at night, generally reaching a low point just before dawn. Decreasing body temperature seems to be a trigger, signaling the body that it's time to sleep. Now consider that engaging in normal vigorous exercise can raise the body's temperature as much as two degrees.

The body then starts to cool down and, just like with Og Mammoth-tail or Wendell, the body begins a process of rest, relaxation, and repair.

There are varying theories on why that happens, just like there are for why we need to sleep or what happens when we do. Suffice it to say that anything you can do to improve "sleep hygiene," the term that clinicians use for healthy restful sleep promotion, is a good idea. Your immunity, mood, concentration, and physical fitness and more will be better if you do.

Generally, the National Heart, Lung, and Blood Institute recommends

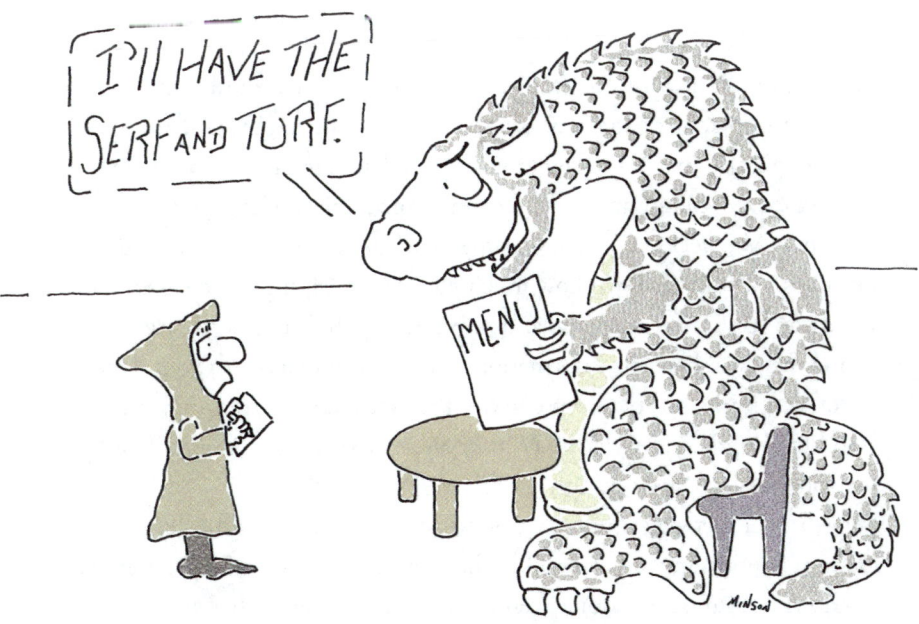

that if you think you are experiencing a sleep disorder or if you often feel sleepy during the day, don't wake up feeling refreshed and alert, or are having trouble adapting to shift work, you should talk with your healthcare provider.

In my first book I talk a lot about communicating the way your healthcare provider thinks. On that note, to get a better sense of your sleep problem, he or she will probably ask you about your sleep habits.

Before you see him or her, think about how to describe your problem. Here are some items to consider:

- How often you have trouble sleeping and how long you've had the problem
- When you go to bed and get up on workdays and days off
- How long it takes you to fall asleep, how often you wake up at night, and how long it takes you to fall back asleep
- Whether you snore loudly and often or wake up gasping or feeling out of breath
- How refreshed you feel when you wake up and how tired you feel during the day
- How often you doze off or have trouble staying awake during routine tasks, especially driving

Your doctor also may ask questions about your personal routine and habits. For example, he or she may ask about your work and exercise routines. Your doctor also may ask whether you use caffeine, tobacco, alcohol, or any medicines (including over-the-counter medicines). Keep a sleep diary for a couple of weeks. Write down when you go to sleep, wake up, and take naps. Also write down how much you sleep each night, how alert and rested you feel in the morning, and how sleepy you feel at various times during the day. Share the information in your sleep diary with your doctor.

You can find a sample sleep diary in the National Heart, Lung, and Blood Institute's *Your Guide to Healthy Sleep* (www.nhlbi.nih.gov/files/docs/public/sleep/sleep_healthy.pdf). Even better, it's free.

Just remember, age is not a reason to accept a lack of restful sleep. If you are experiencing anything like what you have read, get help. After all, you don't have to suffer alone even if you choose to sleep that way.

Summary

So I said it at the beginning, and I think it's really evident now. We are what we eat and do. If anything, our behaviors have as much to do with what we are and what we become. They can extend our lives, and regardless of our biology and genetics, they can make all the difference in the quality of what years we have left. The topics I mentioned in this chapter are far from all of the behaviors that may be applicable, but they provide a starting point for some self-examination. Hopefully, it has made you more aware of some things that you may not have considered before. Regardless, I'd ask that you keep one thing in mind. If you are going to help yourself to a big thick juicy mammoth burger, serve it on a whole-grain bun.

CHAPTER 3

YOUR PHYSICAL ENVIRONMENT

THE BIG TOXIC ELEPHANT

IN THE ROOM

The year was 1962, and a groundbreaking literary work was having its first impact on the public and industry. It warned that that Earth's long-term prospects were bleak, and it communicated a pervasive sense of warning in what would become a new phrase, "civilization malaise." The book was *Silent Spring*, and its author, Rachel Carson, an educated, considered, and eloquent scientist, had dedicated her life to the study and protection of our physical world. In what would become her best-known and arguably most important work, she would help to define—by virtue of the arguments and positions taken—the sides of an environmental debate and movement that continues to this day.

Some members of industry accused her of overstatement, inaccuracy, and socialism. Environmentalists and the public viewed it as a call to action. Regardless of their position, everyone was suddenly more acutely aware of the importance of their physical world and a need to remain vigilant in assessing and protecting it.

There is a lesson in her work for this book.

We've talked about your biology and we have talked about your behavior, but almost as importantly, your environment asserts a huge influence on both.

Webster's defines an environment as either the complex of physical, chemical, and biotic factors (such as climate, soil, and living things) that act upon an organism—*that means you and me; I'll be organism number one, and you can be organism number two*—or ecological community and that ultimately determines its form and survival. Or it can be the aggregate of social and cultural conditions that influence the life of an individual or community.

This chapter is dedicated to the first part of the definition. We'll get into the second in the next chapter.

A Real Fish Story

Most people think of the environment as a great global enterprise way beyond the influence or control of any one person. While that is somewhat true, each of us has an immediate environment—a room, an efficiency apartment, or a house—that is very much subject to our control.

I've always been kind of fascinated by the environment in the sense of hills and trees, ponds and lakes. Especially ponds and lakes. When I was a boy I was insane for fishing. More accurately, I was obsessed. I read every fishing magazine and article published by the Department of Fish and Wildlife that came out. I memorized those weird little drawings of every finned creature native and naturalized to the state. In no time I knew the differences between the spotted bass, the white bass, the largemouth bass, and even the nuanced differences of the famed Guadalupe bass. None of which were anywhere near where I lived. It was a strangely cruel twist of fate that had placed me in the Texas Panhandle, the most semiarid part of Texas, which is pretty semiarid to start with. In that way, I was very much like the character Phillip Nolan in *The Man without a Country,* destined forever to move from ship to ship and never set foot on land, except I was the boy without a fish. Oh, there were stock tanks and little artesian shallows where I could drop a line, but what they held was nothing like that glorious game fish that occupied my thoughts.

Then one day an opportunity was afforded to go down to East Texas, the greenest, most lake-ridden part of the state. And I had a wonderful idea.

I would catch some of those prized fish, and I would transplant them back to the barren aquatic confines of the flattest place in the world.

Now the great writer and philosopher George Bernard Shaw said, "The reasonable man adapts himself to the world. The unreasonable man persists in trying to adapt the world to himself. Therefore all progress depends on the unreasonable man."

It was a very solid bet that in those days I was the unreasonable boy. You'll see why in a second. My plan was pretty ingenious. First, I started studying about the requirements of transporting fish. They needed water, of course, but the water needed oxygen. I managed that in an aquarium bubbler affixed to a large Styrofoam cooler. Admittedly, it took some work on my part. Soon my bedroom resembled a low-rent extension of NASA with plastic tubing and batteries, a filter, and variously altered large white containers that had the look of a fishy lunar module. It also made my room look a little like a satellite location for the city dump.

My mother, a patient and generally nonplussed woman, walked by at one point and, upon glancing in, uttered a phrase that I would hear repeated by her many times in the years to come.

"What are you doing now?" she asked.

"Building a fish transporter," I said.

She sighed, I think.

"You are not going to keep fish."

"No," I answered confidently. "I am going to transplant them."

And so I did.

The trip was everything I had hoped. The dry caliche plains gave way to rolling green and then thick stands of trees that almost made me feel claustrophobic. The low brush in the east was soft and lush and welcoming, not like the prickly pear or bayonet-like yucca that ringed the poor estuaries I dealt with back home. This was some great Eden-esque source of life. The water into which I cast the hook, line, and bobber was an aquamarine promise of dissolved oxygen and microscopic stuff that fed the slightly bigger creatures that were gobbled up by the king of the cove, the largemouth bass. I did not have long to wait. By then end of the day I had two perfect five-pound specimens languishing in the fish lunar module. Right before we started home, I filled it with East Texas bayou water and fired up the bubbler. Now came the interesting part.

I learned two things on that trip home. Bayou water gets pretty fragrant after about a hundred miles, and largemouth bass don't like rumble strips on a highway. Every time the car's tires vibrated, those two bass went ballistic and hammered their displeasure in a tail-flapping pounding that threatened to rupture the Styrofoam survival craft. In a drama reminiscent of Apollo 13, it somehow held out and we finally made it home.

That night, I walked up the driveway to my waiting mother with the lunar module almost dragging the ground.

"We have to get this to the pond." I said with complete urgency.

"Welcome home," said my mother.

So out we drove with the reeking coolers full of bayou water. With great care I deposited the bass into the lovely little stock pond, and there they stayed. The next day when I returned, they were still there, alive and everything. The next day I found the same thing. And so it went.

Success.

I had transplanted fish.

I had made a deal with myself that if this worked, I would give myself a reward, so on Saturday, overloaded with tackle boxes, fishing poles, and more gear than a High Plains, freshwater version of Jacques Cousteau, I arrived ready for something like what I had experienced hundreds of miles to the east. I was all ready for a glorious day of catch-and-release.

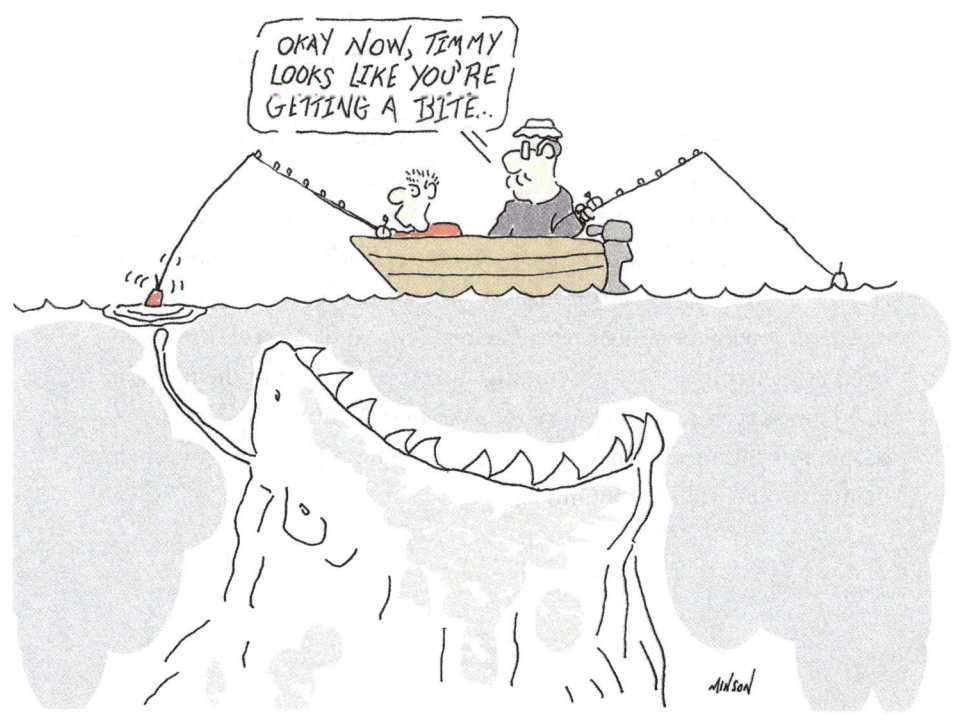

Instead, I found two old cowboys sitting on the bank with a cast iron skillet over a small fire. They were *frying fish*.

"Hey, kid," one of them said, "what do you know, we've been fishing here for years and we never caught anything before."

You can just imagine what went through my head.

And that is the story of my first real experience with addressing and shaping my environment.

I'm much, much older now, and I am still at it—challenging my environment, even though I am no longer kidnapping fish. I am also still of the philosophy that I, organism number one, and you, organism number two, should always be taking stock and protecting and improving our own environment.

Again, the very word environment conjures up a lot of things to a lot of people, but it's not prescriptive about dimension. It simply means everything constituting any space around us: the housing in which we live (e.g., residential or institutional homes), the air we breathe, the water and food we consume, the products we use, the workplaces where we are employed or volunteer, the institutional or public spaces where we spend time (such as hospitals, shopping malls, recreation centers, or parks), and the communities we populate. It can be as closed in as a seat on public transit and as wide as the ocean.

So that seems like a lot to consider, I know, but before you check out on me or throw up your hands and say, "This is way too much to worry about. I think I'll just watch an episode of *Somebody in America Might Have Talent* or *The Strangest Things People in Oklahoma Ever Ate* or *Really Awful Housewives of Wherever* instead," I want to suggest something.

First, though, remember what George Bernard Shaw said, my disastrous fish enterprise notwithstanding? If you keep in mind the thought that I am suggesting and you try to make *your* environment better adapted to your needs, then these concepts defining our dynamic environments become really important.

Factors That Make Seniors Vulnerable to Their Environment

So where do you start? Well, fortunately there are a lot of educated people who have given this a lot of thought and by virtue of that they have given us a head start.

According to an International Symposium on Environmental Factors and Seniors as a Vulnerable Population, there are five factors that contribute most to seniors' vulnerabilities to environmental risks:

1. Physiological changes that occur during the process of aging and how they relate to the physical requirements of our environment. What this is talking about is the changes to our individual bodies that may make adjustment of the environment necessary for a continued optimal quality of life. Remember, you may not be able to change *you* to adapt to the environment of your home or workspace, so "unreasonably" you may just need to adjust your environment to suit you. We covered a lot of the physical changes to our bodies after 50 in chapter 1, but the impact of those changes affecting the hospitability of your home environment, and beyond, is just as individualized. As joints calcify and muscles lose their strength, the arduous nature of negotiating a house, an apartment, or a neighborhood can become a real struggle. Just take stairs, for example, or if you can't, don't take the stairs.

If you live in a three-story row house and have progressive arthritis in your knees, either you will have to become relegated to remaining in one-third of your dwelling or you will have to endure a lot of pain or maybe you will need to adjust the way you are transported upstairs. Think of those lift chairs or other elevating technology. Then again, you may consider relocation. That is *really* changing the environment. You get the idea anyway.

2. Living arrangements or the quality of the housing environment. This factor may be one of the most individually actionable environmental features discussed by the group.

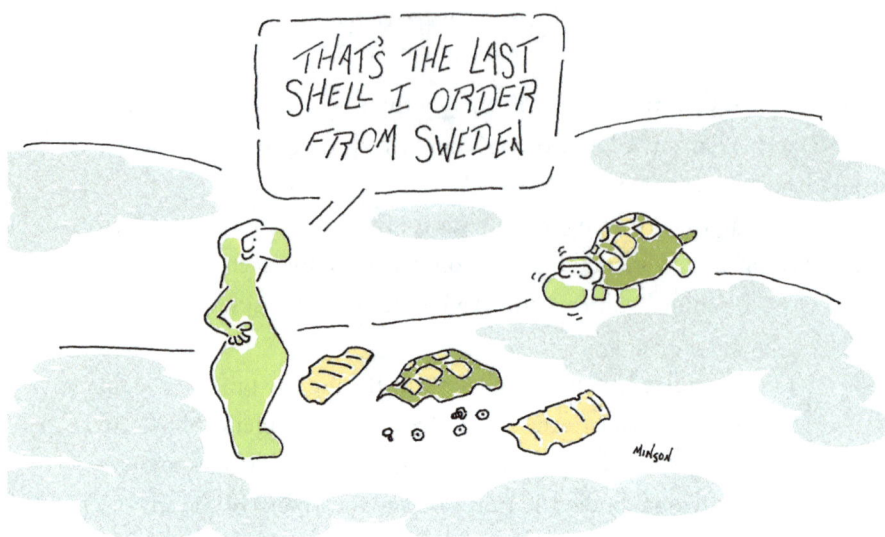

That idea is especially true when you consider indoor and outdoor air quality and your home's location. To say this issue is huge is an understatement. Recently, there has been a lot of conversation in the media about the impact of climate change on health. Regardless of your political leanings, climate change, whether intermittent (like a thermal inversion or an ozone alert day) or longer term (as in drought and increasing heat waves), has been well documented by current events that feature climate and climate-related effects impacting the old and the very young most severely. Imagine for a second that you have progressive respiratory illness and you see the "it's not a healthy day to be a breathing mammal" notification from your local weather station. Sure, you can stay inside, maybe, but unless you have some air-cleaning mechanism in place, eventually you will be required to breathe, and it's not like the air in your home will be trucked in from out of state. At least not yet.

And that is just one part of our local environment. There are many others and you will want to make sure they are all optimal.

So what can you do? Well, you can get an assessment of your home. This sounds expensive, but it doesn't have to be. There are many tools online that allow you to self-evaluate. A good one is the USDHHS checklist in its Healthy Housing Inspection Manual (http://www.cdc.gov/nceh/

publications/books/inspectionmanual/healthy_housing_inspection_manual.pdf), which will help you organize your own home evaluation and can advise where to go next in correcting any issues.

The manual provides tools, checklists, and even resources for additional assessment and action. It also covers some of the toxins and threats to health that can arise from your garbage, pet-borne contaminants and illnesses, vermin and their control or removal, and much more. I know all those things sound pretty unpleasant—and maybe even a little Dickensian—but better to think about them and know what to do than have to suffer because of them.

If the air quality because of some pollutant or, say, mold is a concern, items such as home mold-testing kits are cheap and easy to obtain. If you need them, high-efficiency particulate air (HEPA) filters are also reasonable considerations. The assessment I mentioned may help determine if you do.

Filters meeting the HEPA standard have many applications, including use in medical facilities, automobiles, aircraft, and homes. The filter must satisfy certain standards of efficiency, such as those set by the US Department of Energy (DOE). To qualify as HEPA by US government standards, an air filter must remove (from the air that passes through it) 99.97 percent of particles that have a size of 0.3 microns or larger. Good luck finding the ruler to confirm that. You'll just have to trust the product insert.

3. Socioeconomic status. So I am sure you are thinking, now here's a "what you can do" section that will really come in handy. How can I make a million dollars? Well, I don't have that answer. Suffice it to say that how much you can spend affects how many protective or reconstructive efforts you can address.

4. Body burden of environmental contaminants and historical environmental exposures. This is a measure of cumulative effect by the toxins and elements on you. This also isn't something you can determine on your own. It takes a team: you, your healthcare provider, and maybe an environmental specialist like an industrial hygienist. They can be found in the phone book or online and really aren't that expensive. What

you also need to do is listen to your body. If you feel bad, "get checked" and voice your concerns to your healthcare provider.

5. Seniors' level of awareness on environmental health issues and environmental health literacy. Hopefully, this book is a helpful starting point.

So what we are talking about are the physical issues of your environment, such as doorways, stairs, and the like as well as the more "metabolic" aspects like air, water, earth, and fire. Sounds kind of alchemical, huh?

In some cases, the environment may even be, dare I say it, metaphysical. Here's an example.

An environmentalist dies and reports to the pearly gates.

St. Peter checks his dossier and says, "Ah, you're an environmentalist—you're in the wrong place."

Thinking that Heaven could never make an error, the environmentalist reports to the gates of Hell and is let in. Pretty soon, the environmentalist gets dissatisfied with the environment in Hell and starts implementing eco-friendly improvements. After a while, he addresses global warming in Hell (no small feat), and air and water pollution are soon under control. The landscape becomes covered with grass and plants, the food is organic, and the people are happy. The environmentalist has become a pretty popular guy.

One day, God calls Satan up on the telephone and says, "So, how's it going down there in Hell?"

Satan replies, "Hey, things are going great. We've got clean air and water now, the temperature is 75 degrees, and the food tastes better, and there's no telling what this environmentalist is going to fix next."

God replies, "What? You've got an environmentalist down there? That's a mistake—he should never have been sent there. Send him back immediately."

Satan says, "No way. I like having an environmentalist on my staff. I'm keeping him."

God says, "Send him back up here right now or I'll sue."

Satan just laughs and answers, "Yeah, right. And just where are you going to find a lawyer in Heaven?"

Which leads me to the concept of environmental law and what you can do.

First, get smart. There are a lot of laws and regulations, intended to serve and protect you, that are already in place. Who executes them depends on whether you are talking to your local jurisdiction, a state office, or the federal government.

At the federal level it is the Environmental Protection Agency (EPA). Each state, however, has specific offices and agencies that are responsible, and at the county, local, or community level it is likely that there will be another office or department that addresses this, too. That is where you are most likely to see actual immediate advocacy and response. If you live in a rural area or small community, it may be your state. So let's start there.

The EPA has a helpful online tool (http://www2.epa.gov/home/health-and-environmental-agencies-us-states-and-territories) to identify state offices of the environment. In case you don't know who your resource is locally, the state office can be an invaluable assistant in identifying it.

Why do you need to know who's in charge?

For one thing, it can help keep you aware of environmental issues, like spills or toxins, product recalls, and more. Here's a nice resource for keeping track of releases and contaminations: http://www.epa.gov/epahome/r2k.htm#tri. You just enter your zip code. Secondarily, if you have a specific question, complaint, or worry, they can advise. This is especially applicable in the event of a release or contamination of air, water, soil, food, and more. In many cases, like food issues, both the environmental agency and the local health agency may interact and have joint responsibility.

Environmental Risks

To capture the types of general environmental elements and the kinds of hazards that you might encounter, I have included a brief list below. For some of the components mentioned, I'll go into greater detail later in the chapter.

Outdoor air quality. Some of the major risks include particulate matter and heavy metals from industries and power plants, volatile organic compounds (like benzene or styrene), sulfur oxides, nitrogen oxides, ozone, and smog. There is abundant research that associates outdoor air pollution with adverse health effects, including premature mortality and aggravation of existing respiratory and cardiovascular conditions.

Indoor air quality. Tobacco smoke in indoor environments, wood smoke, mold, formaldehyde, synthetic materials, and cleaning chemicals are some of the key risks identified in indoor environments. Indoor air pollutants can exacerbate asthma and chronic obstructive pulmonary disease.

Water quality. Microbiological contaminants in water have been identified as one of the major environmental risks for seniors, especially those who have immune problems. The presence of some compounds such as manganese and arsenic in drinking water is also important since it may have potential neurological impacts. Additionally, seniors are also more likely to experience a more severe and/or longer lasting illness from aqueous environmental contaminants.

Food. Exposure to a high level of mercury and persistent organic pollutants (POPs), such as dioxin and polychlorinated biphenyls, as well as possible exposure to pesticides residues in food products are two of the major environmental risks for seniors in this category. In addition, seniors may be more sensitive to microbiological contaminants like viruses or bacteria in food, such as Salmonella and *E. coli* due to reduced immune function.

Consumer products. There are a number of major environmental risks in consumer products, such as pesticide exposure when gardening or in products used on pets, respiratory irritant compounds in cleaning supplies, or combinations of cleaning supplies and laundry and personal care products, such as ammonia, chlorine, formaldehyde, and fragrances. Even older toxic products kept in the house, such as pesticides, moth balls, and other respiratory irritants, can degrade, morph, or liberate to make your home toxic. A classic example of liberated materials can be found in the environmental issues of certain structures immediately after the inundation of New Orleans following Hurricane Katrina.

As a medical director of a search and rescue team, I have seen a lot of contaminated and polluted scenes. None more so, however, than in the aftermath of Katrina. The interesting thing for me was the change that took place between the first couple of weeks when the water was still in the city and then the change in pollutants as the levy breach was plugged and the water was pumped out.

In the first two weeks, we worried about the dirty water with material from submerged cars, houses, storage tanks, and gas, petrochemical, and sewer pipes. Later, the threats came from saturated houses and build-

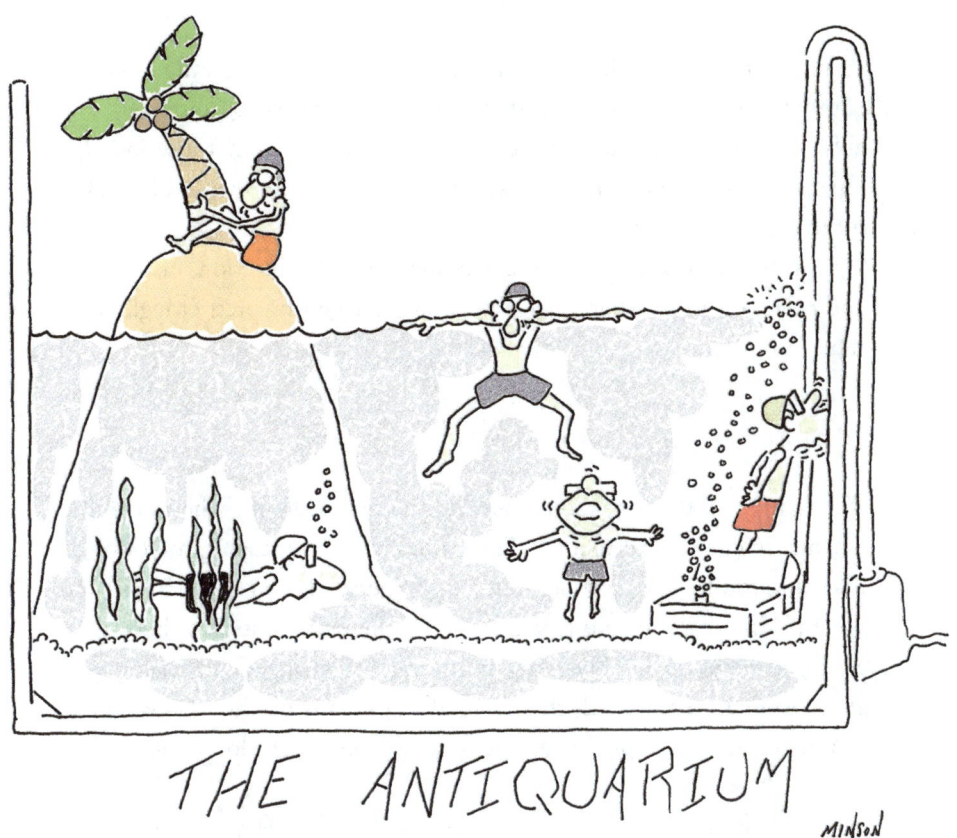

THE ANTIQUARIUM

MINSON

ing materials that began to degrade and gave off compounds as the wet materials dried or deteriorated. As we entered the second two-week phase, we suddenly found individuals suffering from headaches, blurry vision, and more. Our hazardous materials specialists determined that cyanides, hydrogen sulfides, and other compounds were being liberated.

What does that have to do with you? Well, it illustrates that sometimes the threats are obvious and sometimes they are much more subtle. Also, the effect of the *external* environment impacting your *home* environment can create new problems. You have to be aware.

Extreme temperature events. The impact of extreme temperature events on seniors in general and especially those with existing chronic conditions has been recognized as an important environmental concern. During the 2003 European heat waves, increased mortality among elderly populations was significant across a number of European countries. In the United States, seasonal temperature extremes are becoming regular enough threats that public service announcements are becoming more common. A WHO study in 2005 looked at the impact of "unseasonably" hot weather and its impact on seniors and showed that it seriously affected those with chronic illnesses and correlated with the numbers of deaths attributed to same.

This speaks to issues of adequate home thermal protection, insulation, and more. Or to put it another way, "things are getting pretty tough out there!"

Housing

We change. All the time. Sometimes it is incremental, like when we pull a hamstring or cut our toenails. Sometimes it is chronic and progressive, like all the stuff I talked about in the first chapter. I know I am coming off like the king of doom and gloom here, but there's a point. By acknowledging some of the hard facts about our physical changes and getting ahead of them as we build, choose, modify, or ready our homes—a concept better known as *planning*—we make the outcome a lot less gloomy.

Table 3. Jefferson and Franklin Inventions and What They May Have Led to Today

Jefferson	Revolving Book Stand	Multiple open windows on a computer screen
Jefferson	The Great Clock	The Automatic Clock or Time and Temperature maybe?
Jefferson	The Polygraph	The copy machine, not the lie detector*
Jefferson	The Wheeled Cipher	Enigma
Jefferson	The "Turning Machine" for Clothing	The revolving hanger at the dry cleaner's
Franklin	The Franklin-Pennsylvania Stove	Central heating
Franklin	The Lightning Rod	The surge protector for your house
Franklin	The "Long Arm"	The reach extender
Franklin	Bifocals	The same ones you may be wearing to read this

*I am pretty sure my mom invented that.

Additionally, by having your home already configured when you eventually do experience a physical change or infirmity, you will have a lot less to adjust to under stress. If anything, our homes may well be the most commonly changeable environment any of us can control. As I have already intimated, this includes elements of architecture, building, and the qualitative stuff that offsets our physical decline.

Which brings us back to my Founding Fathers fixation again, specifically Franklin and Jefferson. Now, here were two guys who were big on affecting their environment. They did it in ways that impacted architecture, civil engineering, and even the effects of weather (see table 3). Everyone has heard about the Franklin stove, but did you know that he also created the lightning rod to displace strikes and minimize the threat of house fires? He also created a "long arm" to facilitate reaching top shelves. Jefferson created a rotating hanger system to make reaching clothing simpler, and he also created a lazy-Susan-style book wheel so he could spin back and forth between pages in different reference tomes. Think of this as the 18th-century version of having several pages open on your laptop.

Now, I am not advocating that you try to meet those guys' standards, but to age in place safely and comfortably you will probably need to modify your house as you mature to increase access, maneuverability, and functionality. To better frame this idea, we should go think for a second on how we interact with and process our environment.

How We Process the Environment

There are really four commonly encountered physical challenges. Understanding them determines how your home design or alteration needs to match them. They are vision, hearing, dexterity and strength, and cognitive function.

DECREASED VISION

Decreased vision (you'll notice I emphasized that) among seniors is most commonly due to conditions like glaucoma, cataracts, and macular degeneration. The most commonly cited complaints include sensitivity to glare and reduced accommodation or adjustment to changing light levels. Similarly, reductions in visual acuity or sharpness of vision, reduced vision in low light, and reduced fields of vision are other common complaints.

Now why should we concern ourselves with that? Two words: "broken hip," the two most dreaded words in my late grandmother's lexicon.

When I was a kid growing up, I spent my summers with my grandparents in a small town in Oklahoma. Every summer was a strange kind of indentured servitude to my grandfather, who had a laundromat and a miniature golf course, also known as a "putt-putt." He also had a philosophy that the reason that boys existed in the world was to be used as an adjunct labor force, and so I had a number of jobs, most of which, if attempted nowadays, would have landed us all in some kind of child labor court. In retrospect, it probably did me a lot of good. My grandparents were not wealthy people by any stretch, and for a time we lived in a prefabricated, modular home, also known as a trailer. There are lots of stigmas about trailers, but I was pretty happy. What I remember most about it—and that is germane to this book—is an almost nightly occurrence involving my grandmother. Without fail sometime right before she fell asleep, she would imagine or remember some unplugged appliance that was certain to set fire to the place before dawn. She would get out of bed and, in a post–Great Depression generational phenomenon, not turn on the light as she searched throughout the house. Inevitably she would make it some distance before ramming her great toe into some immovable piece of furniture. Then the still night would split as she viscerally, reactively uttered a single-word expletive in a way that would have made a stevedore blush.

I won't say the word, but for the longest time I thought she was invoking President Nixon using a contraction of his first name.

What I think this story really illustrates is the orthopedic dangers of navigating your home in the dark . . . and that was just a story about a toe. Now imagine if that had been a hip.

So what can you do? Well, look into lighting. Use the tools and referenced links in this book to get an assessment. First illuminate your mind and then illuminate your home.

Just remember, mood lighting may work if you have a hot date planned, but it doesn't generally cut it when you are trying to assure safety. If you are of a green philosophy and don't want lights burning all the time, illumination can be set by motion detection so that they aren't on all the time but are there when you are.

I suddenly just imagined Patty Duke in *The Miracle Worker* groping her way down a hallway in black and white. Don't do that!

HEARING LOSS

While some hearing loss is inevitable, as we saw in chapter 1, some reduced hearing ability can stem from a number of things that might be correctable, and for those things there is something you can do. If this book ever makes it to an audio version, I'll have them repeat that line.

WHAT YOU CAN DO

- Maintain and address hearing aids. Malfunctioning hearing aids often can be a subtle failure, but regular maintenance and servicing can prevent unwarranted heartache. It will also make you less annoying to friends, partners, and passersby.
- Make sure you get regular hearing assessments. Audiograms are inexpensive and very helpful, and yet they are one of the most overlooked forms of medical testing for seniors. Ask your healthcare provider for one. At the very least you'll have a baseline for comparison, and if there is a deficiency or a progressive deficiency, you will know and can take action.
- Pay attention to any difficulty or changes in filtering out background noise. I think this is one of the most common patient complaints I have experienced—and one of the most frustrating because it is so often ignored. You can hear just fine at home or when you are in a quiet part of a restaurant talking one on one, but the second the place becomes busy or the background music comes on, it is a struggle to distinguish what is being said. According to every rock and roll station I have heard, "If it's too loud, you are too old!" Well, not necessarily. It may be that too much rock and roll has led to this. Then again I am pretty old. In any case, get checked.

Physical changes, including a loss of dexterity and strength, are probably some of the most emotionally traumatic changes associated with aging. It's sort of a confronting reminder that we are not who we used to be or who we were when we liked what we saw in the mirror the best. I understand it, and in a very caveman, DNA-bound, evolutionarily hard-wired kind of way, it makes sense. There really is nothing like that unappreciated youthful gift of strength and mobility for most people. It's the sheer physical joy of exertion and execution. It is the closest most of us come to leaving the earthbound constraints of gravity to take flight.

With concession to all that, this indictment of self is really tragic, because if Google and the information age have reinforced anything about us, it is that we are much more a cognitive creature and the "self" is something reposed in a calcified vault right above our eyebrows. I think that is important to remember, because physical strength is going to go sooner or later.

As we age, we can expect a loss of muscle strength (up to 40–60 percent from our peak) and concurrent losses of flexibility and coordination. It's sort of like adolescence, in reverse, just with pre-cancerous skin lesions and age spots instead of acne. Add to that reductions in balance, reflex, and reaction time, some reduced dexterity and fine-motor coordination, increased irritable response to environmental vibration, and lowered tolerance to temperature extremes, and you can see that you are—as my grandmother also used to say—"in for a big old time."

So what can you do? Well, for the medical things see your provider, and for the home environment things consult an expert. They can suggest or even implement home modifications—from the installation of bath and shower grab bars and adjustment of countertop heights to the creation of multifunctional first-floor master suites. You might need an automated power chair for ascending and descending stairs. If your healthcare provider advocates for it, you may find that it is a covered expense and costs you little. Then again, if you are rich, there is always the installation of private elevators.

Where do you find these experts?

Certified Aging-in-Place Specialists

To help with this, the National Association of Home Builders recommends that when considering new construction or assessment of an existing structure for someone planning to age in place—that is, to try to remain in their traditional home as long as possible—a Certified Aging-in-Place Specialist should be consulted.

To be honest, before I started research for this book, I didn't know such specialists existed. They do, and the things they have to offer can be very valuable. A Certified Aging-in-Place Specialist (CAPS) has been trained in the following:

- The unique needs of the older adult population
- Aging-in-place home modifications
- Common remodeling projects
- Solutions to common barriers

Keep in mind that when you hire a Certified Aging-in-Place Specialist, you are buying a service rather than a product. Each CAPS professional draws from a different knowledge base and will approach your project in a different way. You can find out more about them here: http://www.nahb.org/en/consumers/homeownership/aging-in-place-vs-universal-design/learn-about-aging-in-place-and-what-a-professional-can-do-for-you.aspx and http://www.nahb.org/en/consumers/homeownership/Find a Certified Aging-in-Place Specialist.aspx.

These folks can advise on a number of things, like exterior home designs that require low maintenance (such as vinyl or brick), low-maintenance landscaping, and decks and patios that are flush with entryways into the house. Their expertise addresses overall floor plans and dimensions of hallways that can accommodate conveyance (think 36 inches wide at a minimum) and enhance or improve lighting to minimize impediments to mobility.

They will also consider "little" things that affect the livability and functionality of a home, like thresholds that are flush (or quarter-inch at the maximum) to eliminating trip hazards, easy-operating, well-placed windows to maximize natural illumination, covered garages and porches, and ramps and handrails, if needed. There is a lot more, but you get the idea.

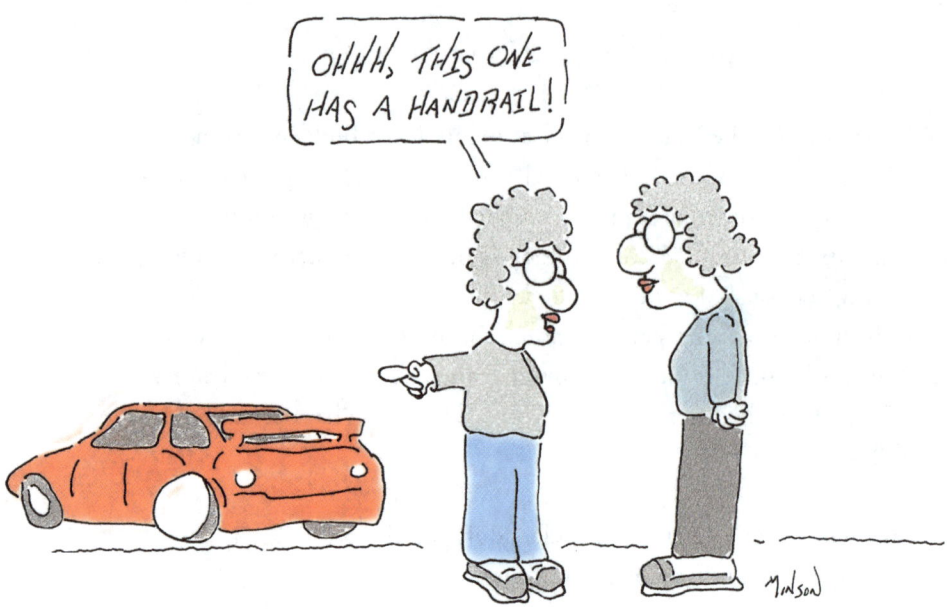

Which reminds me of a story.

I think you have already gotten an idea about the kind of person my mother is: patient, whimsical, candidate for sainthood. . . if you are a fish sympathizer. A few years ago she was in the market for a car. She did her due diligence and shopped around and looked at consumer guides until she thought she knew what she wanted. So off to the car dealership she went. When she came back, she had something that was safe, reliable, and, to my surprise, fairly sporty-looking. It even had an airfoil on the back. When I pointed that out, she happily told me that she had a choice and just really liked the one with the "handrail."

So when I talk about handrails, think airfoils for the home, I guess.

Other parts of the home that can be designed or modified with optimal senior living in mind include lever- or pedal-controlled faucets, built-in thermostatic and anti-scald controls, adjustable countertops, and enhanced stripes on counters to enhance visual orientation. There are also glass-front cabinets to minimize unnecessary effort and the perpetual Easter egg hunt that goes on at my house when I have to find the maple syrup. Enlarged lettering on appliance controls, color-coded outlets that correspond to breaker switches, front-loading laundry machines, leveled appliances to minimize postural changes and to enhance ergonomics, and scald controls on water faucets—the list goes on and on. To really appreciate this, consult the Certified Aging-in-Place Specialists' checklist of home considerations at http://certifiedaginginplacespecialist.com/checklists/.

Household Products and Materials

When you consider the qualitative or habituating aspects (air, water, and hygiene) of our homes, it is an ironic fact that a number of the items designed and marketed to improve it actually may have some harmful aspects. For starters, most of the hazardous ingredients in household cleaning products fall into three main categories:

Carcinogens. Carcinogens cause cancer and/or promote cancer's growth.

Endocrine disruptors. Endocrine disruptors mimic human hormones, confusing the body with false signals. Exposure to endocrine disruptors can lead to numerous health concerns including reproductive, developmental, growth, and behavior problems. Endocrine disruptors have been linked to reduced fertility, premature puberty, miscarriage, menstrual problems, challenged immune systems, abnormal prostate size, ADHD, non-Hodgkin's lymphoma, and certain cancers.

Neurotoxins. Neurotoxins alter neurons, affecting brain activity and causing a range of problems from headaches to loss of intellect.

Here are some compounds that you may also want to note specifically:

Disinfectants. One of the most counterintuitive health threats is that of products that are designed to disinfect. Common sense tells us that killing household germs protects our health. However, disinfectants are sort of biological poisons. In many cases, they should not be in contact with the skin or inhaled as we merrily clean away.

Pesticides. The ingredients in pesticides often include carcinogens and endocrine disruptors. Pesticides are fat-soluble, making them difficult to eliminate from the body once ingested. Pesticides and disinfectants may also include alkylphenol ethoxylates (APEs).

APEs. APEs act as surfactants, meaning they lower the surface tension of liquids and help cleaning solutions spread more easily over the surface to be cleaned and penetrate solids. APEs are found in detergents, disinfectants, all-purpose cleaners, and laundry cleansers. They are also found in many self-care items, including *spermicides*, sanitary towels, and disposable diapers. APEs are endocrine disruptors.

Formaldehyde. Formaldehyde is commonly known as a preservative. Many people do not know that it is also a germicide, bactericide, and fungicide, among other functions. Formaldehyde can sometime be found in household cleaners and disinfectants. It is also present in nail polish and other personal care products. Formaldehyde is also a potential carcinogen.

Organochlorines (OCs). Some types are highly deadly, such as DDT. OCs are also bioaccumulative, meaning we can store up more and more as we are exposed. OCs are present in pesticides, detergents, degreasers, and bleaches. OCs can also be present in dry-cleaning fluids. OCs are carcinogens and endocrine disruptors.

Styrene. Styrene is a naturally occurring substance derived from the styrax tree. Styrene is most commonly used in the manufacture of numerous plastics, including plastic food wrap, insulated cups, carpet backing, and polystyrene plastic. Styrene is also found in floor waxes and polishes and metal cleaners. Styrene is also a known carcinogen as well as an endocrine disruptor. Significant exposures may affect the central nervous system, liver, and reproductive system.

Phthalates. Phthalates are most commonly used in the manufacture of plastics. Phthalates are also used as carriers for perfumes and air fresheners and as skin-penetration enhancers for products such as moisturizers. These chemicals are classified as inert, and, as such, no product-labeling requirements exist for phthalates. Some laboratory studies suggest they may be potential endocrine disruptors and related to hormonal and reproductive abnormalities.

Volatile organic compounds (VOCs). VOCs are emitted as gases that suspend in the air. VOCs include an array of chemicals, some of which may have short- and long-term adverse health effects, and are present in perfumes, air fresheners, disinfectants, and deodorizers. VOCs commonly include propane, butane, acetone, ethanol, phthalates, and/or formaldehyde. These compounds pose a variety of human health hazards and collectively are thought to be reproductive toxins, neurotoxins, liver toxins, and carcinogens.

So how do you know and what can you do? Well, you can consult two sources.

SAFETY DATA SHEETS

The first is the Safety Data Sheet (SDS), most of which can be found at the online Household Products Database maintained by the National Library of Medicine (NLM) at the NIH (http://householdproducts.nlm. nih.gov/). I should point out that the NLM does not test products nor does it evaluate information from the product label or the SDS, but it is a reliable source for information about many items.

This site provides great information on everything from auto products to household cleaning products to pesticides to landscape and yard care, personal care items like antiperspirant, home repair items, pet care, home office items like toner ink, and even arts and crafts supplies. It also gives reference to the SDS.

A Safety Data Sheet (formerly called a Material Safety Data Sheet) is a fact sheet developed by manufacturers describing the chemical and physical properties of a product. Safety Data Sheets include brand-specific information such as physical data (solid, liquid, color, melting point, flash point, etc.), health effects, first aid, reactivity, storage, handling, disposal, personal protection, and spill/leak procedures. As required by the Occupational Health and Safety Administration (OSHA), the target audience for information in an SDS is the occupational worker who may be exposed to chemicals at work. However, much of the information is also relevant to consumers.

HAZARDOUS SUBSTANCES DATA BANK

There is also the Hazardous Substances Data Bank (HSDB), provided by the National Library of Medicine at the NIH http://toxnet.nlm.nih.gov/cgi-bin/sis/htmlgen.

HSDB is a toxicology (the study of poisons) database that focuses on the effects of potentially hazardous chemicals. It provides information on human exposure, industrial hygiene, emergency handling procedures, environmental fate, regulatory requirements, nanomaterials, and related areas. The information in HSDB has been assessed by a Scientific Review Panel.

And if that is not enough, there is also TOXLINE, a bibliographic database with an assortment of citations from specialized journals and other sources. It provides references covering the biochemical, pharmacological, physiological, and toxicological effects of drugs and other chemicals. Most of TOXLINE's bibliographic citations contain abstracts and/or indexing terms and Chemical Abstract Service (CAS) Registry Numbers.

Consumers may find it cumbersome or time-consuming to research all of the ingredients in the cleaning products under the kitchen sink. In that case, product warning labels can be a useful first line of defense and information. All chemical products are required, by law, to include warnings if harmful ingredients are included as ingredients.

Interpreting them is a whole other matter.

Most people think of the warning label in terms of ingestion, as in tipping the bottle of cleanser or pesticide and taking a big swig.

"Really?" you may be asking. "We need a label for that?"

Actually, sadly, apparently . . . yes.

Suffice to say, you should not be drinking things that were not created for ingestion. Period.

Exposure—How Do I Know If It Is Indecent?

Given the title of this subheading, whatever you are about to read will undoubtedly be disappointing. We are exposed to potentially toxic materials all the time—chemical, radiation, biological contaminants. The difference in when they present a danger relies on the concentration, the nature of the offending material, and how long you are exposed. So what about the stuff in those bottles under the sink?

Well, because industrial exposures, as mentioned earlier, are the most likely settings for safety label concern, the language of safety labels, as required by federal law, are fairly technical. They are also the same labels you'll find on the material you use in your home. They apply depending on whether the exposure is by ingestion (swallowing), dermal (absorbed through the skin), or inhalation (breathing it).

Table 4. Oral/Ingestion Toxin Exposure

Toxicity Category	Signal Word	Statements
I	DANGER—POISON Skull and Crossbones required	Fatal if swallowed. Wash thoroughly with soap and water after handling and before eating, drinking, chewing gum, using tobacco, or using the toilet.
II	WARNING	May be fatal if swallowed. Wash thoroughly with soap and water after handling and before eating, drinking, chewing gum, using tobacco, or using the toilet.
III	CAUTION	Harmful if swallowed. Wash thoroughly with soap and water after handling and before eating, drinking, chewing gum, using tobacco, or using the toilet.
IV	CAUTION (optional)	No statements are required. However, the registrant may choose to use category III labeling.

Table 5. Dermal (Skin) Toxin Exposure

Toxicity Category	Signal Word	Statements
I	DANGER—POISON Skull and Crossbones required	Fatal if absorbed through skin. Do not get in eyes, on skin, or on clothing. Wash thoroughly with soap and water after handling and before eating, drinking, chewing gum, using tobacco, or using the toilet. Wear (specify appropriate protective clothing). Remove and wash contaminated clothing before reuse.
II	WARNING	May be fatal if absorbed through skin. Do not get in eyes, on skin, or on clothing. Wash thoroughly with soap and water after handling and before eating, drinking, chewing gum, using tobacco, or using the toilet. Wear (specify appropriate protective clothing). Remove and wash contaminated clothing before reuse.
III	CAUTION	Harmful if absorbed through skin. Avoid contact with skin, eyes. or clothing. Wash thoroughly with soap and water after handling and before eating, drinking, chewing gum, using tobacco, or using the toilet. Remove and wash contaminated clothing before reuse. Wear (specify any appropriate protective clothing, if appropriate).
IV	CAUTION (optional)	No statements are required. However, the registrant may choose to use category III labeling.

Table 6. Respiratory Toxin Exposure

Toxicity Category	Signal Word	Statements
I	DANGER—POISON Skull and Crossbones required	Fatal if inhaled. Do not breathe (dust, vapor, or spray mist). Wear (specify appropriate respiratory protection). Remove and wash contaminated clothing before reuse.
II	WARNING	May be fatal if inhaled. Do not breathe (dust, vapor or spray mist).Wear (specify appropriate respiratory protection). Remove and wash contaminated clothing before reuse.
III	CAUTION	Harmful if inhaled. Avoid breathing (dust, vapor or spray mist). Remove and wash contaminated clothing before reuse.
IV	CAUTION (optional)	No statements are required. However, the registrant may choose to use category III labeling.

These industrial definitions are captured in tables 4, 5, and 6. You'll notice that the tables don't explicitly describe an amount. That information is available in the links previously provided, if you care.

I am guessing by now that you do.

You can learn more about all of this and how it applies to specific cleaning products at the Household Products Database mentioned earlier.

Bear in mind, not all chemical compounds are required to be so described.

Certain ingredients (such as fragrances or certain recipes) are considered trade secrets, and government regulations are designed to protect proprietary information. Without full disclosure, consumers can't always be sure of the unhealthy exposures to these chemicals to themselves and their families.

The safest course of action you can take is to get smart! Become informed. Here are some suggestions:

- Read product labels. Limit the use of products with a signal word stronger than "Caution."
- Wear protective clothing. If they have to do that at a plant or factory, why shouldn't you at home? Now it is a little over the top, but think of the fun you will have answering a sales call at the door in a hazmat suit. I'm kidding, of course.
- Research the chemicals listed on product labels through the

Household Products Database. This includes the stuff we use to clean our environment and ourselves. To that end, there is also the Cosmetics Database (http://www.cosmeticsdatabase.com), Toxnet (http://www.toxnet.nlm.nih.gov), and Scorecard (http://www.scorecard.org).

The Bottom Line?

In some cases the fragrance in a product may actually affect the sensory ability to pick up other odors. It may also have some mild neurological (in the nose) effect. Most of these actually overpower our natural ability to detect the unpleasant odor. That is not always good. It is technically having a chemical effect on us rather than an addressing the odor proper.

Here's another way of saying that: something in a bottle made by a chemical plant that supposedly makes your home smell like a pine forest or a floral garden or a gigantic piña colada should give you pause. Or, to put it yet another way, if something makes your home smell like an air freshener in a New York City cab, beware.

WHAT YOU CAN DO

- Consider using homemade cleaning solutions made from common ingredients such as vinegar, baking soda, lemon juice, and borax.
- You might also consider cleaning solutions that bear the Green Seal logo. Green Seal is a nonprofit environmental standard development and certification organization. Green Seal certifies cleaning products to be effective at cleaning yet safer for human health and the environment.
- Interview cleaning services and hire one that is committed to safe product use. Many national cleaning services and local cleaning companies are now making the switch to green products, but make sure you ask exactly what they are using. Make sure the cleaning supplies that are used by your cleaning service are recognized as being free of toxins. Taking a greener approach to cleaning can help you feel better physically, but you'll prob-

ably also feel better mentally, knowing you are creating a safer environment for yourself, your family, and your pets.

Bottom line? A clean home really should smell like nothing at all.

Cleanliness Is Next to . . . Impossible?

One additional thought for consideration. After all the warnings about cleaning products and chemicals assailing our homes, you might be thinking, "My crazy, filthy Uncle Al may have been on to something with his semi-hoarder, unhygienic lifestyle." Well, not so fast. As we learned, especially as we started dating, hygiene matters. It's even truer as we age.

While there are many "natural" or generative hazards that can be found in a home, the ones that are most prevalent are molds, asbestos, lead, and radon. There have been numerous articles on toxic mold. I want to take just a second and talk about that.

MOLDS

According to the CDC, mold organisms like *Stachybotrys chartarum* do not always present a health problem indoors. However, some people are sensitive to it. If you are one of them, you may experience symptoms such as nasal stuffiness, eye irritation, wheezing, or skin irritation when exposed. Some people have even more severe reactions to molds. Severe reactions are sometimes seen among workers exposed to large amounts of molds in occupational settings, such as farmers working around moldy hay. Severe reactions may include fever and shortness of breath. Immunocompromised persons and persons with chronic lung diseases like chronic obstructive pulmonary disease (COPD) are at increased risk for opportunistic infections and may even develop fungal infections in their lungs.

In 2004, the Institute of Medicine (IOM) found there was sufficient evidence to link indoor exposure to a variety of molds with upper-respiratory symptoms like coughing and wheezing in otherwise healthy people. While it looked at children and others, it found exacerbated asthma symptoms in people with asthma and with hypersensitivity pneumonitis (lung inflammation) in individuals susceptible to that immune-mediated condition.

Generally, it is not necessary to identify the species of mold growing in a residence, and the CDC does not recommend routinely sampling for molds.

If you are susceptible to mold, and mold is seen or smelled, however, there may be a potential health risk. Therefore—no matter what type of mold is present—you should arrange for its removal. Furthermore, reliable sampling for mold can be expensive, and standards for judging what is and what is not an acceptable or how much is tolerable have not been established.

Take-home point? You should really listen to your body, and if you are suffering, see your healthcare provider and have the material tested.

WHAT YOU CAN DO

- Identify areas of mold growth. The key to mold control is moisture control. It is important to dry damaged areas and items within 24–48 hours to prevent mold growth. If mold is a problem in your home, clean up the mold and get rid of the excess water or moisture.
- Fix leaky plumbing or other sources of water.
- Wash mold off hard surfaces with an appropriate cleanser and water and dry it completely. Absorbent materials (such as ceiling tiles and carpet) that become moldy may have to be replaced. This is especially true if flooding or wastewater—as in Katrina—has contaminated the materials.
- If the saturation exposes the areas to microbial growth, consult with an environmental professional about adequate protective measures. If you have suffered flooding, a free resource can be found at www.disasterassistance.gov to register with FEMA. To talk with FEMA, call 1–800–621–FEMA (3362). You can also consult the EPA guide titled *Mold Remediation in Schools and Commercial Buildings* (http://www.epa.gov/mold/mold_remediation.html). Although focused on schools and commercial buildings, this guide also applies to other building types.

If your home was built before 1978 and no remediation has been performed, it may have some sources of lead. Lead paint is still present in millions of homes, sometimes under layers of newer paint. Here's a chart that illustrates my point.

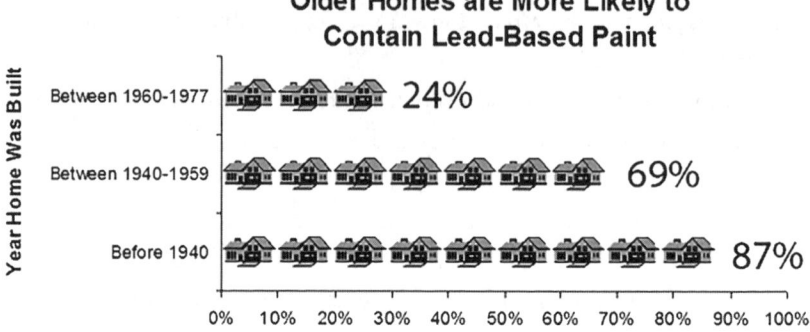

If the paint is in good shape, the lead paint is usually not a problem. Deteriorating lead-based paint (peeling, chipping, chalking, cracking, damaged, or damp) is a hazard and needs immediate attention. It may also be a hazard when found on surfaces that children can chew or that get a lot of wear and tear, such as windows and window sills, doors and door frames, stairs, railings, banisters, and porches.

You can also find lead in household dust resulting from indoor sources such as deteriorating lead-based paint. Lead dust can also be tracked into the home from soil outside that is contaminated by deteriorated exterior lead-based paint and other lead sources. Even during renovation, repair or painting activities can create toxic lead dust when painted surfaces are disturbed or demolished.

You can get more information at the following EPA website: http://www2.epa.gov/lead/renovation-repair-and-painting-program-consumers.

ASBESTOS

According to the Consumer Product Safety Commission, asbestos is a mineral fiber. It can be positively identified only with a special type of microscope. There are several types of asbestos fibers. In the past, asbestos was added to a variety of products to strengthen them and to provide heat insulation and fire resistance.

Where is it found? Houses built between 1930 and 1950 may have asbestos as insulation or in siding or shingles. Asbestos may be present in textured paint and in patching compounds used on wall and ceiling joints, even though its use was banned in 1977. Artificial ashes and embers sold for use in gas-fired fireplaces may contain asbestos. Older products such as stove-top pads may have some asbestos compounds. Walls and floors around woodburning stoves may be protected with asbestos paper, millboard, or cement sheets. Asbestos is found in some vinyl floor tiles and the backing on vinyl sheet flooring and adhesives. Hot water and steam pipes in older houses may be coated with an asbestos material or covered with an asbestos blanket or tape. Oil and coal furnaces and door gaskets may have asbestos insulation. Many types of common building materials such as floor tile, sheet flooring, joint compounds, or textures may contain asbestos.

The health risks are often associated with chronic exposure. The risk of lung cancer and mesothelioma increases with the number of fibers inhaled. The risk of lung cancer from inhaling asbestos fibers is also greater if you smoke. People who get asbestosis have usually been exposed to high levels of asbestos for a long time. The symptoms of these diseases do not usually appear until about 20 to 30 years after the first exposure to asbestos. While that may not matter so much to a senior, you might well consider loved ones and children who are around.

RADON

Radon is a naturally occurring radioactive gas. It is usually found in igneous rock and soil, but in some cases well water may also be a source of radon. It is heavier than air and therefore often accumulates in basements or lower areas of homes. It is not produced as a commercial product.

In 2005 the US surgeon general, Richard H. Carmona, issued a health advisory warning Americans about the health risk from exposure to radon associated with indoor air. The chief physician urged Americans to test their homes to find out how much radon they might be breathing. Dr. Carmona also stressed the need to remedy the problem as soon as possible when the radon level is 4 picocuries per liter (pCi/L) or more, noting that more than 20,000 Americans die of radon-related lung cancer each year. In 2009 the WHO estimated that 15 percent of lung cancers worldwide were related to radon exposures.

For concerns about radon and information on testing, assistance, and remediation, you can contact the EPA's hotline for radon, 1–800-SOSRA-DON (1–800–767–7236).

So what can you do?

Well, first consider the source, the risk, and the issues as described. Then take action and get help. There are a lot of resources out there, as you can see, and many of them are free.

Senior-Friendly Communities

So now I have completely terrified you about all the lurking hazards in your home to the point that you will probably never want to set foot back in the house. Having accomplished that, let me take a minute to talk about the next most immediate environment, your city or town.

Is your city a senior-friendly city? Here's how you can tell. In general, a senior-friendly city is one that structurally and operationally accommodates the specific requirements of seniors and provides services to address those needs or make the activities of daily living easier, such as driving, shopping, walking, and functioning. As I said earlier, older adults who regularly participate in physical activity and social interaction are more likely to enjoy a better quality of life. Open, safe, well-maintained, and well-lit parks, green spaces, and sidewalks encourage everyone to be more physically active. Features such as pedestrian crossings, traffic islands, crossing lights, and audio signals make those streets safer.

There are a lot of resources for evaluation. Most specifically, there is a program established by CDC known as a Health Impact Assessment (HIA). Through its Health Impact Assessment to Foster Healthy Community Design Initiatives (HCDI) grants, HCDI helps cities and towns determine whether proposed planning and policy changes will have a positive health impact in general. A CDC-funded HIA conducted in Davidson, North Carolina, for example, resulted in rewriting street design standards to improve street construction and add more signs, sidewalks, and bike lanes.

These changes help improve health equity across all ages and abilities by increasing physical activity, mobility, and even access to services.

Other aspects that are inherent but that bear mentioning include economics, seasonal or climate variation, temperature, snow, light variation, urban sprawl or distances, the natural environment, physical space (suburban, vertical, and longitudinal housing spread), familiarity with the physical space, cleanliness, and safety. That's a lot, I know, but every one of those things can make an environment inhospitable or even hostile for a senior.

If you'd like to know how senior-friendly your city is, you can use the criteria established by the HIA and contact your local chamber of commerce or government center to see.

An excellent source of information and assistance in evaluating your community, specific to issues that may concern seniors, can be found in the AARP's *Livable Communities: An Evaluation Guide* (http://assets.aarp .org/rgcenter/il/d18311_communities.pdf).

WHAT YOU CAN DO

- Look at crowding and allocation of resource matters. If the majority of a population is over 50, then that group likely has a political voice.
- For census information, try the public library or your city or county planning office. (Complete accuracy is not as important as getting a general idea of locations with concentrations of older residents.)
- For zoning and preservation information, try the city or county planning office.
- For regulations (such as snow removal), try the relevant local government agency responsible for that issue (for example, the city manager's office or the department of public works or parks and recreation).
- To find out whether other groups are conducting similar surveys, check with the relevant local government agency responsible for that issue, look for coverage in your local newspaper, ask citizens groups that may be concerned about the issue, or ask members of your group.

Enlist allies and partners. There is safety and power in numbers. The support and collaboration of others can go a long way toward making your efforts go smoothly—from gathering information before you start your research and evaluation.

Think about it. The physical aspects of your city may affect your navigation and enjoyment of it. In a city where the geographic space is limited by a mountain range, coastline, wetland, or marsh, the architecture has nowhere to go but up. The plus side is that most of the locations that you want to visit are probably closer together, but without facilitation to the climb, like ramps, elevators, or escalators, access may be arduous or impossible. Similarly, areas unrestricted by geography tend toward wide area sprawl, and while that may mean less climbing, getting to a location is often a greater challenge.

Here's an example. Let's say you just love canned rutabaga soup. We'll assume you have had a mental status examination that shows that, no, you are not insane and that this is just some inconceivable culinary peculiarity of yours. The only place to get it is at Rutabagas R Us. If you live in Baltimore, Maryland, then the physical distance to your rutabaga-lovin' heart's desire may be just three or four miles as the crow flies, but that might be across the harbor, making the trip an actual seven or eight miles. Or it could be close, but when you get there, it is on the third floor of the mall, which had to be built that way to accommodate parking garage development. Or it may be in a building that is a converted historical structure that was designed before Americans with Disabilities regulations were part of the equation. Or it's a cold and snowy day. In which case, knowing Baltimore, you will get your soup but won't be able to find toilet paper, bread, or milk on a shelf anywhere.

Yes, I *do* know Baltimore.

Now flip that consideration to Houston, Texas.

Sure, you can get your rutabaga soup, but it is 35 miles away. Granted, you won't have to climb too many stairs when you get there, but now you are at the mercy of cyclical traffic constraints and jams in a place where the automobile culture is king and mass transit is less prevalent. Granted, you will not see a whole lot of ice and snow, but the climate can often make Purgatory look temperate, and at times torrential rain or hurricane threats are part of the equation.

You get the idea. If you don't, here's a little story that illustrates it even better.

I went to medical school in Galveston, Texas, at the University of Texas Medical Branch (UTMB), the oldest medical school west of the Mississippi (sounds like a stereotypical Texan boast, I know, but it is true). It's a medical school that has sustained a lot of climate challenges, including a major hurricane in 1900 and another in 2009 that threatened to respectively wipe the campus off the map. My exposure first came about when I interviewed for medical school on a beautiful October day in the 1980s. I arrived on the island to temperatures in the mid-60s, humidity below 40 percent, and a gentle breeze that made the waves on the beach a beautiful shade of blue-green.

What I didn't know then was that this was a climatic event that occurred roughly one week a year and as rarely as the migration of unicorns. Nevertheless, I was sold on the place.

Fast-forward to the next August and the beginning of classes. I arrived to a place that seemed kind of like the one I had visited, only now it was a study in the number 90—90 degrees and 90 percent humidity. That meant that even though it was 90 degrees, it *felt* like a million degrees.

It was like I had been stretched out on the anvil of the sun and God was trying to make a horseshoe. From that moment on, I was acutely appreciative of the concepts of both weather and climate. For the record, I graduated from UTMB and it was a great experience, but I definitely had some adjusting to do.

Climate and Weather

I have sort of alluded to these concepts a couple of times already, but to formally explain the difference in climate and weather, let's go with some folks who really know what they are talking about.

According to the National Aeronautics and Space Administration (NASA), "the difference between weather and climate is a measure of time. Weather is what conditions of the atmosphere are over a short period of time, and climate is how the atmosphere 'behaves' over relatively long periods of time."

When we talk about climate change, we talk about changes in long-term averages of daily weather. Today, children always hear stories from their parents and grandparents about how snow was always piled up to their waists as they trudged off to school. Well, if they didn't believe it, then the winter of 2014 changed that.

If summers seem hotter lately, then the recent climate may have changed. In various parts of the world, some people have even noticed that springtime comes earlier now than it did 30 years ago. An earlier springtime is indicative of a possible change in the climate.

Some scientists define climate as the average weather for a particular region and time period, usually taken over 30 years. It's really an average pattern of weather for a particular region. When scientists talk about climate, they're looking at averages of precipitation, temperature, humidity, sunshine, wind velocity, phenomena such as fog, frost, and hailstorms, and other measures of the weather that occur over a long period in a particular place.

For example, after looking at rain-gauge data, lake and reservoir levels, and satellite data, scientists can tell if during a summer an area was drier than average. If it continues to be drier than normal over the course of many summers, then it would likely indicate a change in the climate.

In addition to long-term climate change, there are shorter-term climate variations. This so-called climate variability can also be represented by periodic or intermittent changes related to El Niño (which is not Spanish for the number 9) and La Niña (not Columbus's ship), volcanic eruptions, or other changes in the Earth and atmosphere.

From my limited perspective, climate matters in a very concrete way. It impacts how I garden. I have for many years somehow managed to keep a small Concord grapevine alive in my backyard. It has, if you will forgive me, become almost like a pet. Only instead of licking or purring, it gives me grapes once a year for all my affections and efforts. Next to it is a small garden space that I utilize to keep a ready supply of salad fixings. For that reason, I pay attention to the USDA planting advisory and growing chart and act accordingly.

Know what?

Those climate and planting zones have changed.

This last year the US Department of Agriculture (USDA) and the National Oceanic and Atmospheric Administration (NOAA) came out with big comparison maps. The map below shows how the climate growing zones have moved "up," or if you are a map purist, north. Pretty interesting, huh?

Now, weather is basically the way the atmosphere is behaving, mainly with respect to its effects upon life and human activities. Most people think of this in terms of temperature, humidity, precipitation, cloudiness, brightness, visibility, wind, and atmospheric pressure, as in high and low pressure. That is a pretty good way of thinking about it.

In most places, weather can change from minute to minute, hour to hour, day to day, and season to season. Climate, however, is the average of weather over time and space. An easy way to remember the difference is that climate is what you expect with some assurance, like a very hot summer, and weather is what you get with uncertainty, like a hot day with pop-up thunderstorms.

You can get reliable contemporary information at the NOAA website: http://www.ncdc.noaa.gov/cag/mapping/global.

This matters from a practical standpoint, as these recent problems with drought, disease, wildfires, and more have correlation to these cyclic

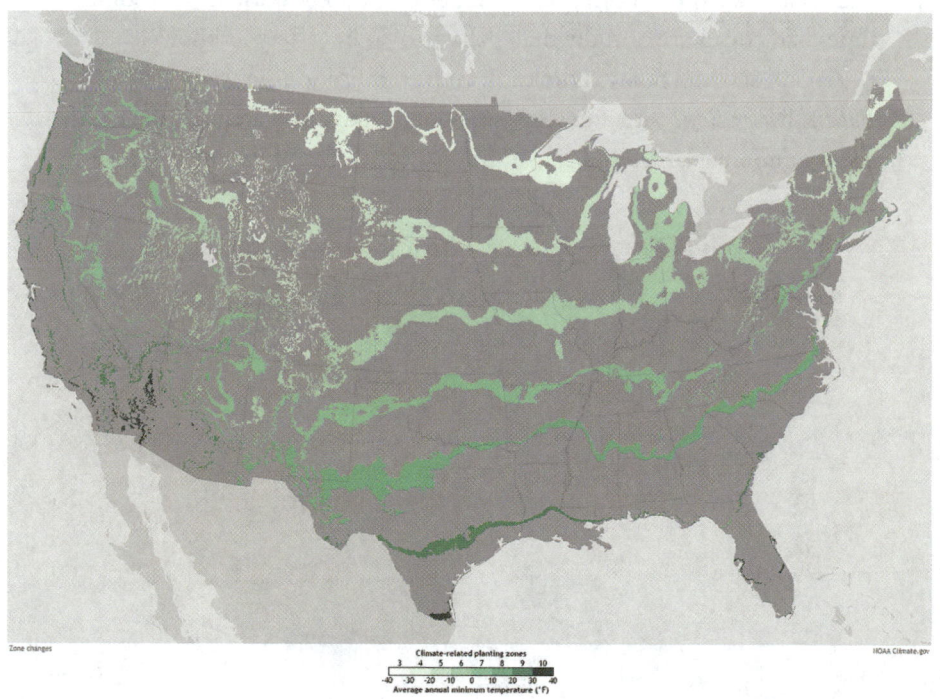

Zone changes

Climate-related planting zones

3   4   5   6   7   8   9   10

-40   -30   -20   -10   0   10   20   30   40

Average annual minimum temperature (°f)

NOAA Climate.gov

and longer-term changes. The ability to survive or endure these climate changes can change drastically as we age. So pay attention.

To further illustrate my point I have included another map, this one provided by NOAA. It shows the relative warmth and cooling alterations against normal. As you can see, many of the areas with the most significant changes are oceanic. Think our global kitchen and air conditioning system. This is significant and will warrant efforts to minimize these changes and the associated impact on seniors for generations to come.

Water, Water Everywhere, and Not a Drop to Drink

In the chapter regarding behaviors, I covered the habitual issues of water consumption and dehydration. Remember my gastrointestinal After School Special song about hydration? Unfortunately, you'll probably never forget it.

Well, that is all based on the assumption that the water coming through the pipe in your home is clean and healthy. But is that an assumption you can make? Most of the time, yes, but we live in a crowded and dynamic world, subject to human error, natural disasters, and sometimes bad corporate or individual behavior. So how do you know?

A good starting point is the EPA. In its publication on water health, *Bottled Water Basics*, it addresses issues of consumable water and the differences in nomenclature and classification. Now some of you may choose to

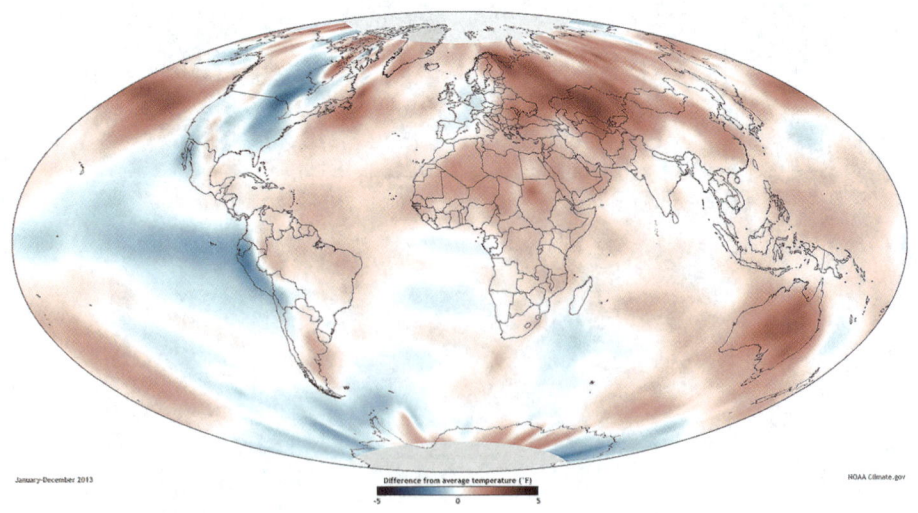

January-December 2013   Difference from average temperature (°F)   NOAA Climate.gov
                                          -5   0   5

drink tap water, while some may want to employ filtration or "end of use" processing of municipal or well-provided tap water. Others may wish to take additional precautions or use bottled water because they have medical problems such as weakened immune systems, chemotherapy, or organ transplants.

Biologically speaking, the biggest issue aside from bacterial or coliform elimination is the treatment of water to eliminate a particular organism called *Cryptosporidium*. This microscopic protozoan has a protective shell that makes it resistant to most chemical cleansers. It is found in most lakes and streams and recently has even been linked to some public swimming pools. It can be removed by reverse osmosis, distillation, ultraviolet light, sustained boiling of water, and certain grades of filtration. The grade of filtration is actually one micron pore size and is designated by the American National Standards Institute (ANSI) and the National Science Foundation (NSF).

In the affected, it causes a diarrheal illness and in those with health problems like I just mentioned, it can even cause death.

WHO'S TO SAY IT'S SAFE TO DRINK?

Tap water is regulated by established standards for water provided by public water suppliers. Bottled water is under the jurisdiction of the FDA. Specifically, it addresses the identity and quality established by the FDA as a packaged food according to the Federal Food, Drug, and Cosmetic Act. There are also state and local agencies that have a role.

Any bottled water that is sold in interstate commerce must meet FDA standards for physical, chemical, radiological, and microbial contamination. However, if the water is bottled and sold in a single state, that state's health department presides solely. To be certain, contact your state health department.

So whether you are facing an incoming hurricane, or just learned that a spill occurred at a local factory making tap water unsafe, or just want to know what you are getting when you look at the myriad of "waters" on the grocer's shelf, here is a breakdown as described by the EPA.

Drinking water. Also known as potable water, this is just what the name implies. It is water that is intended for drinking. It is safe for human consumption. There are no added ingredients besides what is considered usual and safe for any tap water, such as fluoride. If you notice, this does not speak to the source of the water.

Distilled water. Distilled water is a type of purified water. This water is processed by boiling with the steam reconstituted by condensation. It is then bottled. Distilling water kills all microbes and removes all dissolved materials like minerals. For that reason, it often has a fairly flat taste.

Purified water. Purified water is water that comes from any source but has been treated to meet the US Pharmacopeia's definition of purified water. Purified water can be made using any suitable method to remove any chemicals or contaminants. Types of purification include distillation, deionization, reverse osmosis, and carbon filtration. Like distilled water, it has its advantages and disadvantages: potentially harmful chemicals may be taken out, but beneficial minerals may be taken out as well. Want to read more? Try this: http://www.fda.gov/ICECI/Inspections/Inspection-Guides/InspectionTechnicalGuides/ucm072925.htm.

Sterilized water. This is water that can come from any source, but it has been treated to meet the US Pharmacopeia's standards for sterilized water. This is water generally used for mixing dry medication so that they can be administered through an intravenous line or as an injection. Sterilized water is completely free from all microbes.

Spring water. This is what you often find in bottled water at the store. It's from an underground source or aquifer (also known as ground water) and may or may not have been treated and purified. Though spring water sounds more appealing (like many others, I imagine my spring water coming from a gushing fresh spring at the base of a tall snow-capped mountain), it's not necessarily the best water for drinking if you have other options.

Studies done by the Natural Resources Defense Council (NRDC) have found contaminants in bottled water, such as coliform, arsenic, and phthalates. For a discussion of these contaminants, see http://www.nrdc.org/water/drinking/bw/chap3.asp#table2.

Much of bottled water is labeled as spring water when in fact it is coming from a municipal source and is nothing more than glorified tap water.

This topic has been a popular one in recent years, sparking a great deal of discussion and even controversy.

Mineral water. This is ground water that naturally contains 250 or more parts per million of total dissolved solids. Sounds yummy, huh?

So, how do you make sense of this? To check the quality of your local tap water, check with the EPA's site for local drinking water at http://water.epa.gov/drink/local/index.cfm/drink/local/index.cfm.

To check the water quality of your favorite bottled water, you can consult a variety of consumer sites like the Environmental Working Group's report on bottled waters (http://www.ewg.org/research/ewg-bottled-water-scorecard-2011). Additionally, you can start by reading the label on the bottle. In addition to the volume of water, any pertinent nutritional claims, and any contact information for the bottler, the label may include the type of bottled water, its source, and the way in which it is treated. If you still have questions you can also contact the bottler. And with a nod to the hilarious Lewis Black, you may notice that under nutritional information, water bottles even quantify the fat content.

If there is *any* fat, maybe you should rethink your hydration strategy!

One additional note: carbonated water, soda water, seltzer water, and sparkling and tonic water are actually considered soft drinks and thus are not regulated as bottled water.

Summary

If you didn't realize it already, the physical environment has a huge impact on our health and quality of life at any age. As we grow older, our ability to survive or endure is reduced. That doesn't mean we are helpless. In fact, as you have seen, there are lots of resources out there for you to get smart and get ready. I'll offer that the best time to do it is before you encounter a problem. That way, you'll be in at least a much better frame of mind, which is the subject of the next chapter.

CHAPTER 4

THE SOCIAL AND PSYCHOLOGICAL ENVIRONMENT
I THINK, THEREFORE MY HEAD HURTS

This chapter is about adaptation and psychological survival. It is also about some of the very destructive things that seniors sometimes do—to themselves and others. I'm talking depression, isolation, ageism, and drugs, or as I like to think of it, dinner at Eugene O'Neill's house.

Actually, the better or at least the more intellectual way of starting off this chapter in the proper tone is with my third-favorite quote by Albert Einstein, who said "Once you can accept the universe as matter expanding into nothing that is something, wearing stripes with plaid comes easy."

It really is all about perspective.

With perspective in mind, I just have to say that I like the movie *Harold and Maude* a lot. If you haven't seen it, then—to bastardize Shakespeare terribly—get thee to a theater quick or use On Demand or the Internet or something. It's a great story about a boy obsessed with the allure of the darker aspects of human existence who comes into the company of, and falls in love with, a septuagenarian who has endured all sorts of terrible things but who is still entranced with the beauty and joy of life.

So I am going to suggest we try to remind ourselves about all this in terms of perspective, because at the end of the day perspective and outlook is what we have at our disposal, right? I mean, life gives you lemons… and you make a garnish for a fish, right?

It is a sad fact that, according to the Substance Abuse and Mental

Health Services Administration (SAMHSA), a part of the US Department of Health and Human Services (HHS), substance abuse, particularly of alcohol and prescription drugs, among adults 60 and older is one of the fastest-growing health problems facing the country. Yet even as the number of older adults suffering from these disorders climbs, the situation remains underestimated, underidentified, underdiagnosed, and undertreated. Until relatively recently, alcohol and prescription drug misuse, which affects up to 17 percent of older adults, was not discussed in either the substance abuse or gerontological literature.

There are a lot of reasons for this: insufficient data, shame, bias toward and against the elderly, very little research dedicated to the subject, and an ever time-pressured healthcare system that encourages less and less time between provider and patient. In cases of psychological illness and problems, or getting to the truth about overuse, abuse, or addiction and the contributing, underlying issues, a quick "what brings you in today?" just won't cut it.

Seniors and Depression, a Different Shade of Blue

Now, I have been accused of being a little obtuse at times and even kind of existential. Okay, yeah, maybe so, but it's existentialism in the practical Haggar polyester Sansabelt slacks kind of way, limited only by one's own definitions of "it fits" and the imagination of some engineers at Monsanto. When it comes to psychological disorders and maladaptive conditions—all jokes aside—this is a gargantuan problem among seniors, one that needs much better attention and action from all of us.

Depression among seniors is actually different from depression in younger demographics. Depression in the elderly is often frequently confused with the effects of multiple illnesses and the medicines used to treat them. It often occurs with other medical illnesses, and it generally lasts episodically longer than in younger people. Roughly 25 percent of people age 65 or older suffer from depression. More than half of doctor visits by the elderly involve complaints of emotional distress. In 2008 the Geriatric Mental Health Foundation reported that 15–20 percent of older adults in the United States have experienced depression. And just in case I'm not being depressing enough with all this, here's another fun fact. The

National Institute of Mental Health estimates that for cases of "late-life" depression, affecting roughly 6 million, only about 10 percent will actually be diagnosed and get care.

That is just sad! No pun intended.

Even worse, depression often exacerbates other conditions and can increase the likelihood of other medical problems like heart attacks. It also increases the likelihood that those types of events will result in death. Depression reduces immunity and slows rehabilitation from injuries, illnesses, and surgeries. According to the Journal of the American Geriatric Society, depression is also one of the major causes of decline in the health-related quality of life for senior citizens.

You could have figured that out on your own, huh?

Depression also increases the risk of suicide, especially in older white males. In fact, the suicide rate among people ranging from 80 to 84 years is more than twice that of the general population. In this county 20 percent of suicides are committed by seniors, with the highest success rate belonging to older white men.

So by now you are thinking, where the heck are the cartoons about this

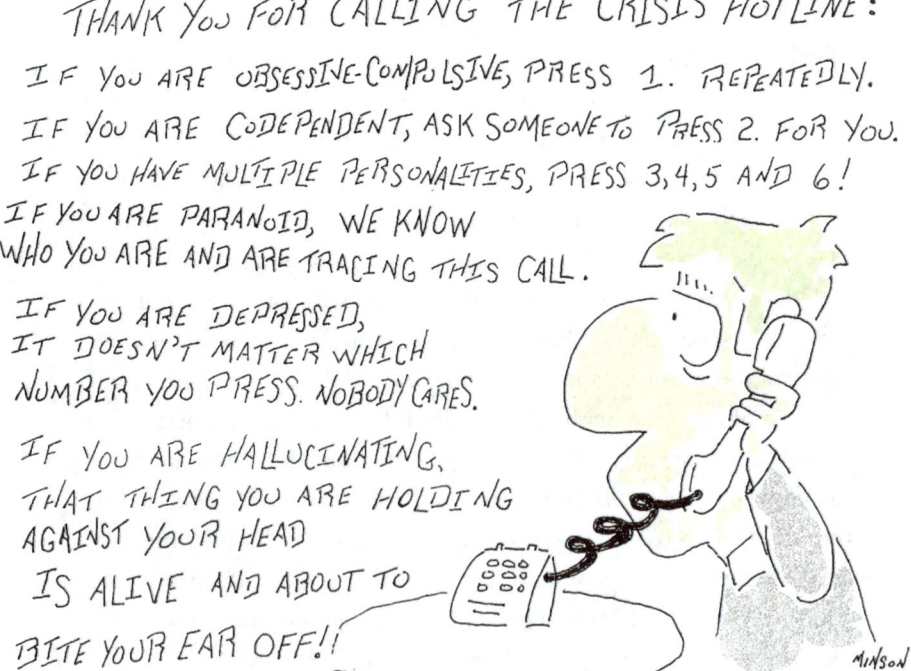

THANK YOU FOR CALLING THE CRISIS HOTLINE:

IF YOU ARE OBSESSIVE-COMPULSIVE, PRESS 1. REPEATEDLY.

IF YOU ARE CODEPENDENT, ASK SOMEONE TO PRESS 2. FOR YOU.

IF YOU HAVE MULTIPLE PERSONALITIES, PRESS 3,4,5 AND 6!

IF YOU ARE PARANOID, WE KNOW WHO YOU ARE AND ARE TRACING THIS CALL.

IF YOU ARE DEPRESSED, IT DOESN'T MATTER WHICH NUMBER YOU PRESS. NOBODY CARES.

IF YOU ARE HALLUCINATING, THAT THING YOU ARE HOLDING AGAINST YOUR HEAD IS ALIVE AND ABOUT TO BITE YOUR EAR OFF!!

MINSON

stuff? And how bad are they going to be? Well, they are coming—just in the nick of time.

Stigma

A lot of people, of every age, don't seek help for a psychological disorder because they fear the potential of associated shame and stigma from a misinformed world. That is what's really sad. I mean, think about it. If you had a broken leg, you'd get nothing but sympathy unless it happened while in the act of felony commission, and yet mental health and substance issues are still erroneously viewed, even by some medical professionals, as a character flaw. I mean, nobody criticizes a fracture patient for not having stronger bones, right? That is stigmatization, not to be confused with an astigmatism, which still gets you sympathy unless you are driving or skeet shooting!

Stigma has been defined as an attribute that is deeply discrediting. The stigmatized trait can set someone apart from the rest of society and bring with it feelings of shame and isolation. That is downright wrong. At its very worst, a person with a stigmatized trait is unable to perform an action or live a normal life because of the condition, and others may view the person as the problem rather than viewing the condition as the problem. More recent considerations include the results of stigma—the prejudice, avoidance, rejection, and discrimination directed at people believed to have an illness, disorder, or other trait perceived to be undesirable. Stigma causes needless suffering, potentially causing a person to deny symptoms, delay treatment, and refrain from daily activities. Stigma can exclude people from access to housing, employment, insurance, and appropriate medical care. It can also interfere with preventive and maintenance health efforts. It can even kill. Thus, examining and combating a stigma can even become a health priority.

See, I had a point after all.

Seniors are often stigmatized based on general misunderstandings or ageism, but when you add to that the additional misunderstanding and erroneous conceptions about mental or emotional illness, the problems become more than just cumulative. They actually amplify one another, or are considered "comorbid."

Remember the old chestnut "Sticks and stones may break my bones, but words will never hurt me"? Of course you do. It's one of the greatest social lies ever told. And, even worse, it rhymes, making it catchy.

I think what it is meant to communicate is perspective. You'd have to be pretty Zen-like, almost to the point of being emotionally bulletproof for cutting words not to hurt. That said, giving in to it actually empowers the offender.

With respect to a slightly better poet, William Shakespeare, I'll offer this from *Antony and Cleopatra*, "Their tongues rot that speak against us."

So there.

Risk Factors

For seniors, there are definitely some common factors, situations, and conditions that can lead to depression or at least that should put you on the lookout for the development of depression.

They are

- Being female
- Being single, unmarried, divorced, or widowed
- Lack of a supportive social network
- Stressful life events
- Certain medicines or combination of medicines
- Bodily changes like amputation, cancer surgery, etc.
- Family history of major depressive disorder
- Fear of death
- Living alone, social isolation
- Illness
- Past suicide attempt(s)
- Presence of chronic or severe pain
- Previous history of depression
- Recent loss of a loved one
- Substance abuse

If you are experiencing some of those things, get help. Start with your healthcare provider and, tough as it may be, make him or her listen to you. Tell him or her up front, "I have an issue that isn't going to be quick."

Here is something interesting about the cause of depression in seniors. In some cases, brain scans of people who develop their first depression in old age reveal areas of ischemia (decreased blood flow) that show up as "spots" in the scan. These ischemic areas may be due to a number of causes, including small strokes resulting from untreated hypertension (high blood pressure) or other blood-vessel-ravaging diseases like diabetes. Subsequent chemical changes in these brain cells may enhance the likelihood of depression separate from any life stress. So, you see, it may not always be mental after all. Notice I didn't say it wasn't always all in your head, but anatomically speaking, I could have.

So what does that have to do with the environment? Glad you asked.

Why Rhino Abstinence Bothers Me

I recently read an online article that, while it has to do with rhinoceri, also illustrates a point about another interesting species that sometimes does things for "no apparently good reason." Rhinoceri, or rhinoceroses if you prefer, are endangered because of poaching, habitat loss, and more. In an attempt to save them, captive habitats have been set aside in several areas to encourage an interest in mating and breeding. Now, despite creating what conservationists considered to be the ultimate rhinoceros love nest, they were finding that—for no apparent reason—the animals didn't seem to be in the mood.

Now, I imagine, if you are like me, it's the very definition of irony that rhinoceri, given the constant, keratinaceous prominence on the front of their faces, weren't feeling amorous, but it was true. This was a real problem, but try as the conservationists might to create a conducive environment, the rhinos just wouldn't breed. Then some Texas researchers started to look at the sonic environments of the habitat and found that while they had not shown a direct relationship between ultrasonic sound and behavior disruption, they did find that a considerable ultrasonic soundscape existed. Some of it was natural in origin, but much came from civilization-generated sources like jet plane engines, traffic, and even the electronic signatures from human habitat visitors. The researchers from

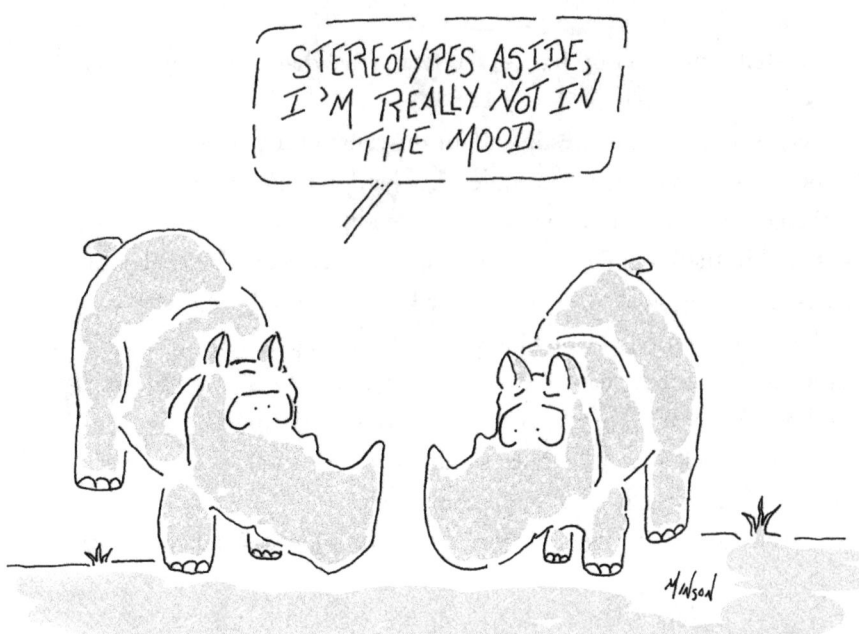

Texas State University noted that rhinos can hear sounds at much lower frequency ranges than humans, and rhinos in the wild use their infrasonic hearing to detect predators based on the vibrations their footsteps sent through the ground. It made sense, but to me the most interesting point was that this habitat wasn't in the middle of a downtown area. This one was 90 miles out in the country. As it turns out, what seemed pastoral and quiet to human ears was actually a surrounding sphere of chronic, constant infrasound.

Currently, the researchers are still trying to draw definitive conclusions about the relationship between subsonic influences and rhinoceros health. Even if there is no direct correlation between that kind of sound and rhino mating, one thing is for sure. Things that unsettle or make any creature feel unsafe or irritated have a psychological impact. As humans, we are also influenced by the psychological and social environment around us.

Now, am I saying that seniors are getting depressed because of invisible, consciously inaudible sound waves and that they should start walking around wearing aluminum foil hats? No. I am saying that, as with many psychological factors, there are a lot of subtle and unidentified triggers that can affect—not cause, but affect—our mood and psychology. Of course, if aluminum foil hats are a good look for you, well then, knock yourself out. Just be prepared for the occasionally awkward moment as you board public transportation.

In all seriousness, there are some things you can do to foster a positive psychological environment. In a recent article in *Psychology Today* the psychology of color, privacy, and even design indicated that significant subconscious benefits can result from an aesthetically conducive environment.

Of course, it is all relative and very subjective. If you are Morticia Adams, for example, then a bright and happy yellow decor is not likely to be as positively received as if you are Doris Day. Just the same, the devil in me would really like to see the reality show resulting from those two having to room together.

The Environmental Setting

Everyone needs a combination of private, semiprivate, and public spaces, but your personality can affect what that really means exactly. There is a book called *Some Place Like Home: Using Design Psychology to Create Ideal Places*, written by a psychologist named Toby Israel. I found it really interesting. She maintains, as you might expect, that extroverts like openness and place high value on rooms in which to gather and socialize. They may not want curtains on the windows. An extrovert may position his or her desk facing a window for the stimulation of people walking by. Conversely, introverts may think more clearly in a den-like home office or may feel more relaxed in smaller, intimate rooms. They may be more likely to close a door to a room than an extrovert would and may prefer more acreage around a house.

Where it can get really interesting is when you have an introvert living with an extrovert. This can actually significantly impact the quality of life of both of the cohabitants. Imagine a residential or congregate living setting. Wouldn't it be better if the psychological profile of the residents were considered and matched before assigning living arrangements? Or it might be wiser to design the dwelling or room to accommodate both. This may involve compromise, but almost every human encounter does.

It Isn't Easy Being Green—The Effect of Color

With all due respect to Kermit the Frog, like it or not, humans are emotional animals, and color affects everything from our moods to our heart rates. For most people, blue is generally calming and red stimulating. However, in a recent article published in *Color, Research & Application*, participants in two different studies had such cerebral arousal in red rooms that it paradoxically lowered their heart rates. In a third study, multicolored rooms lowered participants' heart rates more than gray ones. Introverts were the most strongly affected.

In one study a group of people reported feeling more positive in a red room than in a blue one. Those who started out in a bad mood worked faster on a routine task in a red room than in a blue one, and they wrote longer creative essays. But they made more clerical errors.

No, I did not write this book in a red room, despite what the copy editors will tell you.

So what? Get out the red paint? Well, no, because color is also one of the most subjective design elements because our past experiences, the associations of colors within our culture, and a bunch of other things that affect our preferences. A Francophile, for example, might feel energized around navy blue because of the widespread use of the color in France.

I am suddenly reminded of that kid in *The Shining*, croaking "REDrum" over and over.

The point is that it pays to look at color in terms of your individual history and experience. The same can theoretically be said for smells—like with Proust's madeleines—or textures or, of course, music, which, as we all know, differs for everybody.

On that note, if your best years were in the disco era, well, then get out your Bee Gees albums and—I mean this wholeheartedly—you have my sympathies.

Fêng Shui or What This Room Needs Is Some Throw Pillows!

Now, if your experience with Chinese culture ends with "I'll have the Kung Pao, extra spicy," then you are going to want to pay attention here.

Fêng shui is a Chinese philosophical system of harmonizing a person with his or her environment. The words literally translate as "wind-water" in English. So if you have been reading this with a smirk as you listen to your sound machine emulating electronic waves crashing on a beach, well then, the joke's on you!

I'll admit that I was initially incredulous when I first considered the merits of this design concept, but an architecture colleague of mine who designs buildings that literally make my jaw drop told me that it really is a concept of infusing a psychological binding of energy and flow. He challenged me to try writing in one of his creations, and I had to admit, I "felt" better about what I had written.

Need more?

A recent Harvard study showed that the amygdala, the part of the brain involved in fear and other emotional processing, is often activated when we're surrounded by sharp objects. This may explain why so many people like traditional furniture with its turned legs, smooth wooden surfaces, and ornamental curves. This also doesn't speak well for my 40-pound, Tykonda, bear-trap-shaped dining room set, I guess.

It really is relative. For some, the spare, uncluttered lines of much modern decor can be relaxing—the shape equivalent of modernism's often unsaturated hues. If you think about our mammoth-burger-eating cave dweller and Wendell the saber-toothed cat, from an evolutionary point of view, openness and space let you see opportunities and threats and, in that way, are sometimes more relaxing because you're not going to be blindsided by the Wendells of the modern world.

Some designers actually advocate for a personality test like a Myers-Briggs to help their clients choose furnishings that suit them. "Thinking" types may prefer cooler colors and a more modern, high-tech space. "Feeling" types are drawn to furniture with warmer colors and materials, such as wood, and to softer forms. Laura Ashley prints might appeal to a Feeling type if, say, you are James Tiberius Kirk, whereas Danish or maybe Vulcan modern would appeal to the Spocks in your house. You get the idea. It's just what works for them.

Art—It's Not Just Some Guy's Name

What should you hang on the walls? While it has been said that beauty is in the eye of the beholder, numerous studies show that most people prefer realistic and natural scenes to abstract ones. People with a high need for structure, in particular, negatively rate abstract paintings, according to a study published in the *Journal of Personality and Social Psychology*. Knowing the title of said abstract painting, however, gave these same sticklers for structure a more positive view. People who like abstract art also tend to be sensation-seekers and more open to new experiences than those who prefer realistic art, according to a 2009 study published in *Psychology of Aesthetics, Creativity and the Arts*.

But not all abstract art is the same, at least according to research done by Richard Taylor, a professor of physics at the University of Oregon. Taylor analyzed the drip paintings of Jackson Pollack and discovered that Pollock's paintings are of a fractal nature—the pattern of the entire painting is basically the same as the pattern of any small section, much the way a single branch of a tree shares the same basic pattern or geometry as the entire tree. This visual repetition and organization is part of what makes gazing at a tree or a cloud—or a Pollock—so pleasing. Thank you, this will be on the test!

Of course, I like cartoons, especially badly drawn but fundamentally well-intended ones, which can also be purchased in the lobby . . .

In any case, if you can get your hands on a Pollock, well, I'd hang on to it, under a tree, on a round couch, down by the ocean. You get the idea.

It's Not the Heat, It's the Humidity

This one I can attest to personally, but don't take my word for it. There have been scores of industrial efficiency and industrial engineering reviews of the effect of temperature on people. Having the thermostat on an inhospitable setting can make a person feel lonely or unhappy. In the work environment, adjusting the thermostat has been shown to reduce emotional dissatisfaction among workers and to result in reduced absenteeism and resignations. Temperature strongly influences how we feel about ourselves, our environments, and the people around us. Don't believe me? Enjoy your Russian winter then let's chat.

Physical warmth can diminish feelings of loneliness and increase feelings of generosity, according to Yale psychologist John A. Bargh. In a recent study in *Emotion*, participants who reported feeling the loneliest also took the warmest, longest, and most frequent baths or showers—"quite literally to compensate for feeling socially cold."

Warm Hands, Cold Hearts?

In two studies by UCLA researcher Geoffrey Ho, people were asked to rate the efficacy of heating pads or ice packs and then answer questions about their employer or a hypothetical company. Those who got their hands warm expressed higher job satisfaction and greater willingness to buy from and work at the made-up companies. If we are psychosocially chilled, then we seek physical connection and warmth. Likewise, if the environment is inhospitable, it affects our mindset.

Just ask the rhinos.

These findings are just the latest to show how someone's psychophysical environment can shape his or her psychological state. There is a fancy term for this. It's called "embodied cognition." In short, it means that social exclusion can make us feel physically chilled.

But you knew that already, right?

Better stated, "Abstract psychological and social concepts—how we think and feel about people, including ourselves—grow out of basic physical concepts like warmth and coldness," according to John Bargh of Yale University.

Some parts of the brain are particularly adept at translating physical sensations into psychological effects. By looking at subjects inside an fMRI machine, Bargh found that activity in the insular cortex, a center for assessing unpleasant stimulation, spikes when participants hold chilled objects and drops when they hold toasty ones. The warmed subjects were also more likely than the cold ones to offer to a friend the prizes they received for participation, suggesting a possible overlap between the neural centers of trust and physical comfort.

Just like with rhinos and the infrasonic affects of their habitat, we perceive triggers and cues from our environment, and these cues register as a physical and thus psychological effect. Things like temperature affect our perception and mood even when we are not consciously aware of it.

This is extremely important when you consider the senior population and the factors that can lead to depression or dysthymic—mood altering—effects.

How Do You Know If You Are at Risk for Depression?

Earlier I listed a bunch of situations and conditions that are often associated with new onset depression among seniors.

According to the US National Library of Medicine, a part of the NIH, there is a screening form developed from the Quick Inventory of Depressive Symptomatology Self-Report (QIDS-SR).

I know. I know what you are thinking. "Really? That seemed like a good acronym?"

Hey, no one consulted me. Just try to get past that because it's a really good tool. In fact, it's a part of a whole bunch of self-checks and tools for a variety of medical conditions—everything from abdominal pain and acoustic neuromas to yeast infections. This treasury of self-help can be found at http://www.nlm.nih.gov/medlineplus/healthchecktools.html.

"SCREENING" FOR DEPRESSION

Only a qualified health professional can truly diagnose depression. There is a reason for that. At the same time, most people need some help on where to start with regard to psychological problems like depression so they know they need to seek out a professional. I have provided a tool in the form of a self-test below that can aid in early assessment and self-reporting. This tool should not be used in place of a consultation with a health professional. If you have any concerns, see your healthcare provider or mental health professional.

If you or someone you know has thoughts of death or suicide, contact a healthcare professional, clergy member, loved one, friend, or crisis line, such as 1–800–273-TALK (8255), or, even better, call 911 immediately.

The following test will help your healthcare provider assess your condition. Fill it out before your next visit with your healthcare provider. He or she will score it and then can discuss what actions to take if any.

Please check the one response to each item that best describes how you have felt for the past seven days.

1. Fall Asleep
   ☐ I never take longer than 30 minutes to fall asleep.
   ☐ I take at least 30 minutes to fall asleep, less than half the time.
   ☐ I take at least 30 minutes to fall asleep, more than half the time.
   ☐ I take at least 60 minutes to fall asleep, more than half the time.

2. Sleep during the Night
   ☐ I do not wake up at night.
   ☐ I have a restless, light sleep with a few brief awakenings each night.
   ☐ I wake up at least once a night, but I go back to sleep easily.
   ☐ I awaken more than once a night and stay awake for 20 minutes or more, more than half the time.

3. Waking Up Too Early
   ☐ Most of the time, I awaken no more than 30 minutes before I need to get up.
   ☐ More than half the time, I awaken more than 30 minutes before I need to get up.
   ☐ I almost always awaken at least one hour or so before I need to, but I go back to sleep eventually.
   ☐ I awaken at least one hour before I need to and can't go back to sleep.

4. Sleeping Too Much
- ☐ I sleep no longer than 3–8 hours/night, without napping during the day.
- ☐ I sleep no longer than 10 hours in a 24-hour period, including naps.
- ☐ I sleep no longer than 12 hours in a 24-hour period, including naps.
- ☐ I sleep longer than 12 hours in a 24-hour period, including naps.

5. Feeling Sad
- ☐ I do not feel sad.
- ☐ I feel sad less than half the time.
- ☐ I feel sad more than half the time.
- ☐ I feel sad nearly all the time.

6. Decreased Appetite
- ☐ My usual appetite has not decreased.
- ☐ I eat somewhat less often or lesser amounts of food than usual.
- ☐ I eat much less than usual and only with personal effort.
- ☐ I rarely eat within a 24-hour period, and only with extreme personal effort or when others persuade me to eat.

7. Increased Appetite
- ☐ My usual appetite has not increased.
- ☐ I feel a need to eat more frequently than usual.
- ☐ I regularly eat more often and/or greater amounts of food than usual.
- ☐ I feel driven to overeat both at mealtime and between meals.

8. Decreased Weight (within the Last Two Weeks)
- ☐ My weight has not decreased.
- ☐ I feel as if I've had a slight weight loss.
- ☐ I have lost 2 pounds or more.
- ☐ I have lost 5 pounds or more.

9. Increased Weight (within the Last Two Weeks)
- ☐ My weight has not increased.
- ☐ I feel as if I've had a slight weight gain.

    ☐ I have gained 2 pounds or more.

    ☐ I have gained 5 pounds or more.

10. Concentration and Decision Making

    ☐ There is no change in my usual capacity to concentrate or make decisions.

    ☐ I occasionally feel indecisive or find that my attention wanders.

    ☐ Most of the time, I struggle to focus my attention or to make decisions.

    ☐ I cannot concentrate well enough to read or cannot make even minor decisions.

11. View of Myself

    ☐ I see myself as equally worthwhile and deserving as other people.

    ☐ I am more self-blaming than usual.

    ☐ I largely believe that I cause problems for others.

    ☐ I think almost constantly about major and minor defects in myself.

I have also included the tool at www.preparetodefendyourself.com.

WHAT DO I DO NOW?

The responses to the above questions may possibly indicate the presence of depression. This is simply a screening tool. If you will notice, I did not provide information on how you could score it yourself. There is a good reason for that. Mark Twain said that a man who represents himself in court has a fool for a client. Well, the same applies for medicine. Especially regarding mental health.

Remember, by filling out the questionnaire in advance, you can make more efficient use of your face-to-face time with your provider.

SO NOW I AM DEPRESSED?

Now, I feel that it is important to point out that everyone is going to feel sadness from time to time. It seems obvious, but there really is a uniquely

American phenomenon, borne in part because of our generally good fortune, that we expect happiness and are shocked when it doesn't occur. Frankly, I blame the movies.

It brings to mind a quote "that Americans expect to be happy all the time and are dismayed when it doesn't happen, and that the rest of the world expects unhappiness and they aren't disappointed."

Gloomy perhaps, but also somewhat credible. So let's be kind of continental for a second and consider or accept that we are going to be sad at times. The difference between sadness and depression is really a matter of magnitude, quality, and duration. If you notice, the qualifier in the questionnaire is over "the past two weeks." This doesn't mean that a person can't be clinically depressed in less time. It just means that if you have a good reason and you feel down correspondingly and it is not of the caliber of hopelessness, you shouldn't go overboard and worry that now you are depressed and probably should be taking a pill. That said, if you really think you are depressed, get help, and if you need to, take the pill your healthcare provider prescribes. Just be sure to talk it through with him or her.

Maybe make your provider look at the results of your test. He or she should be impressed that you put all that effort into making his or her job easier. I would be if my patient did.

Forms of Depression

It always helps to actually know what you are talking about. According to the CDC and reiterated at the senior advocacy site A Place for Mom, there are several forms of depression:

Major depression. This condition is marked by severe symptoms that interfere with your ability to work, sleep, study, eat, and enjoy life. Some people may experience only a single episode within their lifetime, but more often a person may have multiple episodes.

Dysthymic disorder (dysthymia). This condition describes depressive symptoms that last a long time (two years or longer) but that are less severe than those of major depression.

Minor depression. This condition is similar to major depression and dysthymia, but symptoms are less severe and may not last as long.

Of course different people have different symptoms. Some symptoms of depression include the following:

- Feeling sad or "empty"
- Feeling hopeless, irritable, anxious, or guilty
- Loss of interest in favorite activities
- Feeling very tired
- Not being able to concentrate or remember details
- Not being able to sleep or sleeping too much
- Overeating or not wanting to eat at all
- Thoughts of suicide, suicide attempts
- Aches or pains, headaches, cramps, or digestive problems

No one thing accounts for a definitive diagnosis. Often it's a few of the conditions and the information you provide during a medical consultation. Remember what I said earlier about having a fool for a client? While this is not a checklist for self-diagnosis, it does give you an idea of some of the things your healthcare provider will need to know. That will help you help him or her help you.

Other Things Affecting Depression

Several factors, or a combination of factors, may contribute to depression. I have mentioned a few earlier in the chapter, but in keeping with the WHO theme of "health," other factors include

- Genes. If you have a family history of depression you may be more likely to develop it than those whose families do not have the illness. Older adults who had depression when they were younger are more at risk for developing depression later in life than those who did not have the illness earlier in life.
- Brain chemistry. People with depression may have different brain chemistry than those without the illness. That predisposition along with triggering factors may result in the development of a depressive illness.

- Environment and Stress. Loss of a loved one, a difficult relationship, or any stressful situation may trigger depression.

For older adults who experience depression for the first time later in life, the depression may be related to changes that occur in the brain and body as a person ages. For example, older adults may suffer from restricted blood flow, a condition called *ischemia*. Over time, blood vessels may stiffen and prevent blood from flowing normally to the body's organs, including the brain. If this happens, an older adult with no family history of depression may develop what is sometimes called "vascular depression." Those with vascular depression also may be at risk for heart disease, stroke, or other vascular illness.

Depression can also co-occur with other serious medical illnesses such as diabetes, cancer, heart disease, and Parkinson's disease. Remember the term comorbidity? Well, here you go. Depression can make these conditions worse and vice versa. Sometimes medications taken for these illnesses may cause side effects that contribute to depression. A healthcare provider with expertise and who is experienced in treating these complicated illnesses can help work out the best therapeutic strategy.

If you know someone who has depression, first get him or her see a healthcare provider or mental health professional. Be supportive, understanding, and patient. Be attentive and encouraging. This is going to be tough.

Suicidal Talk

Under no circumstances should you ever ignore comments about suicide, and you shouldn't hesitate to report them to your loved one's therapist or doctor. Even offhand remarks or "kidding" should be taken seriously. You may well prevent a tragedy.

WHAT YOU CAN DO

Like I said before, if you suspect that you are depressed, get to a healthcare evaluation and get help. The first thing that a competent healthcare provider will do is rule out a physical or medical cause. In the elderly, the causes associated with clinical conditions are quite numerous. If your healthcare provider determines that you need some kind of clinical care, ask him or her to make sure it is from someone who specializes in geriatric depression. As I also said earlier, there is a big difference in depression occurring in older people and younger populations.

I mean, think about it. Would you go to a pediatrician for an adult problem? Well, your mental health is no less important and influenced by age, so get the right kind of physician or healthcare provider with the right credentials.

What to Expect

Here are some general approaches to psychological or mental health providers' therapies for senior depression:

Psychotherapy. This is often the first line in treatment. Basically it is talking with a trained and licensed therapist. Psychotherapy helps by teaching new ways of thinking and behaving and by changing habits that may be contributing to the depression. Many depressed older people also find that support from family and friends, involvement in self-help and support groups, and their psychotherapy are helpful. Psychotherapy is especially beneficial for those who have endured major life stresses (such as loss of friends and family, home relocations, and health problems) or who prefer not to take medicine and have only mild to moderate symptoms. It also is helpful for people who cannot take drugs because of side effects, interactions with other medicines, or other medical illnesses. Therapy can help you understand and work through difficult relationships or situations that may be causing your depression or making it worse.

Psychotherapy in older adults can address a broad range of functional and social consequences of depression. Many healthcare providers recommend the use of psychotherapy in combination with antidepressant medicines.

Medications. Medicines called antidepressants can often work well to treat depression. They are not fast fixes, however, and can even take several weeks to work. Antidepressants are also serious medications that can have side effects, including headache, nausea, difficulty sleeping, restlessness, sexual dysfunction, nervousness, and agitation.

Certain older antidepressants such as amitriptyline and imipramine can be sedating and cause a sudden drop in blood pressure when a person stands up. This is known as *postural hypotension* and can be really dangerous, as in cases where it leads to falls and fractures. If you have these side effects, take heart, as most of them will lessen over time, but make sure to talk to your physician or healthcare provider about anything you experience.

I mentioned the delay before the medications start to work. This is called latency. Antidepressants may take even longer to start working in older people than they do in younger people. Since elderly people are more sensitive to medicines, doctors may prescribe lower doses at first. In general, the length of treatment for depression in the elderly is longer overall than it is in younger patients.

So what I am really saying is, be patient . . . when you are the patient. Next up: fun with homonyms!

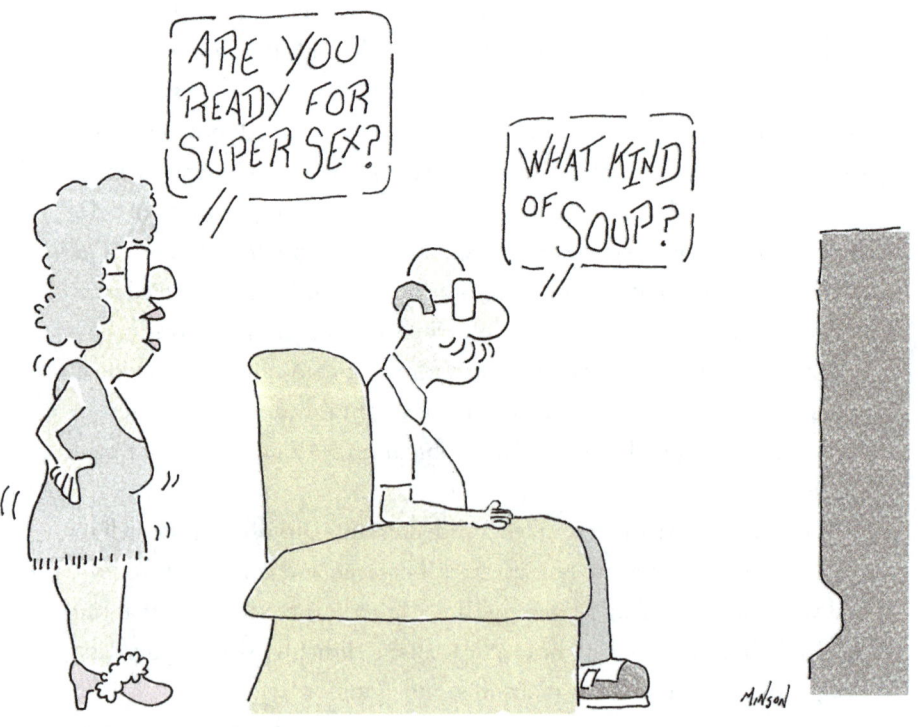

Electroconvulsive therapy (ECT). This type of treatment is some-times used for severe depression that is very difficult to treat and does not respond to medication or therapy or when depression is very severe and interferes with basic daily functioning such as eating, bathing, and groom-ing. Although ECT once had a bad reputation, it has greatly improved as a therapy and can provide relief for people for whom other treatments have not worked. Be aware that ECT may cause side effects of its own, such as confusion and memory loss. Although these effects are usually short-term, they can sometimes linger.

Other options. These include newer forms of brain stimulation, such as repetitive transcranial magnetic stimulation (rTMS), and experimental protocols. Generally you will find these options at university-based medi-cal practices.

One thing you should remember. These things take time, and you may need to try a few different therapies and medications before finding one what works for you.

Self-Help Adjuncts

Now, this next point is really important, and just because I am offer-ing these recommendations, you should not expect that this may cor-rect the problem without additional support and care. It is important to remember that neither you nor someone you care about with depression can simply "snap out of it." Treatment choices differ for each person, and sometimes different treatments must be tried until you find that one, or combination of *ones*, that work.

That said, *there are some things you can do to help improve the situation. That* said, *get that healthcare evaluation first*!

Try to do things that you used to enjoy before you had depression. Studies have shown that doing these things, even when you don't expect to enjoy them, can help lift your spirits. To lighten someone's mood and to be supportive, maybe, after the clinical evaluation, invite him or her out for walks, outings, and other physical activities. And, finally, keep reminding him or her that with time and treatment, the depression can be treated and alleviated or controlled.

If it is you who is affected, go easy on yourself. You should also consider some other strategies, like breaking up large tasks into small ones to experience successful benchmarks, and doing what you can as you can. Just set attainable short-term goals. That will foster a sense of success. You also shouldn't attempt too many things at once. Spend time with other people and consider talking to a friend or relative about your feelings. Once you have a treatment plan, try to stick to it. Remember, it will take time for treatment to work. Also do not make important life decisions until you feel better. If you are facing a time-sensitive issue while in therapy, discuss decisions with others who know you well.

If you know someone who has been diagnosed with depression or you suspect that he or she is depressed, first encourage and help him or her see a healthcare provider or mental health professional.

Who Can Help?

There are specialists—remember, many are in university medical settings—that are looking at these types of issues for seniors. There are also many academic and governmental supportive programs that are collaborating on senior psychological issues.

One example of a collaborative effort at the University of Washington looked at epileptic issues and the comorbid presence of depression. The Prevention Research Center (PRC) at the University of Washington implemented the Program to Encourage Active, Rewarding Lives (PEARLS). Modeled after the Chronic Care model and developed by PRC investigators, PEARLS has proven to be an effective community-based intervention that significantly reduced symptoms of minor depression or dysthymia in homebound older adults by addressing aspects of social isolation, medical comorbidity, physical impairment, transportation difficulties, and stigma.

Between 1999 and 2003, University of Washington investigators at the Health Promotion Research Center (HPRC) and community-based service providers conducted a randomized controlled trial funded by the CDC to test the effectiveness of PEARLS in older adults living in the community. Individuals in this study were relatively housebound and had an average of five chronic medical conditions. Those who were treated in the PEARLS program were three times more likely to experience a reduction in their depressive symptoms than those who were not.

For more information you can go to http://www.pearlsprogram.org/ or http://www.pearlsprogram.org/Our-Program/PEARLS-for-Older-Adults .aspx.

There are also a number of other government and public-private enterprises that can offer some useful information.

NATIONAL ALLIANCE ON MENTAL ILLNESS

The National Alliance on Mental Illness (NAMI) works to support and educate the public about various mental disorders with the goal of improving the quality of life for all persons diagnosed with mental illness. NAMI's website (http://www.nami.org/) provides the latest facts, statistics, and research advances on different types of mental health conditions.

NATIONAL COUNCIL FOR COMMUNITY BEHAVIORAL HEALTHCARE

The National Council for Community Behavioral Healthcare is a nonprofit group with member organizations across the United States. The website (http://www.thenationalcouncil.org/) explains its goal of assisting people with mental illnesses and addiction disorders so they can recover and lead active and productive lives. The website also provides available support services along with inspirational patient stories.

NATIONAL INSTITUTE OF MENTAL HEALTH

The National Institute of Mental Health (NIMH) is the largest research organization in the world that focuses on mental health diseases. The NIMH website (http://www.nimh.nih.gov/index.shtml) provides in-depth information and the latest findings on topics ranging from anxiety, ADHD, and autism to OCD, panic disorder, and depression.

Drug Abuse

As I wrote earlier, this phenomenon is becoming a real public health crisis among seniors, and yet it is also a virtually silent epidemic. According to a

Johns Hopkins Health Alert, the number of Americans over age 50 abusing prescription drugs is projected to rise to 2.7 million in 2020—a 190 percent increase from the 2001 figure of 910,000. According to the US Substance Abuse and Mental Health Services Administration, of 184,000 Americans who started treatment for any type of drug abuse in 2005, 10 percent were age 50 or older.

In order to truly discuss this intelligently, some more definitions are probably in order. I know what you may be thinking.

"Hey, wait a minute! This guy is trying to *teach* me something."

Guilty. Read on.

ILLEGAL VERSUS ILLICIT

These are two terms that get interchanged a lot. While they have some similarity, they actually mean different things.

Illegal drugs are those that are either being used in an illegal pursuit or that have no legal use of application. Heroin is one example. Outside of some really unusual research—and, no, you can't use that with the cops—there is no "legally known" use for the drug. In general, it has to do with how obvious the criminal behavior of unsanctioned use is. The term illicit use is a little more nuanced and really means unsanctioned or improper. It may also be illegal but is not necessarily so.

Here is the difference. If you have prescription for a pain medication that you get filled when you fracture your ankle skiing in March and use it consistent with the prescribing instructions, then that is legal and appropriate. If you break your finger six months later and do not consult anyone and start taking the remains of leftover medications from that ankle injury months before, that may be considered illicit, and also is probably illegal too. If you give a couple to your cousin, Moe, who is down for the weekend and can't find anything good on cable, well, that is illegal for sure. Make sense? Good.

Technically, legally, both illicit and illegal drugs are not lawful. The law enforcement definition of illicit is illegal with an expectation by the perpetrator that the action will not be discovered. For that reason—and many others—you should not try to use this book as a precedent or citation during the legal defense of your drug trial. Seriously, don't!

It's worth making a distinction between drug misuse, which is common among seniors, and drug abuse, which is arguably less prevalent among the older population.

The majority of seniors who become dependent on prescription drugs are being treated for legitimate medical issues such as pain, anxiety, depression, or insomnia. They may do it by increasing their dose—against medical advice—in order to seek greater relief from their condition. This is drug *misuse*.

Drug *abuse* is less common among seniors but is a big issue nonetheless. Abuse involves the repetitive and willful habit of taking drugs for the purpose of pleasure, ecstasy, and euphoria but does not include the repeated use of drugs for therapeutic purposes.

This distinction is important. Seniors who are misusing medications for therapeutic purposes may be doing so because their current treatment plan simply isn't effective in addressing their symptoms. Misuse or overuse can be controlled if physicians reevaluate treatment options so that patients don't rely on more medication than prescribed in order to get full relief.

Drug abuse, on the other hand, can be more difficult to get under control and may require drug treatment.

Most recently, the definitions are being altered slightly, though you may still encounter them as you do your own research.

DSM-5

The *Diagnostic and Statistical Manual of Mental Disorders*, fifth edition (DSM-5), is the 2013 update to the American Psychiatric Association's classification and diagnostic tool. It is what many psychiatrists and healthcare providers use to establish a clinical diagnosis and provides a common vernacular for clinicians.

It has some new language regarding substance use that is slightly different from the preceding language:

Substance use disorder in DSM-5 combines the DSM-IV categories of substance abuse and substance dependence into a single disorder measured on a continuum from mild to severe. Each specific substance (other than caffeine, which cannot be diagnosed as a substance use disorder) is addressed as a separate use disorder (e.g., alcohol use disorder, stimulant use disorder, etc.), but nearly all substances are diagnosed based on the same overarching criteria. In this overarching disorder, the criteria have not only been combined, but strengthened. Whereas a diagnosis of substance abuse previously required only one symptom, mild substance use disorder in DSM-5 requires two to three symptoms from a list of 11. Drug craving will be added to the list, and problems with law enforcement will be eliminated because of cultural considerations that make the criteria difficult to apply internationally.

In DSM-IV, the distinction between abuse and dependence was based on the concept of abuse as a mild or early phase and dependence as the more severe manifestation. In practice, the abuse criteria were sometimes quite severe. The revised substance use disorder, a single diagnosis, will better match the symptoms that patients experience.

Additionally, the diagnosis of dependence caused much confusion. Most people link dependence with "addiction" when in fact dependence can be a normal body response to a substance.

Actually, I am pretty sure that passage was intended as a cure for insomnia.

THE KEITH RICHARDS DIET

Technically, any drug can be harmful if abused. The rock star Grace Slick is reported to have said about medicine cabinets that she kept, "one medicinal, the other for recreational purposes. I was always afraid of getting the mouthwash mixed up with the mescaline or the acid with the aspirin. Hell, that could be dangerous—too much aspirin could be fatal." Similarly, Keith Richards described himself as an alchemist and stated that he used his body like a laboratory.

I chuckled when I first read that, but when I was writing this book, I sobered up pretty fast.

Get it? I sobered up. Anyway…

Many medications are *physically* addictive, such as opioid painkillers like acetaminophen and hydrocodone (Vicodin) or acetaminophen and oxycodone (Percocet). Sedative, antianxiety, and insomnia drugs like alprazolam (Xanax) and diazepam (Valium) can also cause physical dependence when taken daily, even at prescribed doses. Even without any misuse or abuse, a patient who is physically dependent will experience uncomfortable drug withdrawal symptoms if he or she abruptly stops taking the medication. If a patient wants to stop a medication that he or she is dependent on, a doctor will often prescribe gradually decreasing doses (a "taper") to reduce discomfort and physical reaction.

Addiction is more often the result of drug abuse. Addicts, seniors and otherwise, are usually not only physically dependent on the drug or drugs they are taking, but also take them in a clearly compulsive and harmful way. According to the National Institute on Drug Abuse, "compulsive drug use despite harmful consequences—is characterized by an inability to stop using a drug and failure to meet work, social, or family obligations."

Oh and as for Keith Richards, he also has reportedly said that he doesn't regret his "use" as it may have scared off some friends and loved ones from doing the same thing. So, take a lesson from Keith, kids.

I just flashed to a visual of the Keith Richards Children's Hour and both horrified and cracked myself up. Crazy fun for all ages!

WHICH DRUGS ARE THE RISKIEST?

As with any addictive substance, access increases the risk of abuse. Older people are more likely (for a variety of reasons) to get prescriptions for two leading types of drugs with potential for addiction: opioid pain relievers and benzodiazepines.

Drug Abuse with Opioids

Among abused prescription drugs, opioids are the most notorious. These drugs, which include oxycodone (OxyContin), oxycodone/acetaminophen, and hydrocodone, attach to opioid receptors in the brain that block the perception of pain. They also can produce euphoria by indirectly boosting dopamine levels in the parts of the brain that influence our sensing of pleasure—hence their addictive potential.

The most common side effects of opioids are nausea, vomiting, dizziness, sleepiness, constipation, and itching. During an overdose, opioids can slow down breathing, which can be fatal. However, a person who takes pain medication for a legitimate ailment or injury has a slim chance of developing an addiction. The risk increases when opioids are given to someone who has a personal or family history of addiction or has a psychological disorder.

Drug Abuse with Benzodiazepines

Other potentially addictive medications are benzodiazepines, such as alprazolam (Xanax), clonazepam (Klonopin), diazepam (Valium), and lorazepam (Ativan). Doctors commonly use these drugs to treat anxiety, panic attacks, insomnia, and acute stress reactions to traumatic experiences, such as the death of a spouse. Benzodiazepines work by slowing nervous system activity.

When used properly—in limited quantities for a short time—addiction is usually not a problem. But taking a larger dose or even typical dosages on a daily basis for an extended amount of time can easily lead to tolerance, and an individual will soon need larger and larger doses to get the desired effect. In addition, suddenly going off a benzodiazepine can trigger extreme anxiety and discomfort, prompting a desire to keep taking it. The possibility of tolerance is also present with sleeping medications such as zolpidem (Ambien) and eszopiclone (Lunesta), which work at the same place in the brain as benzodiazepines.

The health consequences of benzodiazepine abuse for older people include memory impairment, impaired reasoning, confusion, nodding off, car accidents, and falls, which could be fatal.

SIGNS OF A PROBLEM

Now, let's say you are reading this and you are concerned about a friend, a parent, or other relative. There are some things you should look for. You shouldn't ever try to diagnose or take matters into your own hands, but there are some things your clinician will want to know; if you can provide this information, it will help you both—him or her with diagnosing and treating and you with getting the benefit.

Here are some things to watch for:

- Diminished psychomotor performance (as if the individual's intent and his or her body's physical action are disconnected)
- Impaired reaction time
- Loss of coordination
- Increased numbers of falls
- Excessive daytime drowsiness
- Confusion
- Aggravation of emotional state
- Amnesia
- Dependence

These reactions may be more serious in frail older adults and in those with multiple chronic diseases.

Cognitive Issues and Misdiagnosis

This is a particular concern for me. For that reason I am going to suggest something that really is an observation of a recent trend in American medicine. It's not good. With the pressures of faster patient processing and the growing dependence on "data" like scans, x-rays, and laboratory values to tell the patient's "story," the emphasis on obtaining a proper history and interviewing the patient are arguably suffering. I mentioned earlier that psychological, mental health, and especially substance issues require some methodical and careful inquiry to determine that an individual is at risk. It also requires trust and understanding between the caregiver and the patient. That doesn't come from a 15-minute interaction and a whole bunch of paperwork.

This interview—or conversation, for lack of a better term—is even more difficult when the patient is a senior and probably is on multiple medications that may actually affect his or her ability to communicate and process information. The irony is that in some cases it is the practitioner that contributes to the disorder and the confusion around the diagnosis. The practitioner may assign the cause to something mental when it is actually the drugs he or she prescribed. So what can you do? This is where having an advocate may actually save your life. Take a relative or trusted friend with you. If you are prescribed a new drug or medication, be aware of any changes and tell your provider and advocate as soon as you experience them. And don't be put off.

Alcohol

Here are some interesting facts, according to a healthcare provider's guide to senior alcohol by SAMSHA:

- The normal decrease in body water that comes with age means the same amount of alcohol that previously had little effect can now cause intoxication.
- These changes in body water increase sensitivity and decrease tolerance to alcohol.
- The decrease in the rate of metabolism of alcohol in the gastrointestinal tract means blood alcohol level remains raised for a longer time and an increased strain is placed on the liver.

Now repeat after me… "The bar is now closed."

Seriously though, clinicians should tell clients that these age-related changes, combined with alcohol consumption, can trigger or worsen serious problems, including the following:

- Heart problems
- Risk of stroke
- Cirrhosis and other liver diseases
- Gastrointestinal bleeding
- Depression, anxiety, and other mental health problems

Summary

I know all of this has been pretty heavy stuff. It is serious, but like anything else, one of the best ways to confront a dragon is to laugh at it. With that in mind I am reminded of something that a psychiatrist faculty member of mine once offered when some resident physicians were arguing about the nuances of alcohol use and the trickiness of a diagnosis of alcoholism for a patient. Now, it helps to know that this was an esoteric rabbit hole of a discussion that sprang from an actual case in which an individual was an undeniable alcohol abuser, a veritable Charles Bukowski–caliber consumer. Everyone agreed on his diagnosis, including the patient, but the conversation had drifted to subtleties that did not apply to him specifically.

The psychiatrist looked up and said, "People, if you're drinking like it is still the Civil War and the doctor is coming to saw your leg off soon, then you probably have a problem."

We got the point.

CHAPTER 5

ACCESS TO HEALTH CARE

HOW TO GET A BACKSTAGE PASS

If you've read my first book, *Prepare to Defend Yourself . . . How to Navigate the Healthcare System & Escape with Your Life*, you already know I am a big fan of people being informed, even defensive consumers when it come to their own health and medical care. The fact is, there's been a huge shift in the dynamics of medical care in this country. I'm not talking about legislative actions like the Patient Protection and Affordable Care Act; I am talking about actual business dynamics.

In the past, a patient chose a doctor. The doctor saw the patient and billed insurance or the patient. If the patient needed to be admitted to a hospital, the doctor had privileges and administered care in the hospital. It was far from a perfect setup, and there were abuses and issues associated at times, but the physician functioned professionally as the advocate of the patient. She or he had a relationship with the consumer (the patient) and served as an independent contractor to the patient. To the hospital or healthcare system, the doctor was a referrer, and the influence was in the clinician's favor. This hopefully translated to the patient as well. The physician or the healthcare provider "worked" for the patient. Their accountability was to the patient.

Then things changed.

Now the hospital or healthcare system is more and more the employer of the healthcare provider. The system sets the criteria of what constitutes good care. Priorities are often on efficiency, patient satisfaction, and expedited care.

That all sounds good, right?

Well, if efficiency meant expedited *correct* diagnoses and access to the right prescriptions and follow-up confirmation of a cure, then sure. If it meant getting you out of the hospital as soon as possible, processing you through the system, and a cursory evaluation of your "satisfaction," then that may be better tailored to a car dealership. If you want to make certain that you get good care, there are some things you can do. If your diagnosis and treatment have life-or-death connotations, then these are some things you'd *better* do.

Now, you are probably wondering if this chapter will have insights into paying for care. That is in the next section. This chapter is about getting the best care. You see, access to health care is really about two things: getting to the right practitioner and assuring that the process of diagnosis, treatment, and recovery are right. That is what I am going to cover here.

Habla Medical?

After the first book, I was asked by an interviewer, "What is the *one* thing you would want people to take away from your book?"

My first thought was, "If I wanted them to take *one thing* away, I wouldn't have had to write a book." Instead I said, "Learn to communicate the way your healthcare provider thinks."

I still stand by that.

The pressures of managed care systems, the business of medicine, the "disconnect" between multiple specialists, and the distractions surrounding a medical practice means that a practitioner—who does not already know you—has a finite amount of time to figure out what is going on with you and to formulate a treatment plan. I think it is also going to get worse.

So what can you do?

Well, first, read the first book. You'll see that having your information organized in a way that fits the decision algorithm of a physician or caregiver will help streamline the process and will go a long way in assuring that you get a correct diagnosis and treatment. There are tools for that in the book and at the website www.preparetodefendyourself.com.

Secondly, don't trust that your medical information is maintained by the healthcare system. Take control of your information. It is *your* information, after all. Make sure that you have copies.

I often tell the story of how I experienced a confrontational episode with a clerk at a healthcare system whose computer screen "told" her that I owed a balance. The truth was that the software interfaces between the insurance provider and the clinics did not function well. For that reason, delays in credit to accounts occurred. I knew this, challenged it, and persevered. When later I saw an older woman making a choice between paying an outstanding balance and maybe having enough for food, I realized I had to do something to make people aware. And that is just considering the business end.

The Electronic Medical Record

In 2009 President Obama signed the American Recovery and Reinvestment Act (ARRA) into law. It carried with it a mandate to create a uniform standard and system for an electronic medical record (EMR). The legislation specifically aimed at creating more funding and a network of incentives that would be directly offered to reward healthcare professionals or physicians who were ready to adopt an EMR and would abide by the concept of "meaningful use" of electronic medical records by 2014. Legislation like the ARRA and the entire campaign promoting EMR are based on the principle that electronic records provide the combined benefit of securing patient information and cutting down healthcare costs. This assumes that the information will be readily available to those who need it and protected from those who might abuse it.

That sounds great. The reality, however, as with any enterprise of this magnitude, is that it is still not comprehensively happening throughout the country. Why? In order to answer that, it helps to understand how the system came to be. Years ago, hospitals were altruistic institutions, charitable enterprises supported by faith-based initiatives and other benevolent organizations. Eventually, in part due to legislation, hospitals became businesses. As such, they were subject to mergers, takeovers, closures, and the like. Hospitals had their own systems and software for record retention. When they merged, the software didn't always match. Similarly, physicians' offices and practices maintained their own records. Issues of economics and the dynamics of software evolution meant that incongruences between caregivers, practices, hospitals, and thus healthcare systems meant that in many situations the ability of an electronic record to communicate across a system was a struggle.

Even within some hospital departments, the format and specialty-specific medical information form may not be immediately available to all parties that need it. The recent Ebola cases in the United States illustrated the importance of this and how critical a failure could be.

SO WHY DO YOU CARE?

Well, it means that the comprehensive transfer of your information between providers may not always occur. Also, in 2015, penalties are likely to be levied on businesses, healthcare facilities, medical practices, and other entities dealing with patient healthcare data that are unable to upgrade to approved electronic record technologies. The way this will be compelled is by a proposed penalty of 1 percent. Many experts believe that this is likely to increase incrementally, up to 5 percent in future years. Most of the penalties will be levied in the form of reduced Medicare and Medicaid reimbursements for providers and systems. How and whether that cost will be passed on to the consumer (you) is not fully understood.

What is known is that the EMR vendor chosen by a healthcare provider/clinic or its business associates should comply with regulations that have been put forth in this niche, such as the standards set by the Security Rule of the Health Insurance Portability and Accountability Act (HIPAA).

You can look it up . . . if you are still awake.

This means that your information is subject to some very dynamic uncertainties, like hacking or system failures, and there may be additional fees imposed. They may be passed along to you the consumer, or they may result in more providers withdrawing from certain programs.

SO WHAT?

Well, first, when any kind of system, vendor, or business sees a reduction in reimbursement or an increase in cost, what does it do? It passes it along to the consumer. Guess who that is.

It also means that the days are long gone of being able to say, "Well, my records are at my doctor's office" and have that mean something. I liken it to being in a shipwreck at sea and saying, "Hey, there are lots of inflatable lifeboats"—but they are at back on the dock. If you want to make sure it is available, accurate, and assured when you need it, you better make sure you have access to that lifeboat—or your medical record—yourself.

That means having a *contemporary* and comprehensive copy of your own. Consider now all that we have covered in this book so far about seniors and the potential severity of medication and medical error impact, the compromised ability to bounce back from a mistake, the likelihood that multiple meds or polypharmacy is occurring, and the potential dangers of some medication interactions, and you see why having accurate medical information available may make the difference in life or death. The good news is that this doesn't mean you have to walk around with a wheelbarrow full of medical records. In fact, the smart move is to make sure you have multiple redundancies. This means requesting a copy of

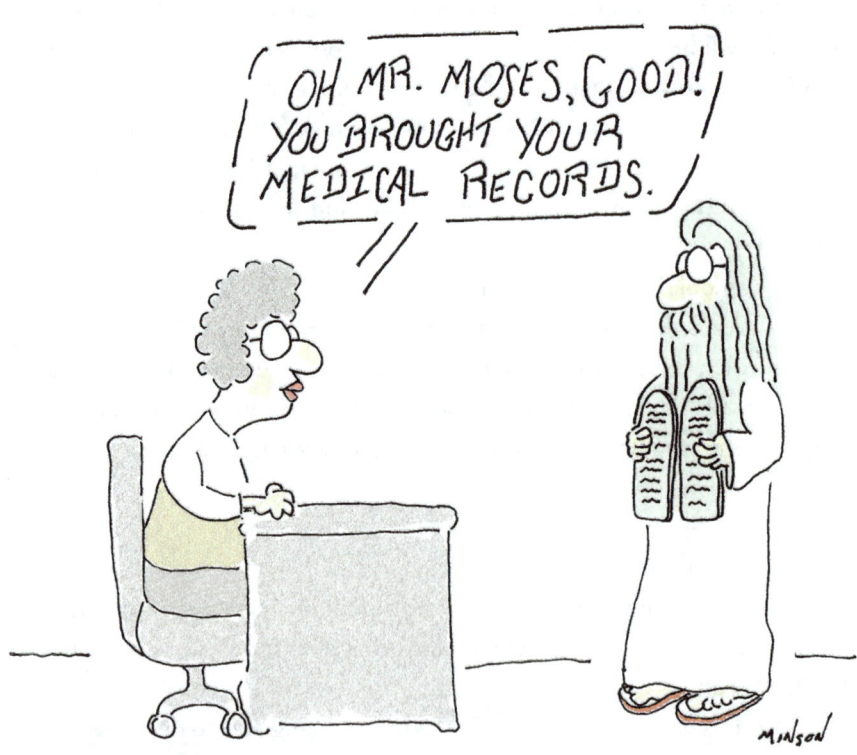

your record for every healthcare visit, for every test, and for every consultation, MRI, diagnostic evaluation . . . you get the idea.

Just writing that makes me feel a little redundant. What I am talking about is backup and backup in different formats.

Now, I like trees. Given the recent advancing massive severe drought in this country, I feel like I need to do trees a little bit of a favor. So I am going to suggest we not kill a billion of them to create static records. I am suggesting it might be really wise to have your records on thumb drives, in the cloud, and reposed on a trusted server.

The Numbers

Here are some statistics and projection provided by the USDHHS *Profile of Older Americans,* 2013, that are going to be really important for the rest of this book.

The older population (65+) numbered 43.1 million in 2012, an increase of 7.6 million or 21 percent since 2002. The number of Americans aged 45–64—who will reach 65 over the next two decades— increased by 24 percent between 2002 and 2012. About one in every seven, or 13.7 percent, of the population is an older American. Persons reaching age 65 have an average life expectancy of an additional 19.2 years (20.4 years for females and 17.8 years for males). The population 65 and over has increased from 35.5 million in 2002 to 43.1 million in 2012 (a 21 percent increase) and is projected to increase to 79.7 million in 2040. The 85+ population is projected to increase from 5.9 million in 2012 to 14.1 million in 2040. What is the application of that to access to healthcare?

According to the American Geriatric Society (AGS), there is a current shortage of geriatricians, physicians specializing in the disease processes and unique physiology of seniors. The estimated ratio in the United States is one geriatric primary care physician to 2,610 seniors. There are only 7,029 certified geriatricians practicing in the United States, roughly half the number currently needed, and those numbers are falling. Now I know that sounds bad, and it is, but get this—by 2030 AGS estimates that the ratio will be 1 to 3,798.

There's more.

There are far fewer geriatric psychiatrists. In 2001 there were about 2,600 geriatric psychiatrists. In 2005, that number was reduced to 2,100, less than half of the 5,000 that are needed to provide adequate care for the current population of older adults. It is now estimated that there are only 1,751. That amounts to one for every 10,865 seniors. That ratio is projected to decrease by 2030 to one geropsychiatrist for every 12,557 Americans aged 75 and older. Only 3 percent of practicing psychologists devote the majority of their practice to older adults, and the current median age of practicing psychologists is 55.

Depressing, isn't it? Get it?

Here is a look at the projected need for healthcare numbers overall:

- More than one million additional direct-care workers will be needed by 2018, according to the latest employment projections.
- Approximately 55,000 social workers are currently needed in long-term care. By 2050, this number will nearly double to approximately 109,000. While nearly 75 percent of licensed social workers work with older adults in some capacity, many have not received training or education in gerontology according to the National Association of Social Workers (NASW).
- In 2009–10, only 2.8 percent of BSW graduates and 6.7 percent of MSW graduates completed a specialization in aging, or an average of 5 percent across all social work graduates according to the Council on Social Work Education (CSWE).

Think that is cause for concern? Check these predictions.

- By 2020, the nursing workforce is expected to drop 20 percent below projected requirements.
- In 2010, physical therapists and physical therapist assistants had demonstrated vacancy rates of 18.6 percent and 16.6 percent, respectively, in skilled nursing facility settings across the United States.

Who We Are and What We Need

According to an analysis of healthcare issues by seniors over 65 by the National Center for Health Statistics, in 2010–12, 42 percent of noninstitutionalized people assessed their health as excellent or very good (compared with 55 percent for persons aged 45–64 years). There was little difference between the sexes on this measure, but older African-Americans (not Hispanic) (26 percent), older American Indians/Alaska Natives (31 percent), older Asians (34 percent), and older Hispanics (31 percent) were less likely to rate their health as excellent or very good than were older Whites (not Hispanic) (46 percent).

Most older persons have at least one chronic condition and many have multiple conditions. In some cases the conditions are not just additive but aggravate each other. As you may recall, this is known as a comorbidity. It sounds as bad as it is.

WHAT'S REALLY WRONG WITH US

In 2010–12 the most frequently occurring conditions among older persons were diagnosed arthritis (50 percent), all types of heart disease (30 percent), any cancer (24 percent), diagnosed diabetes (20 percent in 2007–10), and hypertension (high blood pressure or taking antihypertensive medication) (72 percent in 2007–10).

Let's consider these prevalent conditions for a little bit.

Arthritis

Technically the term simply means inflammation of the joint. There are many types of arthritis: inflammatory (or autoimmune), traumatic, degenerative, and rheumatoid. The most commonly occurring forms of the disease are osteo and rheumatoid. Osteoarthritis is the more common form of arthritis. In fact, rheumatoid arthritis affects about one-tenth as many people as osteoarthritis. The main difference between them is the cause behind the joint symptoms. Osteoarthritis is caused by mechanical wear and tear on joints. Rheumatoid arthritis is an autoimmune disease, meaning the body's own immune system attacks the body's joints.

Table 7. Characteristics of Rheumatoid Arthritis and Osteoarthritis

Characteristic	Rheumatoid Arthritis	Osteoarthritis
Age at which the condition starts	It may begin any time in life.	It usually begins later in life.
Speed of onset	Relatively rapid, over weeks to months	Slow, over years
Joint symptoms	Joints are painful, often swollen, and stiff.	Joints ache and may be tender but have little or no swelling.
Pattern of joints that are affected	It often affects small and large joints on both sides of the body (symmetrical), such as both hands, both wrists or elbows, or the balls of both feet.	Symptoms often begin on one side of the body and may spread to the other side. Symptoms begin gradually and are often limited to one set of joints, usually the finger joints closest to the fingernails or the thumbs, large weight-bearing joints (hips, knees), or the spine.
Duration of morning stiffness	Morning stiffness generally lasts longer than one hour.	Morning stiffness often lasts less than one hour. Stiffness returns at the end of the day or after periods of activity.
Presence of symptoms affecting the whole body (systemic)	Frequent fatigue and a general feeling of being ill are present.	Whole-body symptoms are not present.

Osteoarthritis involves the wearing away of the cartilage that caps the bones in your joints. With rheumatoid arthritis, the synovial membrane that protects and contributes to the lubrication of joints becomes inflamed, causing pain and swelling. Joint erosion may then follow.

Table 7 shows a very general set of differences between the two and will help you better communicate your issues for your healthcare provider.

WHAT YOU CAN DO FOR ARTHRITIS

First, see your healthcare provider. Make sure he or she listens and explains everything to your understanding and satisfaction. Write what you discuss down or use a recording device (of course you should ask first) to assure that you can refer to his or her instructions. Ask if other specialists should be consulted. This could include physical therapists as well as exercise consultants that have training in and awareness of arthritic conditions.

In your daily life, do what you can to minimize stress on your joints. Instead of lifting a heavy pot, maybe slide it across the counter. Use a shoulder to open a door rather than your hand and hold books in the palm of your hands, not with your fingers. You get the idea.

Applying heat to an area with a heating pad or chilling out with an ice pack or ice water can also soothe your joints and muscles. Alternating hot packs with cold ones can also offer powerful relief for some, but, as with exercise, don't overdo it. Talk to your healthcare provider about how to use heat and cold safely. Several studies suggest that people with rheumatoid arthritis (RA) may benefit from fish oil supplements, which contain inflammation-fighting omega-3 fatty acids. They're especially valuable to RA patients, who are said to have a higher risk of cardiovascular disease as well. Of course, ask your provider about all this before you act on any of this. Just use the previous passage as a reminder.

Remember what I said earlier about exercise?

Exercise can give you more energy, improve your mood, and, most importantly, keep joint pain at bay—if you have been cleared for it and feel physically capable of working out. Walking, cycling, swimming, and light weight training done three times a week are options, but check with your healthcare provider to make sure those activities are safe. And just like Dirty Harry always says, "Know your limitations."

Don't exercise when joints are painful or inflamed. Listen to your body. Take a break if you start to feel pain and alternate positions periodically when performing tasks such as gardening or cooking or reading a book— any book—this book, for example.

Smoking is a lifestyle factor that is known to increase the risk of RA. It is also associated with more severe symptoms and joint damage in those who have been diagnosed with the condition. Of course, you shouldn't be smoking anyway.

What can you do?

I like yoga. I know what you are thinking: here goes this guy with the yoga again. It's true, though, and I will state emphatically that I have no conflicting interest in the This Can't Be Yoga outlet chain!

Yoga's emphasis on stretching, whole-body well-being, and group involvement makes the practice especially relevant to some arthritis suffer-

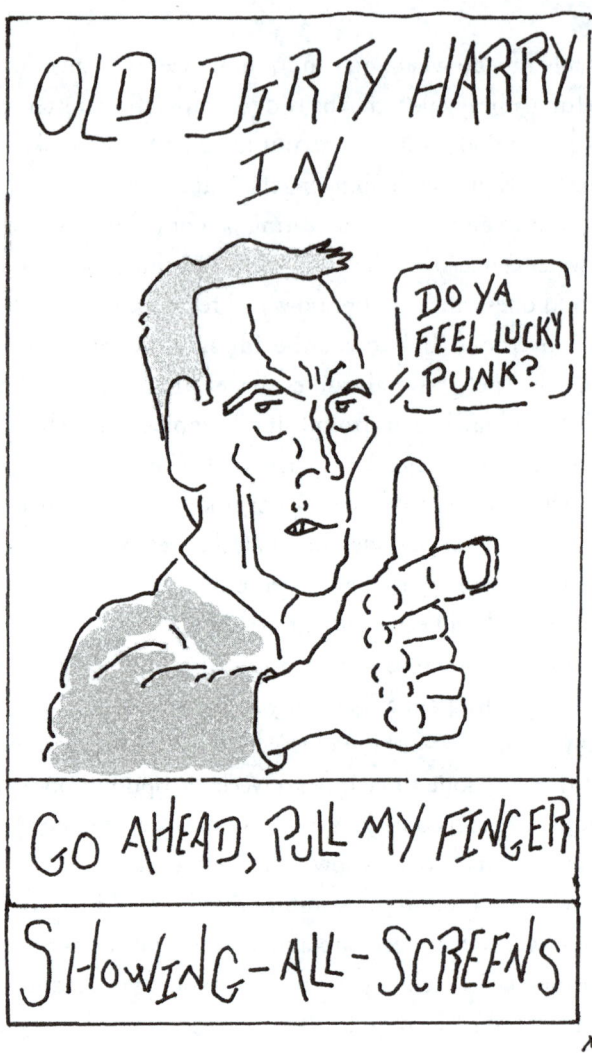

ers. Although the scientific evidence of arthritis-specific benefits is limited, it's still recommended by the Arthritis Foundation. So knock yourself out . . . figuratively.

FUNCTIONING WITH ARTHRITIS, USING ARTHRITIS SPECIFIC TOOLS

Use tools designed for arthritics. There are a bunch of them. In order to do this, you will probably need to get with a physical therapist. As I alluded to earlier, this isn't something medical care providers think about right off the bat, so maybe you can suggest it. If they make the referral, then you'll have justification for your insurance coverage paying for the visit.

Use enlarged handles for food prep to minimize pinch points and flexion. Use cutting boards with nail pegs and raised ledges that help reduce force requirements and secure food during meal preparation. If you're faced with a stubborn jar lid or bottle cap, there are many different types of opening devices that can reduce the amount of stress placed on your hand joints. For cans, use an electric can opener to avoid the finger strain of turning a hand-held model. The same is true for spring-loaded scissors. You might also consider lever enhancements for door latches. There are enlarged handle adjusters for toothbrushes and eating utensils, requiring less stress of your fingers and thumb. There are "turning tools" with collapsible metal pins that depress so they can mold around objects such as oven knobs and the ends of car or house keys. Using the large handle on the tool helps avoid the pinching motion required to turn knobs and keys.

Clothing often requires a lot of fine-motor action that stresses the joints. Consider a buttonhook to help you grasp and fasten buttons on your clothes. Choose clothes with easy-to-close fasteners, such as zippers, large buttons, or hooks. And if you miss a button, blame it on the fastener.

Of course, your arthritis can't be blamed for your wearing stripes with plaid. For that, you can blame Einstein! Just checking to see if you really read chapter 4.

Consider altering your body mechanics. When rising from a chair, use your legs and hips to help you stand up. If necessary, push off on the arms of the chair or a nearby table with your palms—not your knuckles. Another option is to place your palms on your thighs or knees to distribute the force as you push off.

Diabetes Mellitus

As we get older, our risk for type 2 diabetes increases. In fact, in the United States about one in four people over the age of 60 has diabetes.

When you eat, your food is broken down into a sugar called glucose.

Glucose gives your body the energy it needs to work. To use glucose as energy, however, your body must also make insulin, which "unlocks" your cells so they can receive the glucose they need. When you have type 2 diabetes, your body does not use insulin well and may not make enough, either. This means your cells can't use the glucose as energy. The glucose stays in your blood, and that can create problems. Having high blood glucose can cause problems like eye, kidney, nerve, and foot disorders. People with diabetes are also at higher risk for high blood pressure, heart disease and stroke, and other serious conditions.

There is no cure for diabetes, but it can be managed. Balancing the food you eat with exercise and medicine (if prescribed) will help keep your blood glucose in the healthy range. If you'd like to read more, the following site is pretty good: http://main.diabetes.org/dorg/PDFs/living-with-diabetes/living-healthy-with-diabetes-guide.pdf.

Incontinence

Mark Twain is supposed to have said, "One of life's most over-valued pleasures is sexual intercourse, while one of life's least appreciated pleasures is defecation." I think we all just learned a whole lot about old Mark Twain.

I have a patient that likes to say, "Pooping is a celebration of life." Frankly, I prefer Bastille Day, but that's me.

When it comes to your body's elimination of waste, urine or feces, there is one universal truth. You want to go when you want to go and not a second sooner. In a similar thread, not being able to go can be just as unpleasant as going when you don't want to. So let's start with constipation!

In fact, it can be a pain!

CONSTIPATION

Constipation is generally defined as having less than three bowel movements a week, typically with a hard, dry stool that is painful to pass. Which reminds me of a joke. Want to know the definition of an anesthesiologist? It's a doctor that passes gas on a hard stool all day!

In all seriousness, constipation is no laughing matter. If it progresses,

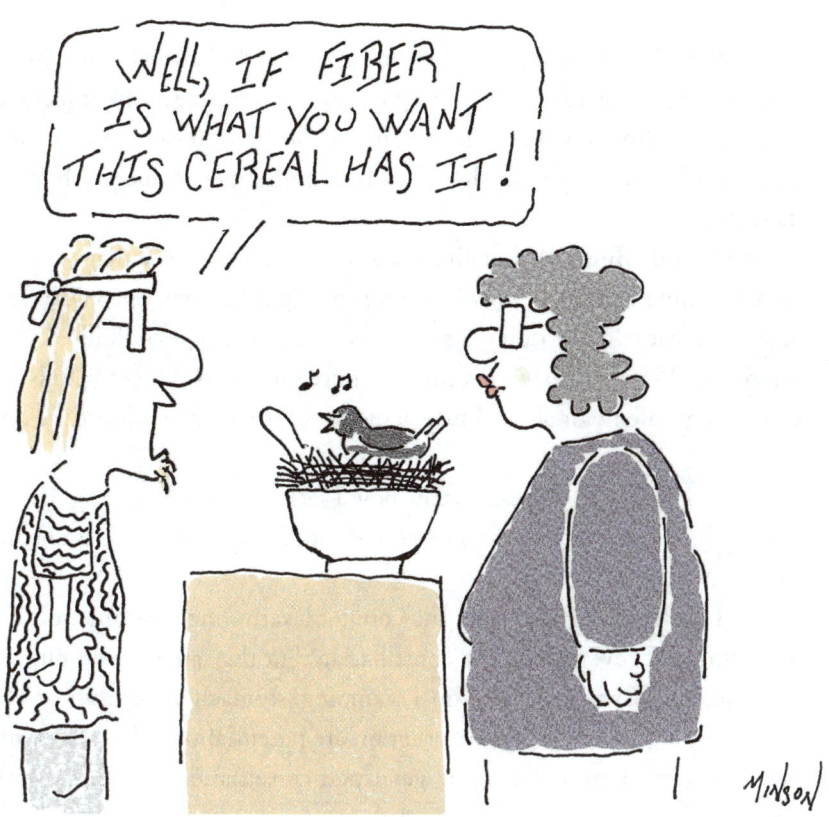

it can lead to a condition known as an impaction, which requires medical care to prevent a life-threatening outcome. It can also be a sign of a more serious condition, such as irritable bowel syndrome, endocrine system problems, cancers, and diseases of the central nervous system. These conditions can be deadly, so it is best to rule out these more critical causes of constipation when possible.

As always, if you are experiencing constipation, first consult your healthcare provider. Once you have done that, here are some options that may be able to prevent the problem and provide some additional relief:

Eat more fiber. I touched on this earlier, but if it's true that you can't get enough fiber, then I can't write enough about it. Eating fiber helps prevent and relieve constipation. There are two different types of fiber: soluble fiber, which helps to soften fecal material, and insoluble fiber, which adds bulk to the stool to help it move through the bowels more quickly. Yee haw! Now you have a plan for your weekend!

Foods that are a good source of soluble fiber include fruits, vegetables, and legumes, while foods that are a good source of insoluble fiber include wheat bran (also known as miller's bran), whole-grain breads, and whole-grain cereals. Ideally, people should include both types of fiber in their daily diets.

Drink more fluids. Although there is no clinical evidence that increased fluid consumption will relieve constipation, many people have reported great relief by doing just that. However, the type of fluid is important. Water and 100 percent fruit juices are good choices. Fluids containing caffeine or alcohol may actually eventually make constipation worse.

Exercise more. You already know how I feel about exercise. Regular exercise has many benefits, and improved motility of the bowels is one of them.

Use laxatives carefully. Over-the-counter laxative medications are sometimes effective at relieving constipation, but they are not without side effects. Bloating, gas, intestinal cramping, stomach discomfort or pain, faintness, thirst, or throat irritation are potential side effects of some over-the-counter laxatives. Again, get expert consultation before you start using these.

Some Risks

Prolonged use of laxatives may also cause an electrolyte imbalance. Oral laxatives can interfere with the body's absorption of certain medications or nutrients. Therefore, while specific side effects of laxatives will vary depending on the person, those considering the use of laxatives should understand these side effects before using them. In addition, some people should avoid laxative use completely. Remember, talk to your healthcare provider and do it REGULARLY. Get it?

FECAL INCONTINENCE

This encompasses a whole host of conditions that amount to an inability to control your bowel movements, causing stool to leak from the rectum. This can be an occasional leak (no biggie, yeah, right) to passing gas uncontrollably (think every long-distance trip with your least favorite uncle) to complete and total loss of bowel control or, as LBJ liked to call it, the nuclear option. I'm lying, actually. He didn't call it that, I don't think.

Causes of fecal incontinence can range from infectious diarrhea like Montezuma's Revenge to structural and nerve damage to the occasional Alfred Hitchcock movie. Regardless, it is always embarrassing and unpleasant. If you are having a problem with this, go see your healthcare provider. Maybe take the high-speed lane.

URINARY INCONTINENCE

This includes a bunch of problems and is worth considering with the specific definitions in mind.

- First there is stress incontinence, also known as effort incontinence. This is due essentially to insufficient strength of the pelvic floor muscles to prevent the passage of urine, especially during activities that increase intra-abdominal pressure, such as coughing, sneezing, or bearing down.
- Urge incontinence is the involuntary loss of urine that occurs for no apparent reason while suddenly feeling the need or urge to urinate.
- Overflow incontinence is a situation in which people find that they cannot stop their bladders from constantly dribbling or continuing to dribble for some time after they have passed urine. It is as if their bladders were constantly overflowing, hence the general name overflow incontinence.
- Mixed incontinence is not uncommon in the elderly female population and can sometimes be complicated by urinary retention, which makes it a treatment challenge requiring staged multimodal treatment. Think a bladder-oriented version of Operation Overlord.
- Structural incontinence is rare. Structural problems are usually diagnosed in childhood (for example, an ectopic ureter). It can also include fistulas caused by obstetric and gynecologic trauma or injury are commonly known as obstetric fistulas and

can lead to incontinence. These types of vaginal fistulas include, most commonly, vesicovaginal fistula (from the bladder to the vagina). These may also be really difficult to diagnose. Often it involves some pretty intense testing like a vaginogram. Now, I am sorry, but that has always sounded like a messenger service that would have probably had people really polarized. I mean, there are telegrams, candygrams . . . just imaging how a delivery person could keep a straight face. Vaginograms can also involve radiologically viewing the vaginal vault with instillation of contrast media or "radio-dye."

- Functional incontinence occurs when a person recognizes the need to urinate but cannot make it to the bathroom. The loss of urine may be large. There are several causes of functional incontinence, including confusion, dementia, poor eyesight, reduced mobility or dexterity, unwillingness to toilet because of depression or anxiety, or inebriation due to alcohol. Functional incontinence can also occur in certain circumstances where no biological or medical problem is present. For example, a person may recognize the need to urinate but may be in a situation where there is no toilet nearby or access to a toilet is restricted.

- Nocturnal enuresis is episodic urinary incontinence while asleep. It is common in young children but can occur in seniors.

- Transient incontinence a temporary version of incontinence. It can be triggered by medications, adrenal insufficiency, mental impairment, restricted mobility, and stool impaction (severe constipation), which can push against the urinary tract and obstruct outflow.

- Giggle incontinence is an involuntary response to laughter. Don't blame this book!

- Double incontinence sounds a lot like a Barbara Stanwyck movie to me, but it's not. At least, I have never seen it on AMC. Due to involvement of the same muscle group, the levator ani— not Lou Reed's old band—in bladder and bowel continence, patients with urinary incontinence are often likely to have some fecal incontinence in addition. This is why it's termed "double incontinence."

- Post-void dribbling is the phenomenon where urine remaining in the urethra after voiding the bladder slowly leaks out after urination.
- Coital incontinence is a type of urinary leakage that occurs during either penetration or orgasm and can be with a sexual partner or with masturbation. It has been reported to occur in 10–24 percent of sexually active women with pelvic floor disorders.
- Additionally, frequent exercise in high-impact activities can cause athletic incontinence to develop. It is usually a component of the deficiency of the pelvic floor.
- Urge incontinence is caused by uninhibited contractions of the detrusor muscle (which squeezes the bladder to expel urine). It is characterized by the leakage of large amounts of urine in association with insufficient warning to get to the bathroom in time.
- Finally, there is also a condition known as polyuria (excessive urine production). The most frequent causes are uncontrolled diabetes mellitus, primary polydipsia (excessive fluid drinking), central diabetes insipidus, and nephrogenic diabetes insipidus. Polyuria generally causes urinary urgency and frequency but doesn't necessarily lead to incontinence

FOR MEN

An enlarged prostate is one of the most common causes of incontinence in men after the age of 40. If you experience incontinence, see your healthcare provider. Sometimes prostate cancer may also be associated with an enlarged prostate. Another common cause of urinary incontinence in men is a side effect of the drugs necessary to treat an enlarged prostate. Additionally, radiation used to treat prostate cancer can also cause incontinence.

WHAT YOU CAN DO

Pelvic floor exercises. Pelvic floor exercises or Kegels are simple to do. You just clench and unclench your pelvic floor muscles. Basically you are using the muscles that stop your urinary stream. Frankly, that just gave me an idea for a new aerobics video. Imagine a bunch of people sitting around in their workout gear. Doing apparently nothing. Then suddenly you hear the sound of walnuts cracking. Maybe I'll save that one for the holiday edition.

Seriously though, I am not suggesting that you do Kegels when you are voiding or urinating. In fact, doing that when you are trying to void can actually damage the musculature. The cool thing is that you can do pelvic floor exercises anywhere and anytime: while online, on hold on the phone, or in the car. Start by clenching your pelvic floor muscles for a slow count of five, then release for a few seconds. Repeat 10 times. As you develop strength over time, aim to hold the muscles for 10 seconds and release for 10. Now let's go for the burn!

Stick to a timetable. Don't feel like you need to urinate? Head to the toilet anyway. Why? Timed urination helps keep the bladder empty. Maybe start off with a schedule that is every two hours.

Fill the void. Don't be in a hurry when you're going. Take your time. Maybe read a book . . . oh, I don't know . . . a book about urinary incon-

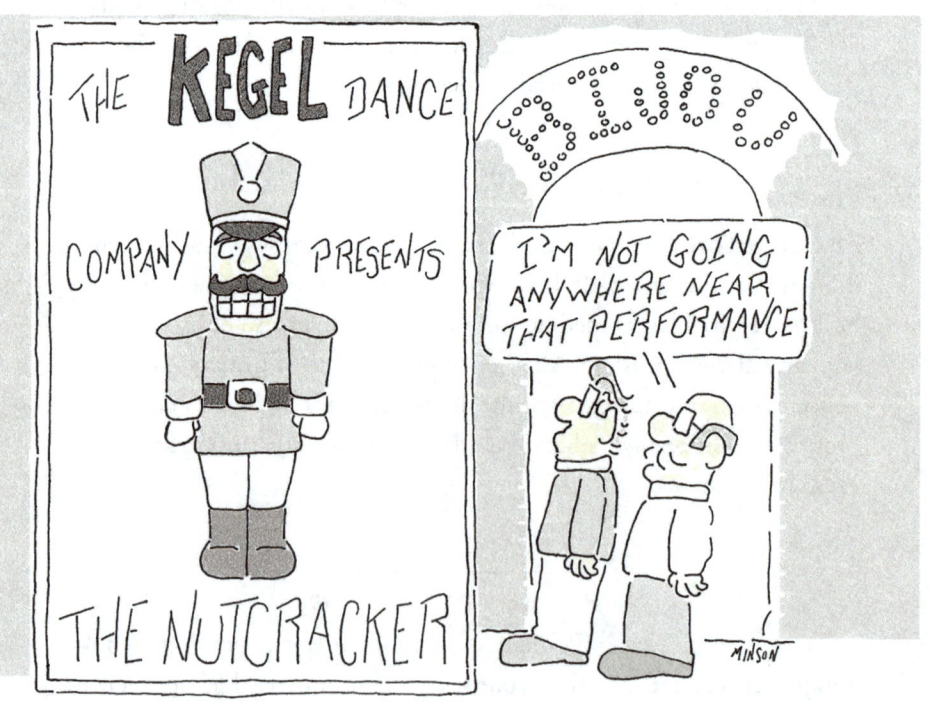

tinence … and senior issues? After you've finished urinating, relax a bit and then urinate again. This practice is called double voiding and helps empty the bladder.

Don't have an accident trying to prevent an accident. Having accidents before you make it to the lavatory? It's time to clear your path of obstacles so you can get there faster. Help yourself once you're there by wearing easy-to-release clothes—think elastic waistbands and Velcro closures. I suddenly had a visual of Clark Kent changing into Superman in a phone booth. Not sure it is the same thing, though.

Go easy with the caffeine and alcohol. To control urinary incontinence, eliminate these diuretics or at least cut back.

Drink up—but not too much. Your body needs fluids, so be sure to drink enough water to stay well hydrated. Refer to the chapter on hydration and you'll be good to go. Get it?

Medication side effects. Speak with your healthcare provider to make sure you're not taking any prescription or over-the-counter medicines that could be making your urinary incontinence worse.

Medication and surgery. Both stress incontinence and urge incontinence can be treated with medication, though bladder training using the tips above is often more effective. Surgery is mainly an option for severe incontinence, though, as with medication, it may not be the most effective initial treatment. This is, for sure, a situation where you want to talk with your healthcare provider.

Hypertension

The Joint Commission released new treatment guideline amendments in 2014 to their treatment guidelines of 2009.

This is one of the most common medical conditions affecting seniors in the United States. It's a fairly insidious problem, too, because it doesn't really warn you that you have a problem until damage is starting to occur. It is a contributing factor to debility, kidney disease, cardiovascular disorders, strokes, dementia, and more.

There are some important ways you can control your blood pressure, some of which I have touched on earlier in the book, but it's worth reminding.

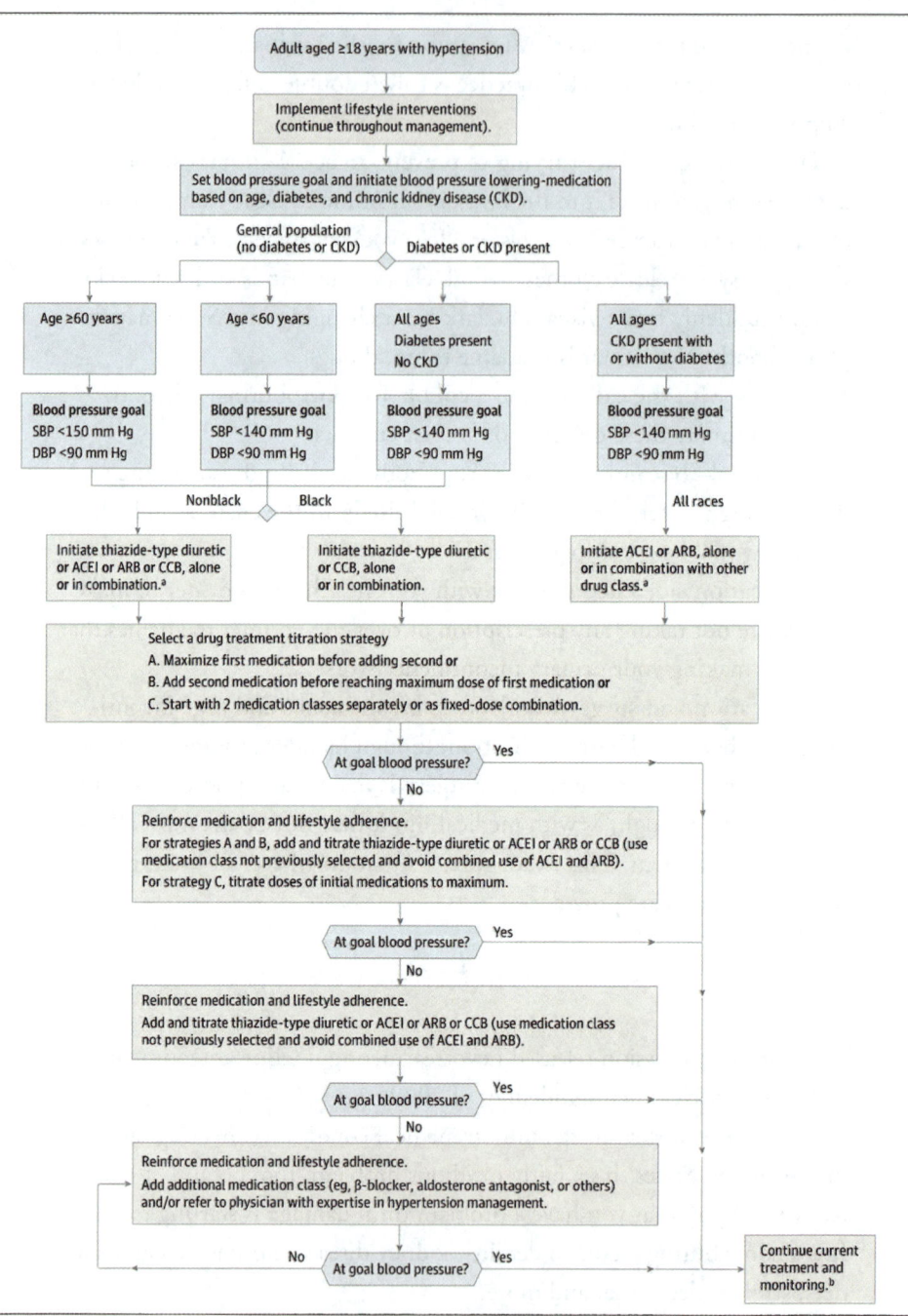

Adult aged ≥18 years with hypertension

Implement lifestyle interventions
(continue throughout management).

Set blood pressure goal and initiate blood pressure lowering-medication
based on age, diabetes, and chronic kidney disease (CKD).

General population
(no diabetes or CKD)

Diabetes or CKD present

Age ≥60 years

Age <60 years

All ages
Diabetes present
No CKD

All ages
CKD present with
or without diabetes

Blood pressure goal
SBP <150 mm Hg
DBP <90 mm Hg

Blood pressure goal
SBP <140 mm Hg
DBP <90 mm Hg

Blood pressure goal
SBP <140 mm Hg
DBP <90 mm Hg

Blood pressure goal
SBP <140 mm Hg
DBP <90 mm Hg

Nonblack   Black

All races

Initiate thiazide-type diuretic
or ACEI or ARB or CCB, alone
or in combination.[a]

Initiate thiazide-type diuretic
or CCB, alone
or in combination.

Initiate ACEI or ARB, alone
or in combination with other
drug class.[a]

Select a drug treatment titration strategy
A. Maximize first medication before adding second or
B. Add second medication before reaching maximum dose of first medication or
C. Start with 2 medication classes separately or as fixed-dose combination.

At goal blood pressure? — Yes

No

Reinforce medication and lifestyle adherence.
For strategies A and B, add and titrate thiazide-type diuretic or ACEI or ARB or CCB (use
medication class not previously selected and avoid combined use of ACEI and ARB).
For strategy C, titrate doses of initial medications to maximum.

At goal blood pressure? — Yes

No

Reinforce medication and lifestyle adherence.
Add and titrate thiazide-type diuretic or ACEI or ARB or CCB (use medication class
not previously selected and avoid combined use of ACEI and ARB).

At goal blood pressure? — Yes

No

Reinforce medication and lifestyle adherence.
Add additional medication class (eg, β-blocker, aldosterone antagonist, or others)
and/or refer to physician with expertise in hypertension management.

No — At goal blood pressure? — Yes

Continue current
treatment and
monitoring.[b]

SBP indicates systolic blood pressure; DBP, diastolic blood pressure; ACEI,
angiotensin-converting enzyme; ARB, angiotensin receptor blocker; and CCB,
calcium channel blocker.

[a] ACEIs and ARBs should not be used in combination.
[b] If blood pressure fails to be maintained at goal, reenter the algorithm where
appropriate based on the current individual therapeutic plan.

WHAT YOU CAN DO

- Eat a better diet. This may include reducing salt. Sodium chloride or table salt is approximately 40 percent sodium. Understanding just how much sodium is in salt is important so you can take measures to control your intake. The amounts that follow are approximations.

  1/4 teaspoon salt = 575 mg sodium
  1/2 teaspoon salt = 1,150 mg sodium
  3/4 teaspoon salt = 1,725 mg sodium
  1 teaspoon salt = 2,300 mg sodium

- Read the ingredients list. Earlier in the book, I mentioned that there is a lot of sodium and salt in processed food. In order to properly calculate your intake of "salt" and sodium, you need to read the ingredients and take those amounts into consideration.
- Enjoy regular physical activity.
- Maintain a healthy weight.
- Manage stress.
- Avoid tobacco.
- Comply with medication prescriptions.
- If you drink, limit alcohol.

Other lifestyle modifications may help reduce your blood pressure without the use of prescription medications, but, as always, talk to your healthcare provider before you plan your strategy. Regardless of whether you have a health issue now or not, adopting a healthy lifestyle is critical for the prevention of high blood pressure and an indispensable part of managing it. Just think of these changes as "lifestyle prescriptions" and make every effort to comply with them.

Whether you have been diagnosed with high blood pressure or are concerned because you have some of the risk factors for the disease, understand this: while there is no real "cure," *high blood pressure is manageable.*

It is estimated that over 20 percent of people with hypertension are unaware of their condition. This symptomless disease could leave them with substantial *health consequences* like I talked about earlier. You don't want to be one of them. If you haven't had a checkup in a year, see your healthcare provider to be tested.

Pain Syndromes

Chronic pain is one of the most common problems experienced by seniors. It can be the result of a number of conditions or a byproduct of incapacity or another comorbidity. Regardless, as with everything else, you should see your healthcare provider. In addition, there are some things you can do.

RELAXATION TECHNIQUES AND MEDITATION

Learn deep breathing or meditation. These techniques help your body relax, which may ease pain. A lot of patients describe the phenomenon of tension and tightness seeping from muscles as their bodies "receive" the message to relax. What we are talking about here is the concept and practice of meditation.

Although there are many ways to meditate, the soothing power of repetition is at the heart of most forms. Focusing on the breath, ignoring negative thoughts, and repeating a word or phrase—a mantra—helps the body to relax. While you can learn meditation on your own, it helps to take a class from a professional. And, yes, saying the word "waffles" over and over is a kind of mantra.

Deep breathing is also a relaxation technique. Find a quiet location, a comfortable body position, and block out distracting thoughts. Then imagine a spot just below your navel. Breathe into that spot, filling your abdomen with air. Let the air fill you from the abdomen up, then let it out, like deflating a balloon.

Reduce stress in your life. Stress intensifies chronic pain. Negative feelings like depression, anxiety, and anger can increase the body's sensitivity to pain. By learning to take control of stress, you may find some relief from chronic pain.

Several techniques can help reduce stress and promote relaxation. Remember the chapter on psychological environment? Well, listening to soothing, calming music can lift your mood and make living with chronic pain more bearable. There are even specially designed relaxation tapes or CDs for this. Mental imagery relaxation (also called guided imagery) is a form of meditation or mental escape that can help you feel peaceful. It involves creating calming, peaceful images in your mind. Progressive muscle relaxation is another technique that promotes relaxation.

EXERCISE

Yes, there's that word again! The fact is that you can boost chronic pain relief with the natural endorphins that are produced with exercise.

Endorphins, as you recall, are brain chemicals that help improve your mood while also blocking pain signals. Exercise has another pain-reducing effect: it strengthens muscles, helping prevent injury and further pain. As always, ask your healthcare provider for an exercise routine that is right for you.

JOIN A SUPPORT GROUP

Meet others living with chronic pain. When you're with people who have chronic pain and understand what you're going through, you feel less alone. You also benefit from their wisdom and experience in coping with the pain. Also consider meeting with a mental health professional. Anyone can develop depression if he or she is living with chronic pain. Getting counseling can help you learn to cope better and help you avoid negative thoughts that make pain worse. Asking for help is a sign of wisdom, not weakness.

DON'T SMOKE

Smoking can worsen chronic pain. It can also worsen painful circulation problems and increase the risk of heart disease and cancer.

TRACK YOUR PAIN

Track your pain level and activities every day. To effectively treat your pain, your care giver needs to know how you've been feeling between visits. Keeping a log or journal of your daily "pain score" will help you keep track. At the end of each day, note your pain level on the pain scale of 1 to 10. Also note what activities you did that day. Take this log book to every healthcare provider visit—to give him or her a good understanding of how you're living with chronic pain and your physical functioning level.

BIOFEEDBACK

Consider biofeedback techniques to decrease migraine and tension headache pain. Through biofeedback, it's possible to consciously control various bodily functions. This may sound like science fiction, but there is good evidence that biofeedback works, and it's not hard to master. Basically, you wear sensors that let you "hear" or "see" certain physical parameters like pulse, digestion, body temperature, and muscle tension. The squiggly lines and/or beeps on the attached monitors reflect what's going on inside your body. Then you learn to control those squiggles and beeps. After a few sessions, your mind has trained your biological system.

MASSAGE

Get a massage for chronic pain relief. Okay, so I wasn't there, but I understand that Aristotle advocated a daily massage. Even if that isn't true, I'm using it. Massage can help reduce stress and relieve tension and is often helpful with all sorts of chronic pain, especially back and neck pain.

So where do you get a massage? Well, it should be somewhere that offers a massage—just a massage.

JELLY DONUTS

Remember the Kennedy story? You are what you do and eat. So eat a healthy diet if you're living with chronic pain. A well-balanced diet is important in many ways. It aids your digestive process, reducing heart disease risk, keeping weight under control, and improving blood sugar levels. To eat a low-fat, low-sodium diet, choose fresh fruits and vegetables, cooked dried beans and peas, whole-grain breads and cereals, low-fat dairy products (cheese, milk, and yogurt), and lean meats.

Get Your Shots

According to the CDC, in January–June 2013, 69 percent of people age 65 and over reported that they had received an influenza vaccination during the past 12 months and 61 percent reported that they had received a pneumococcal vaccination at some point. According to data from the 2012 National Interview Health Survey (NHIS), too few adults are getting their recommended vaccinations (see http://www.cdc.gov/vaccines/adults/index.html).

Why does this matter? Well, every year thousands of adults in the United States still suffer serious health problems, are hospitalized, and even die due to diseases for which vaccines are available.

So what vaccinations do you need? Well, this is a very individualized conversation that needs to occur between you and your healthcare provider. Things that need to be considered include your age, lifestyle (if you are a spelunker or professional rabid bat collector, then maybe rabies is also necessary), whether you have underlying medical conditions like chronic obstructive pulmonary disease (COPD) or emphysema, any immune issues, and more.

Varicella (shingles). This is the chickenpox virus. It is in a class or family of viruses known as herpes viruses. I know what you are thinking, but it's not *that* herpes. Herpes is the term for a big class of viruses.

An estimated 1 million Americans get shingles every year, and about half of them are 60 years old or older. The older a person is, the more severe the effects of shingles typically are, so all adults 60 years old or older should get the shingles vaccine. It is specifically designed to protect people against shingles and will *not* protect people against other forms of herpes, such as genital herpes. The shingles vaccine is *not* recommended to treat active shingles or post-herpetic neuralgia (pain after the rash is gone) once it develops. This is a terrible cause of chronic pain for some, so avoid it by addressing the potential before it occurs.

Even if you have had shingles, you can still receive the shingles vaccine to help prevent future occurrences of the disease. There is no specific time that you must wait after having shingles before receiving the shingles vaccine. The decision on when to get vaccinated should be made with your healthcare provider.

Influenza. For seniors, the seasonal flu can be very serious, even deadly. Ninety percent of flu-related deaths and more than half of flu-related hospitalizations occur in people age 65 and older. In some cases you may have two options for vaccination—the regular-dose flu shot or the higher-dose flu shot designed specifically for people 65 and older. Both vaccines protect against the same combinations of seasonal flu viruses. The higher-dose vaccine should result in a stronger immune response. Again, talk to your healthcare provider about which vaccine is right for you.

Childhood vaccination boosters. Tetanus and Td or Tdap vaccine (tetanus, diphtheria, and pertussis) may be recommended by your practitioner, but should be considered against general health and potential risk.

Hepatitis A and B. This is not generally recommended for seniors, but if you are at risk, your doctor may recommend this.

Meningococcus. This one is now recommended for communal populations like college students or some congregative and nursing home patients.

Pneumococcus. As we get older, our immune systems tend to weaken, putting us at higher risk for certain diseases. According to the CDC, pneumococcal disease, including pneumonia, bacteremia, and bacterial meningitis, is a serious health threat to Americans. Each year, it causes the deaths of approximately 40,000 Americans, most of them over 65 years of age. US Public Health Service data suggest that nearly half of those deaths could be prevented if people 65 and older and others in high-risk groups were given pneumococcal vaccine. Seniors who are 65 and older are two to three times more likely than the general population to get a pneumococcal infection, according to US Department of Health and Human Services.

You will want to discuss this with your practitioner, but for many seniors it is recommended that they get pneumococcal vaccine—which protects against types of pneumonia, meningitis, and blood poisoning—in addition to the flu vaccine.

Pneumococcal diseases can strike at any time of year, but they also can be a deadly complication of the flu. Unlike the flu shot, the polysaccharide vaccine does not need to be administered annually and instead lasts several years. Adults 19 years and older should also get the vaccine if they have heart, lung, or liver problems, HIV, diabetes, asthma, or if they smoke.

Medications

I talk a lot about this in my first book, but there are a few points I want to reiterate here. Medication complications and errors are important, devastating, and completely preventable. They are also, unfortunately, a lot more common in older adults, in part because they are on more medications, a condition known as polypharmacy. Sounds like a really terrible name for a parrot, doesn't it? It is also more common in seniors because those same medications sometimes make them more likely to make a mistake. I have said this before and have insinuated it throughout this book, but it bears repeating at least one more time: *the most important member of your healthcare team is you!*

In order to understand what you can do, you need to know something about the most common forms of medication errors and mistakes experienced or suffered by older patients:

- Incorrect or improper administration (form or concentration) of a medication (i.e., dosage mistakes)
- Taking the wrong medication for a disease or condition
- Taking drugs that are out of date
- Taking drugs at the wrong time or interval
- Taking drugs without considering adverse effects due to drug combinations

Here's what seniors or their family members can and should do:

- Understand the name (and generic name), use, dosage, route of administration, and frequency of each drug, including special instructions such as handling or storage.
- Ask and learn about potential side effects and whether the drug will interact with other prescription drugs, over-the-counter medications, or supplements.

- Question the pharmacist if the bottle looks strange or contains names and dosages that seem different from what they have been told.
- Ask doctors and nurses in medical facilities which drugs are being given and what they are designed to treat.

The key to reducing medication errors is to ask questions when something isn't clear or doesn't seem right.

One more thing. Before you start a new medication, make sure you ask the right questions. I have created a tool for you that will help with that (see table 8). For safety's sake, you might also go over your doctor's answers with the pharmacist when you are getting the prescription filled.

KNOW YOUR PHARMACIST

In my first book I dedicate a great deal of discussion to the importance of the pharmacist as a key member of your medical care team. I'll reiterate that here. These professionals are very likely to be the member of the team you see most frequently. As such, they are incredibly important to you in preventing harmful medical interactions and mistakes, and they serve as a great resource for reducing your costs while maintaining the integrity of your care.

Often they understand the kinetics (bodily absorption, distribution, metabolism, and excretion of drugs) and dynamics (the course of action, effect, and breakdown) of the drug in the body better than anyone. This

Table 8. Checklist of Questions to Ask Your Doctor about New Medications

	Yes	No
Will this interact with what I am already taking?		
How long will it take for the effects to be felt?		
What side effects should I watch for that will indicate a problem?		
If I experience a problem, should I abruptly stop the medication or will that create a problem?		
How can I reach you (provider) during off hours if I experience a problem?		
Are there are any foods that I should avoid?		

is way oversimplified, but kinetics refers to the movement of the drug into and through the body, and dynamics refers to the mechanism of the drug's action on the targeted area of the body. For example, aspirin is chewed and then absorbed through the mucosa and gastrointestinal tract, courses through the bloodstream, and is eliminated by breakdown and excretion by the liver and then the kidneys. That's the kinetics. The dynamics refers to how it binds and works on the cells to impact pain or to "thin" the blood and reduce clotting. Your pharmacist understands this and can anticipate where drugs may interact or create side effects of conditions you will definitely need to know about.

So get to know your pharmacist and talk with him or her just as you would your clinical healthcare provider.

PRESCRIPTION TERMS

Here are some terms you might encounter:

Off-label and approved use. According to the US Food and Drug Administration (FDA), "off-label" use for prescription drugs, biologics, and approved medical devices means any use that is not specified in the labeling approved by the FDA. For cleared medical devices, "off-label" means any use that is not included in the cleared "indications for use." Labeling is considered any written material that accompanies, supplements, or explains the product.

Good medical practice and the best interests of the patient require that physicians use legally available drugs, biologics, and devices according to their best knowledge and judgment. If physicians use a product for an indication not in the approved labeling, they have the responsibility to be well informed about the product, to base its use on firm scientific rationale and on sound medical evidence, and to maintain records of the product's use and effects. Use of a marketed product in this manner, *when the intent is the "practice of medicine,"* does not require the submission of an Investigational New Drug Application (IND), Investigational Device Exemption (IDE), or review by an Institutional Review Board (IRB) according to the FDA. However, the institution at which the product will be used may, under its own authority, require IRB review or other institutional oversight. Your provider is required to explain that to you.

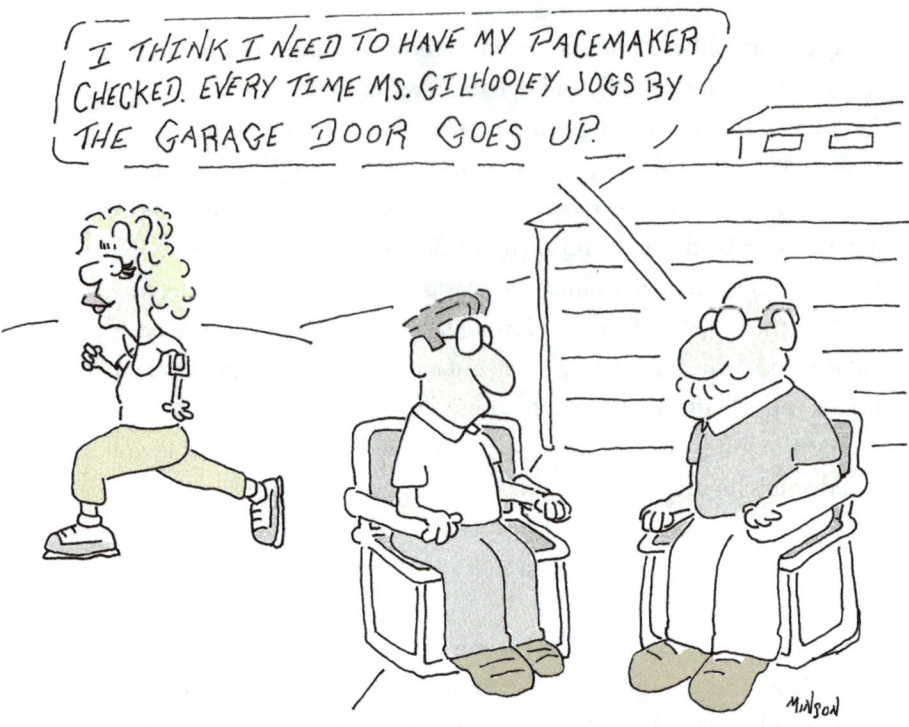

Pill splitting. Recently there has been a lot of discussion in the media and among senior advocacy groups about the practice of pill splitting. In the most basic medical consideration of "Do no harm," I have to say that this is not a recommended practice for everyone. In fact, the FDA considers it a "risky practice" and does not encourage it unless the package insert specifically states it has been approved for splitting. If it does, however, and your doctor or healthcare provider feels you may be a good candidate for this, then there are some things you will want to keep in mind.

First, get clear instruction from your healthcare provider and pharmacist. Make sure you are completely clear about why you are taking the medication and how you should take it. Ask how likely it is to help. Ask if there are any risks.

Know why and how to split the pill. This is often a meticulous and technically difficult procedure. Always use a pill splitter. Do not use a knife! Ask your provider to write a prescription for a pill cutter. That way, your insurance policy or Medicare may cover this. Regardless, you will need the directive and a prescription from your healthcare provider.

Ask your doctor or pharmacist to instruct you. Practice in front of him or her. Make sure you are proficient. If you have doubts or aren't sure, don't do it and communicate that to your caregiver.

Do *not* split medications in advance. The break in the coating for some medications can cause the compound to degrade and render it ineffective or harmful if exposed to air for a period of time.

One more thing...

Access to health care is one of the greatest challenges to seniors. This is due in part to issues of mobility, transportation, financial resources, and a lack of awareness. As with the theme of every other aspect of this book, you can do a lot to facilitate this. Get online. That is where everything is communicated nowadays. If you don't, you are only hurting yourself. Drug recalls, health warnings, outbreaks, and special care issues are almost universally communicated online. The rapid changes associated with health care, including legislation, rules, and trending issues, are all available with a simple click of a mouse. With respect to the physical environment chapter and the idea of rodent abatement, you know I am not talking about the leptospirosis- and plague-carrying variety.

When you consider access to care, the old adage of "knowledge is power" applies now more than ever.

In the next section, "Liberty," I will cover free programs and cost-reducing subsidies that seniors may be able to use to get many of these necessary services and materials along with some helpful material about how you can make ends meet even more effectively.

So stay tumed.

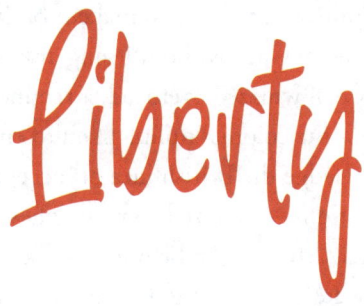

*"Old age is like everything else. To make a
success of it, you've got to start young."*

Theodore Roosevelt

Here's a little story about what one early American thought about his personal liberty.

April 19, 1775.

As strategic retreats went, this one was bad. First, the British had lost the element of surprise. By the time Lieutenant Colonel Francis Smith's command of light infantry and grenadiers had slogged out of the freezing salt marsh onto the road between Boston and Lexington, the minutemen were already gathering in the warmth of the town's tavern and making plans. By the time the British arrived in the town, the colonial stores of cannon powder and shot were not where they had been told. Even as the soldiers searched, the militia had gathered and launched the pitched battle that had gone horribly wrong for the king's troops.

The British strategy had expected to strike quickly, before the colonials even knew they were coming, and to commandeer and destroy their supplies and ability to mount any further armed insurrection. For that reason the British command had decided to carry less ammunition and move like lightning into the town and withdraw before there was any chance of a fight. If it had gone right, Smith and his men would already be back in Boston celebrating. But the secret of their plans had been leaked, and the surprise was on them instead.

Now, all Colonel Smith wanted was to make it back to the safety of the British army under General Gage without losing any more men.

Suddenly, a musket ball whizzed overhead, a reminder of the unorthodox and effective tactics the colonial militia liked to employ. It wasn't just that they didn't acknowledge the British idea of "acceptable" Napoleonic mass-and-march formations of civilized combat. They had also fought in a diffuse, unconventional fashion from behind cover and in smaller, highly organized bands that were not nearly as amateurish as the British command had anticipated. It was enough of a distraction for the exhausted troops that they were not focused on a low stone wall of a nearby farm.

They should have been.

For behind the wall was an 80-year-old farmer, Samuel Whittemore. He was in his field earlier that morning when he saw Smith's company moving toward Lexington. The presence of troops wasn't all that unusual. He had seen British patrols before. When he had seen other reinforcements moving along the road, however, his educated eye told him something serious was going on. You see, Samuel Whittemore was no ordinary farmer. He was a decorated former soldier in His Majesty's army. When he realized what was happening, he had gone into this house, pulled a brace of dueling pistols—a prize of one of his last campaigns, in which he briefly described the previous owner as having "died suddenly"—and a French officer's sword whose past owner also "died suddenly," according to Whittemore. Then, he shoved the weapons in his belt and grabbed his rifle from over the mantle and snatched a powder horn and box of musket balls before heading out to his spot behind the wall.

His neighbors, who had also arrived armed and ready, warned against a position so dangerously close to where the armed regulars would pass by. It might have had to do with their concerns about being too near a counteroffensive by the grenadiers, specialized soldiers, notoriously dangerous, skilled in the use of ordnance, and specifically chosen for their large size and strength. Unfortunately for them, Whittemore was an aggressive fighter and preferred a position where his offensive would be assured of effective range rather than providing a safer option for retreat.

Now primed and loaded, he waited until he heard the sound of jangling tack and the trudge of heavy footsteps. A second later he rose and aimed his rifle. The grenadier in his sights disappeared momentarily in an explosion of black powder. As it cleared, the huge man lay dying in the road. Whittemore did not consider that act for long. This was war, after all, and he was already pulling the dueling pistols from his belt.

As one erupted in a plume of expended smoke and a second grenadier fell, the other spat its lethal carriage into a third soldier, who dropped to his knees. Within minutes that man would be dead as well.

By the time the smoke of Whittemore's third shot cleared, the British detachment had countercharged and was overrunning his position. Without the time to reload, Whittemore drew his sword and prepared to parry the British bayonets.

The large men were on him too quickly, however, and a second later the barrel of a Brown Bessie fired mere inches from his face, destroying his right cheek in a fount of blood and bone. Stunned, the old warrior staggered backward, swinging his sword furiously. From the safer cover positions, his neighbors saw him go down as the grenadiers bayoneted his body 13 times. The other farmers opened up, and the British, realizing that retreat was the better option, fell back to the protection of a grove of mulberry trees beside the road where they could head back toward their lines in relative safety.

Eventually, Whittemore's neighbors moved down to recover his body. Instead of finding him in a pool of blood, however, they saw that he was alive and trying to load his musket to engage again. Recovering from their surprise, his colleagues ripped a kitchen door off a nearby house and fashioned a makeshift stretcher.

He was taken to Dr. Cotton Tufts of Medford, who perceived no hope for his survival. Whittemore's family beseeched the doctor to at least dress his wounds so he could be taken home to die in his own bed. Dr. Tufts did his best, and Whittemore was carried off to await the inevitable.

You'd think after all that they might have known better. Stubbornly, Whittemore refused to die and to everyone's surprise actually recovered his full health, though he was terribly disfigured. He went on to live another 18 years, eventually dying of natural causes at the age of 98. Whenever he was asked about the incident, he was reported to always say, "I would do exactly the same thing again."

For his trouble, Whittemore went down in history as the oldest known combatant of the American Revolution.

Why did he do it?

He, along with many others, had tolerated enough of forced billeting of soldiers, suspension of rights, and imposition of monarchical will. In short, he wanted his liberty and he knew he had to secure it.

"Liberty" is a word that is probably dearer to the American psyche than any other and carries with it as many meanings as there are tongues to articulate it. Regardless, I am pretty sure Sam Whittemore had his own definition of liberty, and given what he went through to secure it for the rest of us, I'd be inclined to give him some credence.

Since I cannot ask him, I went to the dictionary, where I found the following: *Liberty*—the state of being free within society from oppressive restrictions imposed by authority on one's way of life, behavior, or political views. A continuation and associated definition reads: the power to act as one pleases.

So what we are talking about is the idea of self-determination, self-control, and autonomy.

That sounds pretty good. It says I can do what I want and nobody can stop me. Of course, that is not completely true, and it is measured to the degree that I can't do things that will surely endanger others. So if you just got that Junior Scientist Home Nuclear Reactor kit, you might want to rethink setting it up.

More Philosopy

The comedian George Carlin, a personal favorite, used to say that our rights were just a matter of opinion. He is correct. As a society, we decide what we all get to enjoy as far as the limits of government, the limits of individual behavior, and the balance between public safety and the common good. The Founding Fathers obviously agreed. They designed the Constitution to be a philosophical instrument that could be altered and adjusted as technology and mankind advanced and as issues they couldn't have imagined needed addressing. They were also smart enough to not make it easy. Constitutional amendments are possible, but they don't come quickly and require substantial will and industry to create and ratify, which is good.

Thomas Jefferson, who is not as funny as George Carlin but certainly worth heeding, is supposed to have said, "Whenever the people are well informed, they can be trusted with their own government."

Noam Chomsky, in his article "A Well-Informed Populace Is Vital to the Operation of a Democracy," said

If America is to have any hope of one day becoming a true democracy, its populace must be better informed. And if this is to happen, the media must do their part by providing citizens with a more balanced, carefully considered view of the issues.

It is a misguided notion that the populace is too busy watching football and soap operas to care about matters of true import, or that the apparent complacency of the citizenry stems from simple apathy. Many Americans read newspapers. And most of these readers are interested in the front page, as well as the sports page. But a complex web of corporate interests, along with a trend toward fewer companies owning more communications holdings, contributes to a narrowing of views expressed in the papers of record.

This is the perfect lead-in to the fundamental point of this part of the book. Stated simply, *your liberty* requires work and attention. If you and I want to keep the freedoms and privileges/rights we enjoy, we need to read, pay attention, and act when necessary. This is true whether it has to do with the institution of a law, minding our own Social Security accounts, budgeting properly, monitoring those that render our home health care, protecting our personal information, and a host of other things. Now is the time to start. So, roll up your sleeves, put on your readers, and let's all get ready to go to work.

CHAPTER 6

FINANCIAL RESOURCES—HEALTH

WHY SEA MONKEYS ARE A BAD LONG-TERM INVESTMENT STRATEGY

In *Prepare to Defend Yourself . . . How to Navigate the Healthcare System & Escape with Your Life* I use the term *caveat emptor*—let the buyer beware—a lot. When we talk about senior issues, it's even more important to be aware and careful. It's a sad fact that predators prey upon the weak. In many cases seniors are often seen as an easy mark because of their social isolation, cognitive issues, and financial vulnerabilities. Sometimes it is because we don't know any better. In some cases it is because we really want to believe what we are hearing. We trust.

I can completely sympathize. When I was 10 years old, I found the most seductive advertisement in the back of a comic book. It showed a little nuclear family of creatures with tiny crowns growing out of their heads. They were called sea monkeys. Now, while I was a fairly voracious reader as a kid and really liked things like nature and science—insert "nerdy" here—despite my extensive reading, I had never even heard of an animal called a sea monkey. I suddenly felt what I am guessing Coronado felt when he was first told about the golden cities of Cibola or Carl Denham's exhilarating excitement when he first heard the rumor of King Kong.

I asked my mother if she had ever heard of the incredible, heretofore unknown species of civilized sea beings. She admitted she hadn't, but instead of sharing my enthusiasm at the potential of a new frontier in biology, she simply admonished me that I didn't need another pet that *she* would end up having to tend. I tried explaining that they didn't seem to be pets so much as some kind of wonderful aquatic peer. She relented with a remarkable lack of the optimism, and two to six weeks later a package arrived that I was certain would win her over in wonderment.

I opened the box with almost giddy anticipation. Inside was a sea of Styrofoam pellets. I pawed through them and lifted out a small envelope that seemed a little too small for something as remarkable as a whole civilization. That concerned me, sure, but I wasn't yet ready to give up on the impending miracle of discovery and studied the instructions on the packet. Apparently reanimation was a mere 20 minutes and a quart of warm water away. I followed the instructions and carefully measured the temperature of the water that I poured into a wide-bottomed bowl.

They would need that for the development of their society, I guessed.

Then with a Wright brothers sense of imminent exhilaration I opened and poured the contents into the water. It layered out in a sad gray film that could only be described as "scum."

I waited.

An hour later the scum had sunk and formed a sediment across the bottom of the container. Thirty minutes later my mother walked by my room and asked, "So how are things going, Dr. Cousteau?"

Seeing the disappointment, she hesitated and took pity on me. She came into the room and leaned over the fishbowl. A sharp odor of ammonia caused her to draw back instantly. Then she picked up the envelope. In tiny lettering, she read the ingredients.

Brine shrimp.

They weren't just brine shrimp. They were *dead* brine shrimp.

Later, as I scrubbed the fishbowl in the bathroom, the corollary to Coronado and Denham became complete. Denham destroyed half of New York and ended up with a King Kong–sized cleanup problem, and Coronado went broke and was charged with war crimes. Comparatively, I had gotten off lightly.

I also learned the fundamental lesson of this part of the book. Caveat Emptor.

Maybe.

Now, if that is the first principle of self-protection, then the second may well be that before you buy, know what you really need. As the last chapter addressed the idea of the access to health care and the most common issues affecting senior health, we also need to examine what all that will take. Arguably that is a combination of knowing where to go and to whom, but also what resources you may require to get there.

It's a quid pro quo society we live in, so let's quickly examine the way most seniors pay for their care and some resources for prevention, maintenance, and what you can do.

The Facts

According to a statistical analysis by Health and Human Services in 2013, the median income of older persons in 2012 was $27,612 for males and $16,040 for females. Interestingly, median income (after adjusting for inflation) of all households headed by older people rose by 0.1 percent (not statistically significant) from 2011 to 2012. Households containing families headed by persons 65 and older reported a median income in 2012 of $48,957.

The major sources of income as reported by older persons in 2011 were Social Security (reported by 86 percent of older persons), income from assets (reported by 52 percent), private pensions (reported by 27 percent), government employee pensions (reported by 15 percent), and earnings (reported by 28 percent).

According the Gerontology Institute and the National Council on Aging (NCOA), the average senior in good health needs to spend about $381 per month to cover basic health needs. This includes Medicare premiums, supplemental coverage, copays, and out-of-pocket costs. This figure increases to $511 per month for a senior in poor health.

What is the point?

This chapter is about anticipating and preventing fiscal problems or addressing the financial resource question and maximizing how you access your care once you have gotten past the fiscal gatekeepers.

Going back to the Founding Fathers, I'll let Ben Franklin say it in the most economic of terms: "An ounce of prevention is worth a pound of cure."

If you require less corrective care, it costs less. If you maintain your health, you have less of a corrective requirement.

Considering that for most of his life, Franklin generally paid his debts in English currency, the term "pound" has a dual meaning.

So let's look at some financial resources for supporting your health care.

Resources for Health Care

Now, I will start off by saying this is by no means meant to be some kind of comprehensive breakdown of healthcare financial accounting. It's an overview and has some basic recommendations. It should be used as a starting point only. In fact, I am probably the last person on the planet to give any kind of financial advice—and I can back that up with a quick look at my bank balance. That said, here are the basics regarding how most seniors pay as well as some recent developments in insurance and care for the uninsured.

MEDICARE

It is impossible to talk about this subject without acknowledging—with respect to Bob Dylan—that the times they are a-changing. Healthcare choice is becoming a bigger and potentially riskier factor in the lives of preretirees as the Patient Protection and Affordable Care Act (ACA)—also variably known as Obamacare—brings significant change to employer-sponsored and individually purchased health plans. Though a separate federal health insurance system with no connection to the ACA or its online marketplaces, Medicare is also going through its own evolution in terms of plan offerings and customer access. For some people both of these programs are critical for their coverage.

Medicare is a government-provided health and hospitalization insurance program for people 65 and older and for some people under the age of 65 with qualifying disabilities or particular forms of illness.

Though you've likely paid taxes into the Medicare system your entire career, Medicare isn't a completely free program. You'll still have to pay premiums, deducted from your Social Security checks, for some portions of your Medicare benefits. There may also be copays and deductibles for certain services.

If you have health issues already, it's a good idea to investigate coverage based on the services you're likely to need over time. One benefit of the ACA is the prohibition of health insurance based on previous conditions. Also, as of January 2013, an additional 0.9 percent tax is assessed on individuals whose incomes exceed certain thresholds: $250,000 when married and filing jointly, $200,000 for single filers.

When to Apply

Most people apply for Medicare through their nearest Social Security office up to three months before their 65th birthday. If you wait longer than three months after your 65th birthday to apply, you may face a late-enrollment penalty. If you are already drawing Social Security benefits at age 65, you'll generally be enrolled in Medicare.

Medicare Plans

Exploring Medicare particulars can be challenging, but it doesn't have to be. Keep in mind that you can get many current answers to Medicare questions online or in person at your nearest Social Security office. But as of late 2014, here's an overview of current Medicare plans:

Parts A (Hospital) and B (Outpatient). Part A covers inpatient hospital care, and Part B covers outpatient medical care and procedures. Parts A and B are often referred to as "Original Medicare" or "Traditional Medicare"; if you choose to take this option, you'll sign up for them as a pair. You'll get to go to any doctor, hospital, or facility that's enrolled in Medicare and accepting new Medicare patients. You'll end up paying a premium for Part B, which can change from year to year, while Part A is usually free for most people. In short, hospital care is just what it sounds like. It is care rendered when you are *admitted* and treated at the hospital. Outpatient care is clinic-based and considered extramural (to the hospital) care or what you receive in your healthcare provider's office.

Part C (Medicare Advantage). Call this one-stop shopping for your hospital, outpatient (Part A and B), and usually your prescription coverage (see Part D, below). Medicare Advantage policies are *sold by private insurers*. Medicare pays a part of the fee, but you have to pay a premium. This coverage may include differing assortments of services, such as vision, certain prescription drugs or devices, dental, or hearing. Keep in mind that different Medicare Advantage plans have different rules for services and can charge different out-of-network costs.

Part D (prescription drug coverage). Part D adds prescription drug coverage to "Original Medicare" but, as mentioned, may be folded into Medicare Advantage coverage if you elect to take it.

The Dreaded Medigap

What's "Medigap" insurance? If you go with "Original Medicare" (Part A), you'll potentially find some gaps in your Medicare coverage. Medigap insurance is the nickname for Medicare Supplement Insurance, which you purchase privately. Some employers and unions offer Medigap coverage to their retirees, and these plans can vary widely in terms of cost, coverage, and state participation. If you're on Medicare Advantage, it's unlikely you'll need separate Medigap coverage, but it's important to check. Remember the sea monkeys? Read the fine print!

In some cases individuals may want to keep working with their company health benefits after they turn 65. Confer with your financial advisor, human resources department, and Medicare before you make any decisions, but you may qualify for a special enrollment period as a result. You'll need to coordinate with your spouse as well if you share any kind of health coverage as part of coordinating your overall retirement picture. People who continue to work past 65 may also enroll in Part A but bypass Parts B and D if they're already on a company plan.

Who Is Covered?

Now, here is a really critical question you must explore. Are your doctors on your plan? You've probably have some experience with this from checking to see whether your physicians are in-network with whatever health insurance you currently carry. You'll continue to do this on Medicare Advantage. Check availability of doctors and costs on any plan you're considering, particularly out-of-network costs.

Now, please realize that what I am about to say is pretty basic, but the total amount a Medicare covered senior may have to pay is really based on the following:

- The type of care required (in hospital, surgery versus medicine, etc.)
- The type of Medicare coverage
- Whether your physician agrees to charge only the amount that Medicare is willing to reimburse
- Whether you have supplemental insurance as well

One-Stop Shopping

This is an area where a lot of seniors are finding real concerns. The requirements and reimbursements for Medicare are at times onerous for healthcare providers. This is also a fairly dynamic time, with the estimated number of physician providers who are willing to contend with the Medicare requirements dropping. Additionally, Medicare Advantage, which is privately provided, is making changes that could affect whether your provider is still available to you.

The reason? Well, part of it is due to federal funding to Medicare Advantage being pared back by billions of dollars as part of the coming years' cost-containment strategies under the ACA. There are also many other changes coming in the next few years. They are changes you will want to know about and act on. Here are just a few that take effect soon:

- You can get a "Welcome to Medicare" preventative visit *once* while on Medicare. This visit (Medicare billing code G0438) must occur within 12 months of the start of your Medicare Part B coverage. You pay nothing if your doctor accepts assignment.
- An annual "Wellness Visit" is covered once every 12 months *after* the "Welcome to Medicare Visit" has taken place (you don't have to have had Welcome Visit to qualify). Ask for it by name or by the Medicare billing code: G0439.
- There is no deductible or copay for 23 preventive services rated "A" or "B" by the US Preventive Services Taskforce of the ACA.

This is not completely good. In fact it can be quite bad, sea monkey bad. So read the fine print. Talk with your healthcare provider and be prepared to act.

Medicare oversimplified:

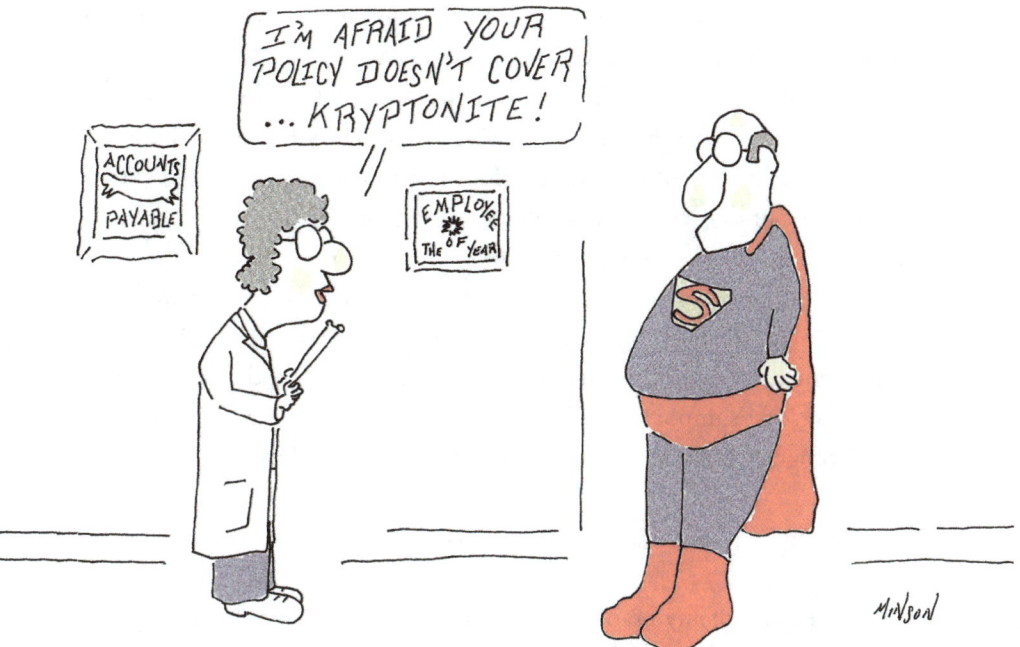

- Part A, which is free for most people, helps cover hospitalization, care in a skilled nursing facility, hospice care, and some home health care.
- Part B, which costs about $100 a month, covers outpatient services such as doctor visits, lab tests, preventive care, some surgeries, clinical trials, mental health care, and durable medical equipment and supplies.
- Part C, also known as Medicare Advantage, varies in cost and allows individuals to enroll in Medicare health plans sold by private insurance companies that contract with Medicare.
- Part D helps cover prescription drug costs.

MEDICAID

Medicaid is a health insurance program run by individual states and partially funded by the federal government. It is the insurance of last resort for many low-income individuals, including seniors. It also has a great deal of variability depending on where you live and your state's laws.

In order to qualify for Medicaid benefits, an eligible senior must have "spent down" most of his or her available assets. Once the financial floor has been reached, Medicaid will pay for most of the costs associated with many types of long-term health care, including nursing home care, skilled care services at home, and hospice care.

As I mentioned earlier, some seniors who qualify for Medicaid are referred to as "dual eligible" because they may also be covered by Medicare. Remember, Medicaid rules vary from state to state and often can be complex, so it is important for low-income seniors to investigate how their state's program works and how to qualify for those benefits.

VETERANS ADMINISTRATION

Senior veterans of any branch of the armed forces who were honorably discharged may qualify for health benefits sponsored by the Veterans Administration (VA). The VA's healthcare system covers all veterans, regardless of age, who have served at least two years of continuous active duty, have a service-related disability, or have served in various theaters of war.

In addition, under the CHAMPVA program (Civilian Health and Medical Program of the Department of Veterans Affairs), eligible beneficiaries, including senior spouses or widows of certain disabled or deceased veterans, may also receive government-sponsored health insurance.

Currently, there are more than 9.5 million estimated veterans older than 65 who are eligible for both Medicare and VA-sponsored health care. These veterans and their qualified dependents can use their VA benefits to complement coverage under their Medicare policies.

The Department of Defense's (DoD) active Military Health System provides health care under its TRICARE program for active-duty service members and their families as well as military retirees of all uniformed branches who have completed at least 20 years of service.

Eligible, retired military personnel who are enrolled in Medicare Parts A and B can apply for the DoD's TRICARE for Life (TFL) program, which, like private Medigap insurance, pays for certain out-of-pocket medical costs not covered by Medicare Part B.

This is a pretty varied subject and again could be its own book, but I'll try to give an orientation that you can use as a starting point.

When purchasing health insurance, your choices will typically fall into one of these categories:

- *Traditional fee-for-service health insurance plans* are usually the most expensive choice. But they offer you the most flexibility when choosing healthcare providers.
- *Health maintenance organizations (HMOs)* offer lower copayments and cover the costs of more preventative care, but your choice of healthcare providers is limited. The National Committee for Quality Assurance (NCQA), a private, 501(c)(3) not-for-profit organization dedicated to a self-described mission of improving healthcare quality, evaluates and accredits HMOs. You can find out whether one is accredited in your state by calling 1–888–275–7585. You can also get this information as well as report cards on HMOs at the NCQA website (www.ncqa.org).
- *Preferred provider organizations (PPOs)* offer lower copayments like HMOs but give you more flexibility when selecting a provider. A PPO also gives you a list of providers you can choose from.
- *Group policies.* Many consumers have health care coverage from their employer. Others have medical care paid through a government program such as Medicare, Medicaid, or the Veterans Administration. If you have lost your group coverage from an employer as the result of unemployment, death, divorce, or loss of "dependent child" status, you may be able to continue your coverage temporarily under the Consolidated Omnibus Budget Reconciliation Act (COBRA). Sometimes I think Dante probably envisioned a particularly punitive level in the Inferno for the creators of some of these acronyms. You, not the employer, pay for this coverage. When one of these events occurs, you must be given at least 60 days to decide whether you wish to purchase the coverage.

In case you have been under a rock or on the moon for the last 20 years, you may not know that if you go outside your HMO or PPO network of providers, you may have to pay a portion or all of the costs of doctors visits, medical tests resulting from that visit, radiological evaluations like CT scans or MRIs, and procedures like surgeries. When choosing among different healthcare plans, you'll need to read the fine print and ask lots of questions. Here are some:

- Do I have the right to go to any doctor, hospital, clinic, or pharmacy I choose?
- Are specialists such as eye doctors and dentists covered?
- Does the plan cover special conditions or treatments such as psychiatric care and physical therapy?
- Does the plan cover home care or nursing home care?
- Will the plan cover all medications my physician might prescribe?
- What are the deductibles? Are there any copayments?
- What is the most I will have to pay out of my own pocket to cover expenses?
- If there is a dispute about a bill or service, how is it handled? In some plans, you may be required to have a third party decide how to settle the problem.

APPEALING HEALTH INSURANCE CLAIMS

This is a big deal. I don't want to sound pessimistic or even combative at the outset, but why mislead you, right? You will probably, at some point, have to fight. Remember Sam Whittemore? Imagine him talking with a representative from Medicare or an insurance company when they had denied a legitimate claim? Frankly, I kind of like imagining that. Well, you might think about channeling his spirit a little. Just remember the rules of engagement. No profanity and no succumbing to anger, though you might think they may deserve it. If you do, they win on a technicality.

If your health insurer has denied coverage for medical care you received, you have a right to appeal the claim and ask that the company reverse that decision. You can be your own healthcare advocate.

Here's what you can do:

Step 1: Review your policy and explanation of benefits.

Step 2: Contact your insurer and keep detailed records of your contacts (copies of letters, time and date of conversations).

Step 3: Request documentation from your doctor or employer to support your case.

Step 4: Write a formal complaint letter explaining what care was denied and why you are appealing through use of the company's internal review process.

Step 5: If the internal appeal is not granted through step 4, file a claim with your state's insurance department. You can find state-specific information through the National Association of Insurance Commissioners website (http://naic.org/state_web_map.htm). To seek help from state consumer agencies, visit http://www.usa.gov/directory/stateconsumer/index.shtml. Just click on your state and start searching for the agency you want to contact.

Step 6: Do not lose your temper, no matter what.

BE BOLD AND MIGHTY FORCES WILL COME TO YOUR AID

What can your state do for you? If you find you're not getting answers on specific Medicare subjects from Medicare (http://www.medicare.gov) itself, your employer, your union, your financial advisor, or Social Security, you can query your state to find out if and which agencies participate in the State Health Insurance Assistance Program (SHIP). SHIP is a national program that offers one-on-one counseling and assistance on Medicare to individuals and their families. Information for all 50 states can be found at www.preparetodefendyourself.com and at http://www.usa.gov/directory/stateconsumer/index.shtml.

My Head Is Swimming, and I Haven't Even Been Drinking

So what's the best way to tie all this stuff together? Stop looking at your health, investment, retirement, and tax issues separately. Medicare is a critical piece of the healthcare affordability puzzle, but it's important to consider choices—and potential worst-case scenarios—within the scope of your broader retirement plan. If you've never had a conversation with a financial planner and have five years or more until you plan to retire, find one and have a broad discussion about where you stand on health, retirement, and estate issues. To find a qualified planner in your community, start with solid recommendations from friends and family and consult organizations like the Certified Financial Planner Board of Standards or the Association for Financial Counseling Planning and Education (http://members.afcpe.org/search).

The Bottom Line

Whether you have retired or you plan to retire at 65 or stay in your career as long as possible, it's important to understand Medicare insurance policies, Medicaid in your state, and how they can both work for you.

THINGS YOU CAN DO

Make sure agencies like Social Security and Medicare will communicate with you or someone you want representing you. I could go into this at length, but just know that there are horror stories about loved ones and even subscribers of Medicare and Social Security who find themselves completely shut out from conversations—vital ones—because they have not established the proper numeric credentials with the agency. I'll cover the SSA "representative payee" in the next chapter

Here is what you can do to save your sanity and maybe even someone's life.

As a caregiver, subscriber, or loved one, you will almost certainly reach a time when you will need to talk to someone at Medicare about a bill, an incorrect ID number, or who knows what. If you are relying on the Medical Power of Attorney form your loved one signed, you will be out of luck. This one was a surprise to me, too, but Medicare will not accept a standard Power of Attorney form. Go figure.

If you want to speak with a Medicare representative on behalf of someone else, either on the phone or in person, you will have to have on file a Medicare Authorization to Disclose Personal Health Information form.

One good thing in your favor is that the Internet is making it a little easier to get your hands on these forms. You can find the Medicare Authorization to Disclose Personal Health Information form at http://www .medicare.gov/MedicareOnlineForms/PublicForms/CMS10106.pdf.

You need to type in the information right online and then print it out, make sure it is signed, and mail it in to Medicare. Make sure to print out two copies, get both signed, and keep one in your file in case you have to do it again. Not saying that will happen, but I'm just saying . . .

I would also recommend that everyone who is signing up for Medicare at age 65 go ahead and prepare this document right then. If you haven't done it and are on Medicare, do it now. You never know when you may have an accident or become ill and need someone to advocate for you, and then it's too late to get this form completed and on file with Medicare. Medicare moves slowly, *think glaciers and plate tectonics*, only not nearly as fast, and you'll realize it can take several weeks to months to get it "into the system." The best time to get these things done is before we need to. Your spouse, your best friend, or your grown child will appreciate that you did it should the need ever arise. Just make sure they are aware and have copies of it and any confirmatory paperwork.

After you've sent in this form, you should wait about 30 days and then start calling Medicare (1–800-MEDICARE) to inquire whether the system has listed your authorized person. If not, call every couple of weeks for another 30 days, and then give up and mail your second signed copy. Always keep a copy for yourself, of course.

I have a patient that actually had to do this four times. She is smart, patient . . . up to a point . . . and, most important, dogged. Ultimately she prevailed, but she was understandably frustrated.

Rules of Engagement

Now I hate to say this, but talking with the government is sometimes a little bit like a game, just like it is with an insurance company (see my first book). Probably most government employees are dedicated, pleasant, and energetic. Unfortunately, the government employee or contractor that you may be contending with on the phone may or may not be very helpful. Whatever you do, no matter how well deserved it may be, no matter how banal or incompetent they come across, don't lose your temper. If you do, you lose. You provide an easy "out" for them to dismiss you and make things much more difficult. Like I said before, it's like they win on a technicality without ever addressing the principle or the issues of your need. Instead maybe make voodoo dolls of them and buy some extra pins, invent clever new innocuous profanities (like "What in the whole grain Cheerios is he talking about?"), or run an extra mile or do an extra rep during your daily workout. Just do not lose your temper.

There, I have said my piece.

Health-Related Care
ASSISTED LIVING

Assisted living is a long-term healthcare option designed for individuals who need assistance with everyday activities such as meals, bathing and dressing, medication management, etc. Currently, it is estimated that there are more than 6,300 professionally managed assisted living communities in the United States, housing more than 900,000 people.

Assisted living costs can vary widely depending upon many factors, including the size of the apartment and the types of services offered. As of 2012, the median monthly rate nationwide at an assisted living facility was $3,326.

More than 86 percent of assisted living residents pay for their rent and services through private, long-term-care insurance or from their own savings, as assisted living is not a service generally covered under Medicare. However, 41 states have waiver programs for low-income seniors to help them afford this option. Check with your state for the particulars. Generally speaking, you should begin with your state's department of health or human services division.

Assisted living coverage assumptions can be dangerous and ones where most people believe they have coverage through a government or private provider program, but don't. The litany of woeful anecdotes is long and sad—sea monkey sad. Don't be part of it. Read the fine print and get the straight story.

NURSING HOMES

Basically defined, nursing homes provide convalescent and/or rehabilitative care for individuals with chronic health conditions or after a hospital stay. The level of care can range from basic (wound care that defies home health) to skilled (medically qualified provision) to subacute (just shy of requiring hospital support). Unlike assisted living, a physician's order is required for admission to a nursing home.

Nursing homes are licensed and regulated at the state level. Care must be provided by registered nurses (RNs) or licensed practical nurses (LPNs). Intermediate care facilities (ICFs) provide eight or more hours of nursing supervision a day, and skilled nursing facilities (SNFs) offer medical services 24 hours a day.

Here are some sobering numbers. As of 2010, the estimated median monthly cost of a nursing home stay in the United States was $7,001. Fees can be paid for out of private funds, long-term-care insurance policies, and/or Medicare and Medicaid.

There are other issues associated with nursing homes, such as financial guardianship usurpment (chapter 7) and physical abuse (chapter 8), but I will get into those a little later. Just in case you were wondering.

Additional Senior Healthcare Options

Now these are not actually endorsed programs, but they are commonly encountered when you are looking for information, so I wanted to provide an overview here.

A State Partnership for Long-Term Care is a program available in 29 states that combines private long-term-care insurance and Medicaid long-term-care coverage. The partnership asserts that it helps potential users of Medicaid retain more of their assets while still being eligible for coverage.

The Program of All-Inclusive Care for the Elderly (PACE) provides integrated Medicare and Medicaid benefits for seniors who wish to continue receiving medical, social and long-term care in their own homes rather than in a nursing home. It is available in 28 states. Information about the state PACE programs can be found at http://www.medicare.gov/your-medicare-costs/help-paying-costs/pace/pace.html.

One resource that many older people do not consider is their local faith-based community. If you read my first book, you'll know I give a kind of goofy historical retrospective on the development of medicine as a charitable or benevolent enterprise arising from theological groups. Goofy I may be, but it is true and a valuable contribution to this discussion.

Many churches and religious organizations offer health screenings. Some have clinic systems. If you recall the first chapters of the "Life" section, I made a strong point about prevention and maintenance. These types of clinics are often critical for people who have chronic illnesses and who need help in monitoring and addressing those problems so that they do not progress or flare up to the point that they require more invasive and severe interventions. Check with your religious center.

If you have a church community, use it. Talk to your minister, pastor, priest, rabbi, imam, shaman, or, if your denomination has a medicine man . . . hey, there you go. I am kidding, of course, but this is pretty serious and heavy stuff, and spirituality for many people is a liberating solution to life's difficulties and challenges. So is humor, infantile though mine may be. Use it.

Also look for health fairs at technical colleges, training centers, and other civic organizations that offer these public services. It's a good way to get overall screening like blood sugar, blood pressure, serum lipid checks, skin cancer checks, and much, much more.

Another resource may be via a community or local government health center. A list of those centers as provided by the Health Resources and Services Administration is found at http://findahealthcenter.hrsa.gov/Search_HCC.aspx.

For resources for home health, visit http://www.medicare.gov/

homehealthcompare/search.html and https://findtreatment.samhsa.gov/locator/home.

Paradise—in a Bowl—Lost

When I got my sea monkeys, I wanted and hoped for a tiny idyllic society in a bowl. Instead I got a hygienic headache and a very valuable life lesson. In a weird way I write these books to help foster that same sort of thing, an idyllic society, not a hygienic headache. A big part of that is fostering your self-protection: in health care, in living conditions, and to prevent abuse. In the next two chapters, I'll go into what you can do to enhance your quality and security of life and hopefully assure a little liberty, too.

CHAPTER 7

FINANCIAL RESOURCES—LIVING EXPENSES

WHY HAZMAT INCIDENTS ARE A LOT LIKE CONSUMER ADVOCACY

Before I get started on the broad subject of living expenses and seniors, I think some context here will be both sobering and helpful. Here are some of that facts about who we—seniors—are financially, as reported by HHS.

Remember what I wrote earlier about the median income of older persons being $27,612 for males and $16,040 for females? It has been estimated that without Social Security 90 percent of older Americans would be (by those numbers) considered below the Federal Poverty Limit (FPL). To better understand what we are talking about, you should know that the FPL is a little over $11,500 a year for a single person (see table 9).

Some Federal Financial Definitions

To make sense of this, some definitions are in order. Bear with me. They matter.

Federal Poverty Threshold. This is a purely statistical determination created by the Census Bureau. It is used for reporting purposes and is for administrative purposes for the government. Think congressional reports and budgets. There is one value for the entire country.

Federal Poverty Guidelines. This is a number created by Health and

Table 9. Federal Poverty Definitions

Persons in Household	2014 Federal Poverty Level (FPL)	Medicaid Eligibility (138% of FPL)	Premium Subsidy Threshold (400% of FPL)
1	$11,670	$16,105	$46,680
2	$15,730	$21,707	$62,920
3	$19,790	$27,310	$79,160
4	$23,850	$32,913	$95,400
5	$27,910	$38,516	$111,640
6	$31,970	$44,119	$127,880
7	$36,030	$49,721	$144,120
8	$40,090	$55,324	$160,360

Human Services and is used to determine eligibility for certain programs like Medicare. It is weighted according to inflation and the cost of living in each of the 50 states and the District of Columbia. The term Federal Poverty Level is often interchangeably with the Subsidy Threshold.
Subsidy Threshold. This is generally a limit over which certain program eligibilities stop.

About 28 percent (12.1 million) of noninstitutionalized older persons live alone (8.4 million women, 3.7 million men). In 2012, about 518,000 grandparents aged 65 or older had the primary responsibility for grand-children who lived with them.

As referenced earlier, Social Security constituted 90 percent or more of the income received by 35 percent of beneficiaries in 2011 (22 percent of married couples and 45 percent of nonmarried beneficiaries). Without it, those folks would have wound up below the poverty line.

What does this mean? It means that with all of the potential threats to savings and fixed incomes, such as inflation, cost of living increases, and healthcare-related costs, seniors are in a particularly vulnerable position. With liberty in mind, this impacts how well you can maintain financial viability and autonomy. There are some things you can do, thank goodness.

The Buddy System

I have to say that after meeting my wife and becoming a doctor, the most gratifying experience of my life has been my involvement in the first responder community. I could never have planned it, but becoming an EMS medical director and then the medical director for an Urban Search and Rescue team has been a career trajectory that has provided more challenge and reward as a physician than I could have dreamed. In addition to being able to respond to a number of disasters and catastrophic events in my state and country's time of need, I've gained experience that has allowed me to participate in developing standards for responders in hazardous materials environments.

Want to know the first rule of engagement in a big HAZMAT scene? It's "know what you are getting into." The second rule is "have backup." More simply put, "have a buddy system in place."

The same is also true of financial management and living resources for seniors. It doesn't matter whether you are financially well off or need some assistance to make ends meet. Backup or support can be in the form of either advice or actual financial aid. Unless you are Warren Buffet, you'll want all the help you can get. The truth is, I am pretty sure Warren Buffet has had some help at times, too, if only in terms of information.

Want an example of what I am talking about? How about Social Security?

Did you know that if something were to happen to you—a stroke, pneumonia, alien abduction, lightning strike, saber-toothed cat attack—unless you have an officially designated, authorized person to receive protected health information, nobody can speak for you or get any information about what is going on with your Social Security situation?

If a designated "buddy" or advocate is necessary regarding Medicare, as mentioned in the last chapter, then it is even more important when it comes to dealing with Social Security. In fact, the two concepts go hand in hand.

FINDING THE ONE

Now, you will want to be careful about your choice. It has to be someone you can trust, really trust. This is also an issue you should address as soon as you can. By the time you need it, say because of an acute debilitation, illness, or a chronic progressive condition like dementia or Alzheimer's, it may be too late.

This is generally the sort of person who will carry a power of attorney for you. Here is something else you will want to consider. There can be broad and limited powers of attorney. And this concludes the extent of my legal expertise. Pretty sad, isn't it?

You should put some time into this and consult a legal authority, a real one, not some guy who watches Judge Judy and eats Cheetos all day. If you don't already have an attorney or legal counsel and can afford one, get one. If you can't, contact the nearest law school. They often have law student volunteers in legal centers and know of other pro bono options that can help.

Some Legal Definitions

Guardianship and powers of attorney are two terms that are very important, and while people like me might think they are interchangeable, a real legal scholar would be right to point out that they aren't. They have some similarities, but they mean very different things with regard to responsibility, accountability, and control.

GUARDIANSHIP

Guardianship is a legal procedure in which one person is appointed by a court to make decisions for someone who can no longer make decisions for himself or herself. For more information, visit http://thelawdictionary. org/article/how-to-legally-declare-someone-as-mentally-incompetent/.

There are *three types of guardians*. A "guardian of the person" is appointed when people cannot take care of their own personal needs, such as medical care. A "guardian of the estate" is appointed if people cannot handle their own business or financial affairs. A "general guardian" is someone who acts in both roles.

A person will be declared *incompetent* and in need of a guardian if he or she lacks sufficient mental capacity to manage his or her own affairs or to make or communicate important decisions about his or her health, property, wishes, or family.

Capacity. Capacity relates to someone's soundness of mind and to the intelligent understanding and perception of his or her action. Regarding legal considerations, it is the power to either create or enter into a legal relationship.

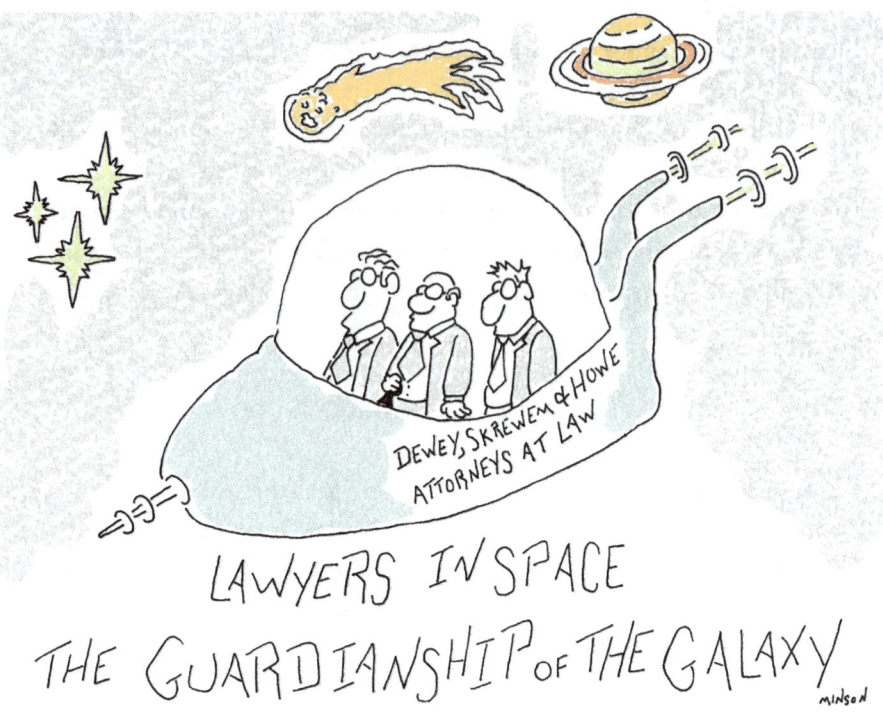

LAWYERS IN SPACE
THE GUARDIANSHIP OF THE GALAXY

Competency. Competency is the presence of those characteristics, or the absence of those disabilities, which render a person or witness legally fit and qualified to give testimony in a court of justice. The term is also applied, in the same sense, to documents or other written evidence.

So your capacity speaks to the more clinical definition (and thus requires some medical validation), which then leads to the latter term of competency, which is a purely legal concept based on the capacity.

Now if you will excuse me, I have to go watch a *Matlock* marathon on cable.

Usually, you do not need a lawyer to serve as someone's guardian. The forms to file a guardianship case are easy to fill out and can be obtained from your local courthouse. The court may require that you get a letter from a doctor explaining why the doctor feels that the person is incompetent, however.

In an acute situation where a guardian is needed, if the incompetent person does not have a lawyer, the court will appoint one to represent the incompetent person at the hearing. This temporary representative is called a "guardian ad litem." The incompetent person also has a right to have a personal lawyer present at the hearing. A jury trial or a broad evaluation of competency may then be requested.

If you are appointed to be a general guardian or a guardian of an estate, you will need the court's permission for many financial transactions on the incompetent person's behalf. A guardian of an estate must manage the business and financial affairs of the incompetent person in a careful manner. The guardian must also give a report each year of the receipts, payments, and other transactions made that year.

If a person is still able to understand legal documents, signing a power of attorney may be preferable to guardianship. With a power of attorney, the person chooses who will handle his or her affairs instead of having the court make this choice. It is handled out of court, and there is no necessary court supervision.

Which leads to the question, "Is my lawyer "competent"? You are on your own with that one.

POWER OF ATTORNEY

A power of attorney can be made for different transactions—financial, medical, and other matters. The power of the agent is limited only to the content of the agreement.

For those who need someone to handle their financial affairs, a power of attorney is very helpful. It must be signed by a person who is mentally competent. As you recall, the person must understand what he or she is signing. This can be done either before a person loses mental capacity or, if this has already happened, during a period when the person has regained capacity, if only temporarily. Again, a doctor could help determine capacity if there is doubt.

If the power of attorney is signed by a person whose competency "comes and goes," it is important to have a written medical determination of competency at the time the documents are signed. A medical opinion is also helpful when the person has a progressive disease—one that gets worse, like Alzheimer's—in case someone later questions whether the power of attorney is valid.

Probably the most useful and powerful type of power of attorney is the *durable power of attorney*. Unless a power of attorney is made durable, the agent (the person who receives the power of attorney) loses power to act if the maker becomes incompetent. For most, that is precisely when the agent's assistance is necessary. A power of attorney can be made durable with clear language in it stating that it remains effective after the maker becomes incompetent.

A word about the agent: It probably goes without saying, but trust in the agent is a crucial issue … which is why I am saying it anyway. The agent has the power to write the maker's checks, sell the maker's property, and incur debt in the maker's name. Sometimes, all that an incapacitated person needs is someone to take care of a Social Security check! Remember the mention of a representative payee earlier. That is the sort of importance we are talking about here.

If your loved one needs someone to make medical and healthcare decisions, a healthcare power of attorney is useful. Your loved one can sign this document as long as he or she is mentally competent or during a period when he or she is mentally alert. The healthcare power of attorney goes into effect when a person lacks the ability to make and understand medical decisions. At that time, the person named in the healthcare power of attorney, the "agent," can make all medical decisions or only those listed in the healthcare power of attorney. The healthcare agent cannot make any decisions related to property or bills. These different roles are shown in table 10.

In any case, when choosing someone to serve as your financial power of attorney agent, trust is paramount. Make sure it is a person who has your best interests at heart. Avoid those who have a history of serious financial issues, and steer clear of anyone who has a personal grudge against any of

Table 10. Guardianship and Power of Attorney

Guardianship	A legal relationship between a ward (a person) and a guardian, who is appointed by a court to make decisions on behalf of the ward. Irrevocable.
Power of Attorney	A legal document made by a person (the principal=YOU) who appoints an agent to act on his or her behalf. May be revoked at any time.
Guardians (Guardianship)	Must account for the money spent on behalf of the ward.
Agents (POA)	Do not have to account for money spent.

your family members. Discuss your financial situation and wishes with the person you choose before you sign the document. The person named as your agent can arrange for investments in mutual funds, stocks, bonds, and property, can claim, sell, or transfer property on your behalf, and can handle taxes and small business operations. Additionally, he or she can pay your day-to-day expenses; can handle mortgage payments, retirement funds, insurance, and more; can deal with government benefits (as long as some additional arrangements are made), interest payments, and bank transactions; and can hire legal counsel to represent you, if necessary.

This is all true with one important exception. Remember what we considered in the last chapter about a Medicare designate? Well, in much the same way, Social Security has a similar requirement. Without having arranged it, if you cannot speak for yourself, real problems can arise.

Interacting with the Social Security Administration

I cover the fact that most seniors in the Unites States receive support from Social Security in a few places in this book. What I am going to speak to next really is for the loved ones of seniors. A lot of people believe that if they have established a power of attorney or designated an agent via some legal action, then that individual can "speak" for them if they become debilitated or noncommunicative. In some situations, that is correct. Regarding the Social Security Administration (SSA) and an awardee's benefits, it is **not**.

The way to do this is to get an *Authorization to Designate a Representative Payee from the Social Security Administration.* This can be a lifesaver. If you don't have it, SSA personnel will not speak to you. Period. They can't, by law.

Now here is an interesting tidbit. Even if you name someone, the SSA will take the request/suggestion into account, but *they* make the final determination about whether a particular individual will be appointed or whether they think someone else would be more suitable.

WHAT'S A REPRESENTATIVE PAYEE?

When people need help managing their benefits, SSA, after a careful investigation, may appoint a relative, friend, or other interested party to serve as the beneficiary's "representative payee." This means the person's benefits are then paid to the payee on the beneficiary's behalf.

HOW IS A REPRESENTATIVE PAYEE CHOSEN?

Appointment to be someone's representative payee isn't automatic. The SSA tries to select someone who knows the recipient, sees the recipient often, and knows his or her needs well. For that reason, if the recipient is living with someone who already knows and is helping the recipient, the SSA usually selects that person to be the representative payee.

WHAT DOES A REPRESENTATIVE PAYEE DO?

A payee acts on behalf of the beneficiary. A payee is responsible for everything related to benefits that a capable beneficiary would do for himself or herself. The SSA encourages payees to go beyond just managing finances and to be actively involved in the beneficiary's life.

A payee also has obligations. They determine the beneficiary's needs and use his or her payments to meet those needs. They save any money left after meeting the beneficiary's current needs in an interest-bearing account or savings bonds for the beneficiary's future needs. They also report any changes or events that could affect the beneficiary's eligibility for benefits or payment amount and keep records of all payments received and how they are spent or saved. They provide benefit information to social service agencies or medical facilities as requested, and they help the beneficiary get medical treatment when necessary.

Administratively, they also complete written reports accounting for the use of funds and notify the SSA of any changes in their own circumstances that would affect their performance or ability to continue as payee. Finally, they also return any payments to which the beneficiary is not entitled.

WHAT CAN'T A REPRESENTATIVE PAYEE DO?

A representative payee can't

- Sign legal documents, other than Social Security documents, on behalf of a beneficiary (this is what a power of attorney is for)
- Have legal authority over income from sources other than Social Security or SSI, such as earned income, pensions, or any other income source
- Use a beneficiary's money for the representative payee's own personal expenses
- Spend funds in a way that would leave the beneficiary without necessary items or services (housing, food, medical care)
- Put a beneficiary's Social Security or SSI funds in his or her own account or another person's account (checking and savings accounts must show the beneficiary as the only owner)
- Keep any funds once he or she is no longer the payee
- Charge the beneficiary for services unless authorized by the SSA to do so

HOW DOES A REPRESENTATIVE PAYEE REPORT TO SSA?

Usually the SSA will send a Representative Payee Report form once a year. If a payee keeps clear records about how the beneficiary's money was spent or saved, the report will be fairly simple to complete.

If you want to get more information or are considering becoming a representative payee applicant, you can learn more at http://www.ssa.gov/pubs/EN-05–10076.pdf or at http://www.usa.gov/consumer-action-handbook/order-form.shtml or at www.socialsecurity.gov/myaccount.

Some Other Financial Considerations
A MATTER OF TRUST

A trust is a legal instrument that allows you to convey property to a trustee, who then manages the property for the benefit of you and/or your named beneficiaries, usually family members. A trustee may be you, another individual, or an institution. The trustee is empowered to manage your property only as permitted by the trust, being legally bound to adhere to its terms. Trusts generally are created to instill and preserve family values and property, protecting your accumulated wealth from creditors, divorce, taxes, and other claims against your estate after your death.

LIVING TRUSTS

A living trust is a legal instrument in which property, whether real estate, bank accounts, or other tangible or intangible wealth (but not IRAs or other retirement accounts) is transferred into the name of the trust while you are alive. The trust provides for what happens to the property in it once the person who contributed the property (called the "grantor" or "settlor") dies. The living trust is revocable and amendable, so if the grantor changes his or her mind about who should inherit or how much, the trust can either be amended or, less frequently, revoked. In effect, while assets have a different title of ownership, the assets remain yours. You can use your assets as you please, and when you die, the assets in the trust are not subject to probate. Here's more: http://www.seniorlaw.com/living-trust-is-it-right-for-you/.

So do I need a will then? Short answer, yes. The will accounts for things that were not spelled out in the trust or for things that are awarded after your death, like an insurance payment.

Why have a living trust? Well, if you have properties in different states, then you will be able to avoid multiple probate costs. There are other reasons, but you really need to talk to a real lawyer about this. One thing more: in some states and situations the grantor may also be a trustee. You'll need to check.

THE LANGUAGE OF TRUSTS

Testamentary trust. A testamentary trust doesn't take effect until after the person is deceased, so it is created by the terms of a will. It must go through probate before the trust is established. This means that the funds must first become public record and will most likely be reduced due to attorney and court fees from probate. The funds entering into a trust are taxed according to the contemporary estate tax law.

Revocable trust. With a revocable trust, the person retains control of all the assets in the trust and can revoke or change the terms of the trust at any time. A living trust is often this type.

Irrevocable trust. Irrevocable trusts typically can't be changed without the beneficiary's consent. The appreciated assets in the trust aren't subject to estate taxes.

Each type of trust has advantages and disadvantages. A trust is a legal entity, so you must follow state rules to ensure that the trust is set up correctly. Have your elderly parent discuss the options thoroughly with an estate-planning attorney before setting one up.

Here are a few other terms for **types of trusts:**

Gift trust. This type is most often used by parents, grandparents, aunts and uncles, or other relatives to gift property and assets to children.

Grantor retained annuity trust. During a set number of years, the trust provides you, the grantor, with periodic payments (usually to satisfy the annuity distribution obligation). At the end of the trust's term, proceeds are distributed to your beneficiaries.

Qualified personal residence trust. You transfer a residence to the trust and retain the right to use it, rent free, for a specific number of years. As trustee, you also may sell the property to reinvest the money in a new residence or to create a grantor retained annuity trust.

Charitable remainder trust, charitable lead trust. These trusts allow a set annuity to be paid for a specific number of years, after which the trust property passes to the beneficiaries. With the remainder trust, you (as grantor) and possibly other family members receive the annuity, with the final trust property passing to a charitable institution at your death. With the lead trust, the reverse occurs—the charity receives the annuity, and your beneficiaries receive the final trust property.

THE JOINT ACCOUNT ACCESS

Even if you don't get into all that other stuff, at the very least you will probably want to allow the people who will be looking out for you when you become incapacitated to access a bank account. This can be as simple as having your child, spouse, or loved one as a signatory or an agent to it. It will allow them to manipulate the funds in the account. Of course, if, say, the SSA accidentally doesn't issue a check or you want to redirect Social Security payments to another new account, the person with joint account access will need to be a Social Security Responsible Payee. Again, this is if you cannot speak on your own behalf.

There Is No Free Lunch

I have written a lot about my motivations about becoming a physician and the financial struggle to get there. I grew up in financially modest circumstances. My first job in a hospital came when I was 16. It was in janitorial services, and let me tell you, if anything will give you a really quick and graphic idea of what you are getting into in medicine, it's cleaning up after sick people. Frankly, I think it should be a prerequisite for any healthcare provider. My next position was washing dishes in the hospital cafeteria, which was kind of the same sort of activity. From there I was promoted to working in the "grill area." That was valuable, completely by chance and because of the woman with whom I worked.

Her name was Esther and she was, I thought, a very peculiar and interesting person. She had wiry hair and wore Irene Ryan–style glasses. She was, among many other things, a voracious reader and a polylinguist. She spoke German, Hebrew, French, English, Spanish, Danish, and a little bit of Russian. Quickly, I started to wonder why someone with her intellectual gifts was satisfied working in the grill with someone like me.

I was young.

Now, it is important to know that I wanted—in addition to becoming a doctor—to someday also be a writer. Maybe it was because of our mutual affinity for the printed word. Maybe it was something much more human, but over the course of one summer, Esther and I began what a casual observer might have considered the strangest of friendships. In truth she was a great friend; wise, patient, and smart as hell. One day as we were working on the grill, the long sleeves she always wore rode up a little, and I saw the tattooed numbers on her forearm.

Esther was a survivor of the Holocaust.

I learned a lot from Esther. I learned you could be injured by the world and somehow not be destroyed. I learned that trauma and hardship, even brutality, are no match for humor and a great spirit. That was one of the greatest things about her—Esther was funny. She had a really great way with a phrase, too. As our friendship matured and she came to trust me, she told me her story. I came to trust her, too.

Eventually, though it took a lot of nerve—in retrospect, it was probably hubris—I let her read a short story I had written. She could have killed me with the wrong choice of words, and I think she knew it.

All she said was, "You know how a Reuben sandwich is no good if the corned beef or pastrami isn't seasoned?"

I said I did.

"Well, people are the same. I think you need to jump a few freight trains and ride the rails a bit, kiddo. Get a little seasoning."

Years later, after a little seasoning, I wrote my first book. It was published, and I took a copy to her. She read it and rendered her review in a single sentence.

"I think you'd make a pretty good Reuben now."

It was better than a Pulitzer.

Among other things, Esther also liked to say, "You gotta eat."

It was a general statement that included the heart, the stomach, and the head. I'm going to plagiarize from her here, but I'll keep it confined to the stomach.

You gotta eat.

Unfortunately, in a country where there is so much wealth and abundance, so many are still hungry. I covered some of the issues of the food we eat in the first section of the book, and now I'd like to offer some resources for people who need some assistance getting food.

SENIOR FOOD PROGRAMS

If you remember my rant from the Behaviors chapter, you know the term "food" is pretty subjective. In terms of financial support, it helps to have some definitions, just so you'll know what you're really talking about.

Congregate meals. These are meals eaten in a group setting. You go there to eat, basically. This can be either governmental or private settings like meal sites or assistance kitchens. Congregate meals are offered in all states. Individuals can choose from meal sites that include churches, senior centers, religious facilities, Area Agency on Aging offices, and housing facilities. Senior citizens can get a free, nutritious hot meal or lunch, and they can also have the opportunity to socialize, attend workshops, and get other support from the community.

Home-delivered meals: This is just what it says, prepared meals are delivered to a senior's home. People who can't make it to a meal site and who are homebound should look into home-delivered meals. To qualify, individuals will need to be unable to shop for food or prepare meals on their own, and they must be homebound. The home-delivered meal programs are also commonly referred to as Meals on Wheels. Volunteers will bring food and meals to homebound seniors, which can help them to remain in their homes for as long as possible. In addition to receiving food and access to the nutrition services, seniors are offered daily contact with staff or program volunteers. They will provide seniors a link to additional services in their communities. A good place to start is by looking up and calling your local Salvation Army, Catholic Charities, St. Vincent De Paul, or a state or local government social service office.

FEDERAL PROGRAMS

Free food is offered to seniors over 60 years of age from the federal government via the Commodity Supplemental Food Program (CSFP). Healthy meals and groceries are offered in partnership with the US Department of Agriculture (USDA) and your state social services agency. Additional nutrition information is also provided in order to help facilitate good health. One of the best is sponsored by Iowa State University's Spend Smart Eat Smart program. You can get free information about low cost, improved nutrition and more at http://www.extension.iastate.edu/foodsavings/.

If you want to learn more about eligibility for the USDA program, check out http://www.fns.usda.gov/csfp/eligibility-how-apply. Additionally, you can find a list of state designates at http://www.fns.usda.gov/fdd/state-da-contacts-csfp-nslp-schools-cacfp-sfsp-nsip-tefap-important.

COOPERATIVE PURCHASING

This is just another fancy term for the buddy system. If everyone on your block or floor in your building or in your neighborhood shares a passion for rutabagas, well, you might consider bypassing a grocer and going directly to a farmers' coop or to a wholesale grocer to buy in bulk. Then you can all divvy up those delicious rutabagas at a fraction of the price. Of course the same holds for other things besides rutabagas, thank God.

MAN'S . . . WOMAN'S BEST FRIEND

For seniors struggling to feed their pets, free dog or cat food may also be available through some home delivery services. Some Meals on Wheels services now provide this for low-income senior citizens and the homebound. It is not yet offered nationwide, but an increasing number of providers are implementing this program. The free food for your pet will free up your income for other basic needs. As for health care for your pet, contact the closest veterinary school or colleges with animal grooming, husbandry, or animal care programs. Often they can provide advice and assistance at a reduced cost; sometimes it's even free. Having a healthy pet can really help a senior citizen or disabled person by providing companionship and other benefits. To get more information, you can also call your local Area Agency on Aging office, which generally has extensive information on many varied resources for the elderly. They are listed in the phone book. Other places to call can include a Salvation Army center, Catholic Charities, or a local community action agency. These are also some nonprofits that can give you information on free cat or dog food as well as other supplies.

Housing Affordability

This is a pretty complicated subject. They used to say that everyone's home is his or her castle. That may still be true, but sometimes it feels like the castle is under siege or that the barbarians are at the gate. Whether you own or rent, you need to consider your changes in aging at home or the need for assistance or even nursing care. There are a number of strategies you will want to address.

By definition, a reverse mortgage is a legal agreement in which a bank pays you an amount of money equal to the part of your home's value that you actually own; in return, you agree that when you sell your home or move or die, that amount of money *plus interest* will be paid to the bank or lender.

This can be tricky. If you own your own home and want to consider the option of a reverse mortgage, there are some reliable sources of information. A good place to start is the National Council on Aging's publication *Use Your Home to Stay at Home* (http://www.ncoa.org/news-ncoa-publications/publications/ncoa_reverse_mortgage_booklet_073109.pdf). Additional information can be found at http://portal.hud.gov/hudportal/HUD?src=/program_offices/housing/sfh/hecm/hecmhome.

This may not be for everyone, and if you notice I am not spending a lot of time explaining, justifying, or championing this. There is a good reason. It really depends on the individual and his or her specific need. Suffice it to say, you should consult the resources above and get with someone you trust before you make the decision.

HELP WITH RENT

Most people don't realize that there are a number of programs that can help with subsidies for seniors who rent. There are qualifications based on your assets and income, but it is worth examining.

If you rent and need assistance, *rent assistance vouchers* can often be provided to seniors and the elderly from programs such as the US Department of Housing and Urban Development (HUD). The precedents are in sections 202 and 8 of the HUD regulations. Your area office on aging can often provide details on housing resources. You can also speak with a HUD federal housing advisor on the phone. A list of those contacts can be found at http://www.hud.gov/offices/hsg/sfh/hcc/hcs.cfm.

The Progression of Living Situations

I have some patients who shy away from the idea of discussing their decline relative to activities of daily living. I often think of this as completely understandable, but a lot like denying that you are going to age or standing on a beach and denying that the tide will come in. You can do it if you want, but pretty soon you are going to have wet feet. And nobody wants that. While it's a really unpleasant consideration, it is one that is completely necessary.

So how do you assess honestly what kind of living situation you need or will need? Sometimes it is easy. Often it is like doing an honest self-appraisal, the single toughest human enterprise of all. A friend of mine, a very funny psychiatrist—and, yes, they do exist—likes to say, "Personally I cling to my delusions. The art is in knowing when the delusion transitions to psychosis and stopping just short."

Keep that in mind.

For purposes of discussion, we might start by considering the types of senior living.

Independent Autonomous Living (IAL). That is what it sounds like. You don't need any help at all. The odds are against us getting to the end in that state.

Aging in place. Sounds like something a rock would do, I know. This is just an extension of IAL. How do you know if you are doing it? Well, here's a test: if you have started buying cereal for the fiber instead of the toy, you are well on your way.

Or maybe you prefer George Burns's definition.

He said, "You know you're getting old when you stoop to tie your shoelaces and wonder what else you could do while you're down there."

Assisted living. This provides help with the activities of daily living—housekeeping, laundry, maybe helping you with errands, etc. I've spent most of my adult life trying to get out of those tasks, but when I can't do them instead of opting not to, it is time to consider an adjustment in my circumstances and living situation. It can either be in a single traditional dwelling or in a communal or group setting. I touched on this earlier in the book, but it is also characterized by how much time the assistance is required.

Skilled nursing. This generally applies to assistance for a medical condition. It can be acute (as in the book *Misery* . . . well, maybe that is not such a good example) but is more traditionally thought of as chronic and progressive care. It is also usually in a facility. A good medical definition is

"an establishment that houses chronically ill, usually elderly patients, and provides long-term nursing care, rehabilitation, and other services."
Nursing homes. This is generally used interchangeably with "skilled nursing facility," though there are differences. It is a place of residence for people who require—as determined by a local hospital social worker and a nursing facility provider—continual nursing care and who have significant difficulty coping with the required activities of daily living. These are the most vulnerable. This is also a situation in which a lot of senior individuals are at risk for neglect, problems, and even abuse.

In the next chapter I will cover some things you can do to help make sure that you are choosing a good one and how to protect yourself from abuse. There is a lot that you and a loved one or advocate can do to protect you. Even if you are pretty functional, it pays to have an advocate. Remember what I said about HAZMAT situations? Well, the same applies in these types of settings. Stick with the buddy system.

Why have I listed these distinctions yet again? Well, because now we are talking about paying and this is an area where a lot of misconceptions come up.

Paying for Long-Term Care

According to HHS, consumer surveys reveal common misunderstandings about which public programs pay for long-term care. So that you don't end up with a problem, it is important to clearly understand what is and isn't covered.

MEDICARE

Medicare pays for long-term care only under certain conditions.

- It pays if you require skilled services or rehabilitative care:
  In a nursing home for a maximum of 100 days (however, the average Medicare-covered stay is much shorter—22 days)
  At home if you are also receiving skilled home health or other skilled in-home services (generally, long-term-care services are provided only for a short period of time)

- It does not pay for nonskilled assistance with activities of daily living (ADL), which make up the majority of long-term-care services.
- You will have to pay for long-term-care services that are not covered by a public or private insurance program.

MEDICAID

Medicaid does pay for the largest share of long-term-care services, but to qualify:

- Your income must be below a certain level.
- You must meet minimum state eligibility requirements (based on the amount of assistance you need with ADL).

Other federal programs, such as those covered by the Older Americans Act and the Department of Veterans Affairs, pay for long-term-care services, but only for specific populations and in certain circumstances. That means you should really consider long-term-care insurance as soon as you read this or think about the words "long-term care."

LONG-TERM-CARE INSURANCE

Now, as little as I know about legal matters, get ready, because I know even less about insurance. Here is what the experts at HHS offer:

Unlike traditional health insurance, long-term care insurance is designed to cover long-term services and supports, including personal and custodial care in a variety of settings such as your home, a community organization, or other facility. Long-term care insurance policies reimburse policyholders a daily amount (up to a pre-selected limit) for services to assist them with activities of daily living such as bathing, dressing, or eating. You can select a range of care options and benefits that allow you to get the services you need, where you need them.

The cost of your long-term care policy is based on

- How old you are when you buy the policy
- The maximum amount that a policy will pay per day
- The maximum number of days (or years) that a policy will pay
- The maximum lifetime amount that the policy will pay (the maximum amount per day times the number of days)
- Any optional benefits you choose, such as benefits that increase with inflation

If you are in poor health or already receiving long-term-care services, you may not qualify for long-term-care insurance, as most individual policies require medical underwriting. In some cases, you may be able to buy a limited amount of coverage or coverage at a higher "nonstandard" rate. This often comes from employer-provided policies or are sustained policies from when you were employed. In any case, check the fine print when you are considering a policy. Some group policies do not require underwriting.

Some Recent Disturbing Trends

Remember the discussion earlier about guardianship? Well, good. That means your mind is still intact and you actually paid attention. There have been a number of cases in which nursing homes have filed—without consultation of the patient or the patient's family—for guardianship of the individual.

"No problem," you say?

Wasn't that kind of them?

To quote the famous coach and sports commentator, Lee Corso, "Not so fast, my friend."

The nursing home may be doing that to take over the payment filings and the financial accounts of the resident. Why would they want to do that? Well, consider this. If the facility submits a bill and the government reimbursement is half, then it has to file the other half for payment by the resident or the resident's insurance or other resource. This cost might be disputed on the "uncovered" amount by the resident or the resident's family member. If the home is also the approving entity with regard to any disputes of the bill, then it can assure that it has complete payment because it also controls the resident's financial authority.

If someone else is the guardian, then the facility has to submit that to the outsider (relative) or the resident, who can potentially dispute the charge or the amount. So the nursing home is eliminating a potential dispute. It also gives them incredible power. Not always good.

Now, hopefully, you are dealing with a reputable bunch of people in a nursing home, but you can assure additional protections by making certain that the same entity that benefits from the payment of a bill is not the same one approving its validity. What this means for families of nursing home residents is that they might consider going ahead and filing for guardianship early on.

So I'll go back to my opening sentence regarding some recent articles about homes filing for guardianship with the courts without discussion with the family or resident. This attempt at usurpment of control assures, at the very least, a huge distraction and legal costs by and for the family of the resident. At worst, it can estrange the family from a legitimate legal say in the determination of the course of care and the quality of the senior's life. So maybe consider getting that guardianship established when you face any big life transitions like moving from your home to a nursing home. Consider discussing this with an attorney at least. Heavy stuff, huh?

Here's another cartoon and just in the nick of time.

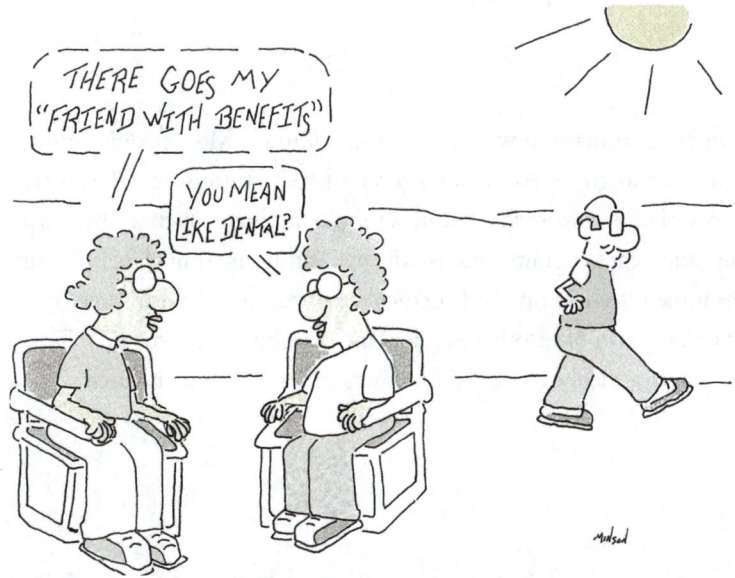

Additional Programs for Seniors

There are way too many resources and programs for one book to comprehensively cover. I said it before and I'll reiterate it here, this book is just a starting point for you. Hopefully, it gives you a good head start. For more information and assistance in financial resources, explore your state or local Area Agency on Aging or use the service Eldercare Locator (http://www.eldercare.gov/Eldercare.NET/Public/Index.aspx).

The programs provide a single point of information and entry into the aging benefits and programs network. Older adults can gain a single place for access or a phone number to call for information on a bunch of services and government benefits. Information is also available for families and caregivers. Some of what can be provided includes information on income and financial aid, transportation, senior citizens centers, pharmacy assistance, daily meals, housing/rent assistance, food pantries, and on and on. Have I sold this hard enough?

Good.

Again, if you need help understanding the ramifications of any of these considerations, look into free or low-cost legal advice. Remember what I wrote earlier about pro bono and law school resources for free or reduced-cost services? They can help with issues, including government disability benefits, income maintenance, and much more.

Senior Centers

These operate in many towns, cities, and counties. Most people think of this as a place to go for social activities and companionship. That is true. It is also a place for workshops and seminars on issues such as low-cost housing, medical programs like Medicare, and budgeting classes. It can be a resource for checkups and medical resources and health screenings. Senior centers also offer other services and can be a place for people to stop by to get a meal or pick up an emergency food box or lunch.

Other Financial Advice and Bill-Paying Assistance

There are many such programs with online resources. Some of these programs are cosponsored by the AARP Foundation. Services will often include money management assistance to help low-income senior citizens and adults with physical disabilities that have difficulty paying routine bills, budgeting, and keeping track of financial matters. The goal of this resource is to also promote independent living for individuals and senior citizens who are at risk of losing their independence due to inability to pay their bills on time and, in general, to help them manage their financial affairs. The program uses a combination of credit counselors and volunteers to assist individuals who may not have relatives or friends who are willing to help.

I would also recommend that you take a look at the website of the National Consumer Voice for Quality Long-Term Care (http://theconsumervoice.org/get_help). This site offers state agency contacts that can provide access to a number of services, including a local Citizen Advocacy Group.

Running Hot and Cold

There are also resources for energy assistance. For example, the federal government's Low-Income Energy Assistance Program (LIHEAP), a part of the USDHHS Office of Community Services, assists low-income households. Priority is usually given to people who are most at risk, such as seniors and the disabled. Assistance can also be offered for households who are experiencing a home energy emergency.

A crisis can be addressed, too. This may result from an unpaid utility or heating bill, the receipt of a shutoff notice, or lack of fuel or wood. Payments from LIHEAP are for home cooling and heating and other emergency energy-related costs during the cooling (April–September) and heating (October–March) seasons. In general, qualified households may be provided a onetime cash benefit per season, up to $600 per heating or cooling season. Payments will be made directly to the vendor or utility company.

You can find out whether you qualify and how at http://www.acf.hhs.gov/programs/ocs/programs/liheap or http://www.aarp.org/aarp-foundation/our-work/income/info-2012/public-benefits-guide-senior-assistance1.html.

Who You Gonna Call for Help with Phone Service?

Did you know that there are programs to help with the payment of a telephone service for seniors? It's true. The Universal Service Fund, provided by the Federal Communications Commission, has a program called Lifeline (https://www.fcc.gov/lifeline) that provides discounts on monthly telephone service for eligible low-income subscribers to help ensure they can connect to the nation's communications networks, find jobs, access health care services, connect with family and loved ones, and call for help in an emergency. See https://www.fcc.gov/encyclopedia/universal-service-fund for more.

Transportation

This subject is interesting. At least in America, we associate mobility with freedom. It's in our very culture and identity. Think about it: for most of our lives we have measured adulthood as when we get a driver's license, and when we have to validate our identity throughout most of our lives, we offer up our driver's license. If you are like me, it is always a humbling experience, as the picture on the ID generally looks like I am coming out of anesthesia after being forcibly groomed with a Flowbee.

At some point though we are going to have to rely on someone else to cart us around. I don't like the idea either, but this is one area that is not just about me. And it's not about you either. There are others who can be affected.

It may not be all at once. It may have to do with your night vision decreasing, depth perception issues, new medical problems, arthritis (can you turn your head properly?), and more. For example, is your hearing what it used to be? Can you hear a car horn? Do you have to turn up the radio so loud that it prevents you from being as aware of sounds outside the car that you might not anticipate a safety issue? There is a lot, I know.

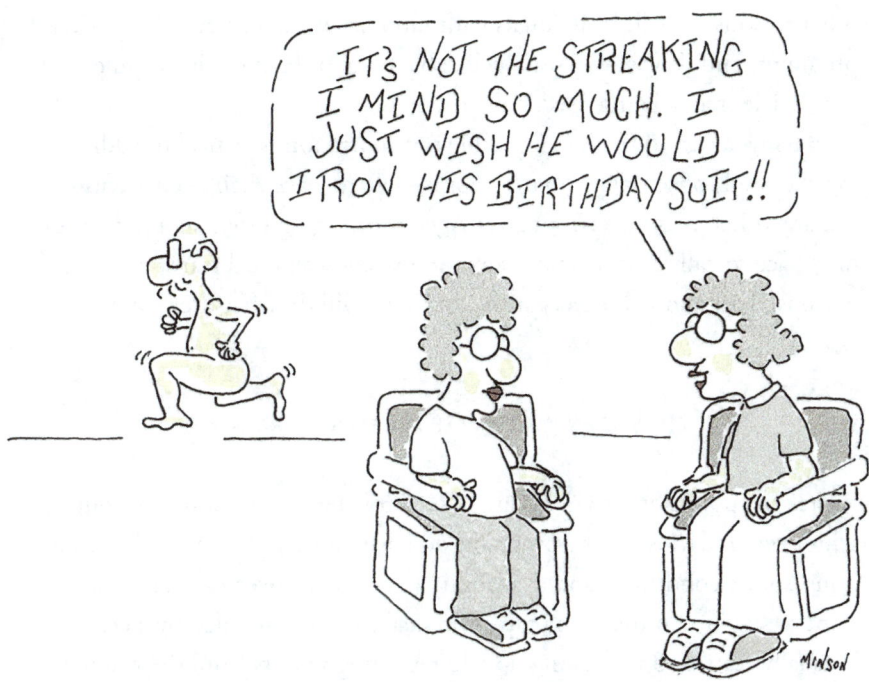

The National Highway Transportation Safety administration and AARP have created some guidance guidelines on this. They can be found and considered at http://www.nhtsa.gov/people/injury/olddrive/ Driving%20Safely%20Aging%20Web/index.html and at http://www .aarp.org/home-garden/transportation/info-05–2010/Warning_Signs_ Stopping.html.

HOLY SMOKE, I'M GROUNDED

When you do give up the keys, it doesn't mean you have to sit home alone interminably. In fact, there are a lot of resources that are available regardless of your financial status.

Transportation can be provided to seniors for appointments, shopping trips, and other needs. Many Agency on Aging centers, nonprofits such as the Salvation Army, and some faith-based organizations offer this service, either for free or a reduced price. A number of needs can be fulfilled by these services. The most common reason will be for a medical appointment or shopping trip for groceries; however, rides can be provided for other reasons as well. Individuals with mobility issues can also access these programs, and drivers will usually be able to help them get into and out of the vehicle that is being used.

Having access to free or affordable transportation is critical to addressing the needs of seniors who may not be able to leave their homes without any other assistance. Your Area Agency on Aging office should be the first place to call for information about low-cost, regional transportation options. Staff and volunteers at the locations will do what they can to assist.

TYPES OF TRANSPORTATION SERVICES

Some transportation programs are offered for the elderly from community senior centers. Most of the programs do have limited funding and restrictions, so the conditions and availability may change over time and you'll want to stay up on that. Any type of transportation provided by a center is usually restricted to picking up and returning seniors from their homes to the senior centers for participation in the activities. They also rely heavily on volunteers, so please volunteer if you can. Call your local center for more information on hours, programs terms, and any fees that may be involved.

Demand-response services will usually involve sending a van or vehicle after a phone request is made from the senior or his or her caregiver. So this type of transportation service does not follow a fixed schedule or route. These rides usually need to be scheduled in advance, and this should normally be anywhere from 24 to 48 hours in advance. Some Agency on Aging centers may make exceptions, but a caller should not expect this.

A key difference in demand-response service is that the driver may pick up more than one passenger at different locations and also drop them off separately. So that is one reason these need to be scheduled in advance. Paratransit and taxicabs may also operate as a demand-response service, but you will want to check on that first.

Transportation vouchers are fairly rare, but they may be an option as well. This can be thought of as a form of financial assistance, and it can be provided to qualified individuals so that they can pay for transportation on their own. Some common uses of a voucher can be for bus tokens, paratransit, taxicab, public transit, or other forms of transportation. Vouchers may be used for either public or private transportation. In addition to Area Agency on Aging centers, other nonprofits that may have a voucher include nonprofits like the Salvation Army or Catholic Charities.

Escorted/assisted transportation programs are options for older individuals with some form of medical condition or disability. It is for individuals who need more hands-on assistance than is offered by other programs. Normally the driver will help you enter and exit the vehicle. He or she may also escort you to your residence or final destination. This type of service may be offered with any form of transportation, whether demand-response or paratransit. It complements these other programs when the senior needs additional support.

Paratransit or fixed route transportation is a service of public transit. This is usually offered for bus, subway, van, or rail services along established routes. This can be coordinated by an Area Agency on Aging, social service agencies, or government resources.

Some of these organizations provide seniors with limited fixed-route services on a regular schedule. This can even include trips to the grocery store, post office, or a local senior center. If it is an automobile-type service, then the paratransit provider will use smaller vehicles such as small buses or minivans to provide the ride. They will also try to accommodate persons with disabilities, offering curb-to-curb or door-to-door service. These tend to be offered at reduced rates, or they may just request a small contribution from the individual.

Some agencies will outsource the transportation to *local taxicab companies*. This is a type of demand-response service that is commonly offered in most states and local communities. In addition, some taxi providers have wheelchair-accessible vehicles and may also be an option available for paratransit users.

Charities and nonprofits like the Salvation Army may also provide transportation assistance. These nonprofit and/or faith-based organizations usually rely heavily on volunteers. Senior citizens may be able to get a ride for a doctor appointment, shopping trip, and socialization purposes. Oftentimes the driver will help people get in and out of the car, if need be. You will need to make a reservation for this type of program.

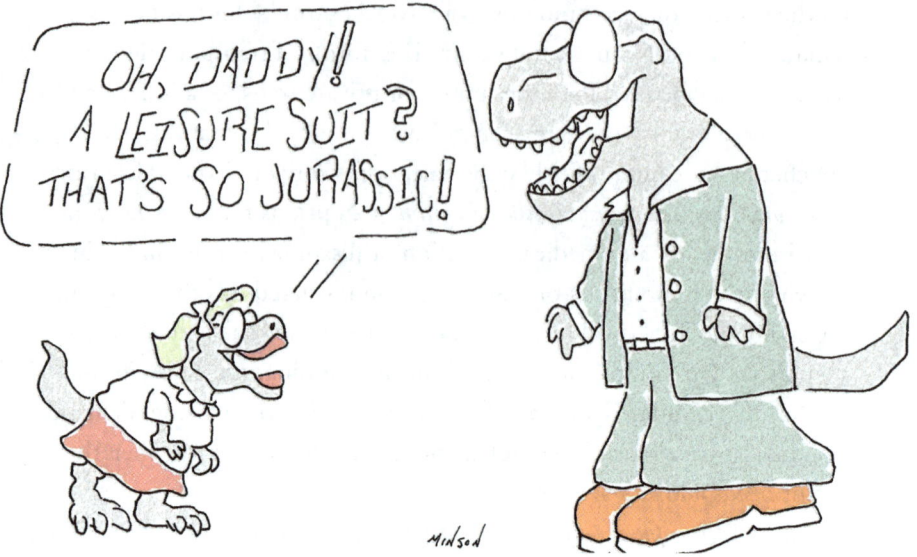

A good place to start for any of these resources is with your local administration on aging.

Should I Move Back In with the Kids?

This is a question that comes up a lot lately. If you have no other financial options or this is something that is desired and mutually beneficial, then of course the answer is yes. That said, if for you as an aging parent or for you as the child of an aging parent, the answer is no, you shouldn't feel guilty or wrong and here's why.

"Just because you're my child doesn't mean we're best friends."

You might reasonably feel that way. You can love your children but not want to live under the same roof. That doesn't make you an awful parent. I mean, think about it: the last time you as a group lived together, one of you was probably desperately trying to get out of the house and on to a new phase in life, like college or a new job. There are gobs of situation comedies about the awkwardness of teenaged amour being thwarted by Dad in his boxers, strolling through the laugh-tracked den of iniquity.

What makes you think it will be better now? For many people the parent doesn't want to be back in a similar situation. Also the roles are going to be very different. That will take some adjustment, at the very least.

In some cases seniors who are thrust back into such a situation experience depression, or they are reminded of their diminished social state in the household (whether true or not), or, worse, they may socially, emotionally, or physically retreat. They may spend more and more time in their room, an environment they do control, and their interactions with peers or adults their own age can suffer. So think about it and have a frank discussion. There is not one answer to that question, and getting the right answer for you is paramount.

Summary

So that is it. At some point we are all going to need a little help.

With mobility in mind, I am reminded of the words of Charles Schulz, the creator of *Peanuts*, who once said, "Once you are over the hill, you pick up speed." The optimism in that seems inherent to your overall view of the world. Personally, I am by nature a tad pessimistic, which will make this a great lead-in to the next chapter.

CHAPTER 8

ABUSE AND SELF-PROTECTION

KEEPING YOUR GUARD UP

In April 1862 the reports from the scouting patrols had General George McClellan worried. He had, for the longest time, harbored a feeling that the reports of the Confederate troop numbers facing him were underestimated, and now what he was reading validated his concerns. On top of that he was a feeling a lot of pressure. President Lincoln was questioning almost every one of his decisions—from the reserve numbers he had left in defense of Washington to his resolve in advancing up the Virginia Peninsula. Even worse, Lincoln had been pressuring McClellan to attack, as he believed that the Confederate army that stood between the Union troops and Richmond to be of a much smaller force.

He was still considering the recent intelligence reports when a courier rode into the camp on a lathered horse at a dead run. The rider pulled back on the reins at the last minute, and his mount skidded to a hard stop right in front of the general. No matter what he might be about to report, the look on the young man's face told McClellan it wasn't going to be good.

"From General Keyes, sir," said the sweating soldier as he leaned out of the saddle with the dispatch.

McClellan took the sealed report and opened it. A second later his eyes widened.

"Is General Keyes sure about this?"

"Yes sir. I saw it myself," said the young rider. "Must be a hundred thousand of them, and they have artillery to match."

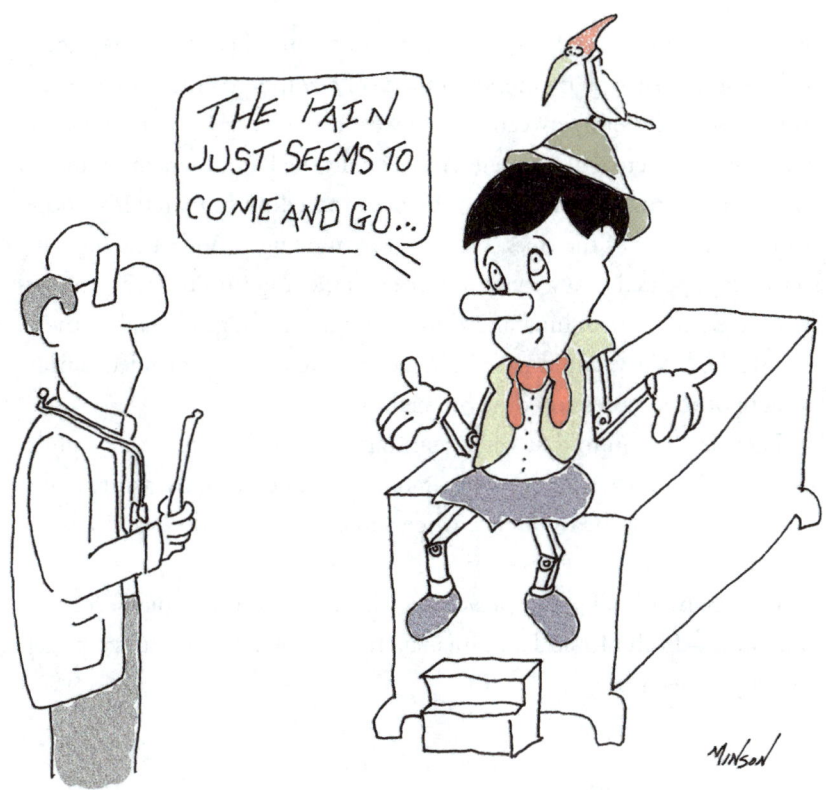

It was worse than McClellan had even imagined. The troops under Confederate general John Bankhead Magruder had massed on his right, and according to Keyes's dispatch, there had to be at least as many cannon as the Union army possessed.

He didn't care what the president or anyone else wanted him to do; this settled the matter for McClellan. Instantly he gave the order to entrench and fortify. The rider wheeled his horse, and a second later he was gone.

Unfortunately, McClellan was wrong.

He had been fooled, the victim of contrived production by a theatrical enthusiast. General Magruder had slightly more than 11,000 men and not even a third of the artillery they suspected. What he did have was imagination and a whole lot of thick woods. His own scouts had reported the massive Union army was slowly, haltingly coming up the peninsula. Days before, he had sent word to General Joe Johnston requesting reinforcements, and in the meantime, with only his small force between the oncoming army and Richmond, he had employed a tactical bluff, one of the greatest in military history. He cut down a number of the trees and had his soldiers shape them like cannons. They then painted them black and positioned them between his real weapons, giving the appearance of quadruple the actual armament. Additionally, he had others mounted on wheels and harnessed the caissons before proceeding to march his troops behind the cover of the trees, momentarily moving in and out of clearings so that it appeared that a massive force was moving into the area. In truth, they were simply marching and riding around in a huge circle, but the ruse worked. What could have been a complete rout was avoided simply because of the impression of invulnerability.

There is a lesson in that when you start to consider senior safety and security. The impression of invulnerability—and conversely, vulnerability—can make all the difference when someone is considering you as a potential victim.

This chapter is all about preventing abuse, by assuring your security and safety—both physical and financially—and where you can go to get help if you need it.

Safety and Security

A lot of my career has been involved in preparing populations for protection against catastrophic stuff. Think outbreaks, terrorism, hurricanes, earthquakes, plagues—real wrath of God stuff. In those settings I often hear the terms "safety" and "security" tossed around and sometimes used interchangeably. Well, that is not correct. They actually mean different things.

Both address the protection of lives, quality of life, and assets and the environment, but while safety is protection against hazards (accidents that are unintentional), security is a state of feeling protected against threats that are deliberate and intentional.

Make sense? Well, if not, try this. Despite the fact that weathermen are always yammering about "nature's fury," they know that *weather* is really just vectors of natural forces, energy encountering air masses. It's a lot like me standing on my porch watching ice creep up the driveway with a slow malevolent resolve. That sounds pretty, but it's really kind of goofy. It's ice for crying out loud, the same stuff I buy at the supermarket, and it hardly has emotion or resolve.

Or try this. I am housetraining a puppy, and what he leaves behind are piles of nature's fury. Ridiculous, right? The only fury is what I am feeling when I discover it.

Now, a person lobbing a hand grenade up the driveway over the approaching ice, mind you, is malevolent. If you recall the story about old Sam Whittemore, then you know that person is also, technically, a grenadier. See? Who says this book didn't teach you anything useful?

Anyway, the point I am making is that sometimes I will use the term safety in this chapter, and sometimes I will use the term security. They are different. It really has to do with the threat. And now you know the difference.

Now, pardon me while I get a poop bag and go scoop up the fury of nature.

Abuse of Seniors

Okay. Get ready for some bad news because, to be honest, this is a huge problem, and as a society we are not very well prepared to acknowledge, recognize, report, address, or correct this. The good news? In the last 10 years a lot of attention has been paid to qualifying the problem and its solution. Some of the solution is going to be in law, some in regulation, and some is purely political. Want more good news? You'll want to hang on to this because what is coming up after this point is pretty disheartening. The good news is that seniors, as I have pointed out before, are the biggest growing demographic in the United States. More than any ethnicity, political doctrine, or other social movement, it is age that defines the biggest growing demographic block. With that potential comes power and the ability to influence change with your representatives. When you read this next part, I think you'll have plenty of resolve to use it, if only out a sense of self-preservation.

The National Research Council defines elder abuse and mistreatment as "(a) intentional actions that cause harm or create a serious risk of harm to a vulnerable elder by a caregiver or other person who stands in a trust relationship to the elder, or (b) failure by a caregiver to satisfy the elder's basic needs or to protect the elder from harm."

According to the National Institute of Justice (NIJ), elder abuse cases tend to be multidimensional. Improving our understanding of the complexity of elder abuse cases can help researchers both develop and evaluate theory-based explanations for abuse. Recent research has shed some light on case characteristics common to different types of elder abuse.

Physical abuse. Contrary to common belief, many elderly victims of physical abuse are high-functioning. It's not the semiconscious senior, but someone just like us. The abuser is often a family member, in many cases the adult offspring of the victim. The abuser may also be a long-term dependent of the victim because of health or financial issues and may take out resentment for this dependence on the elderly victim. These victims are generally aware that they are being mistreated, but their sense of parental or family obligation makes them reluctant to cut off, report, or prosecute the abuser.

Neglect. In cases of elder neglect, the victim may be physically frail or cognitively vulnerable. The caregiver does not take adequate care of the victim, who may acknowledge his or her own shortcomings as a parent and conclude that the tables are being turned—and that he or she deserves no better.

Financial exploitation. Victims of financial exploitation often lack someone with whom they can discuss and monitor financial issues. They may have an emerging, unrecognized cognitive impairment; worry about a future loss of independence; and be overly trusting of a caregiver capable of theft, fraud, and misuse of assets.

Hybrid cases. Cases in which financial exploitation is combined with physical abuse or neglect typically involve financially dependent family members, particularly adult offspring, who have been cared for by the elderly person. As the elderly person declines in health and becomes more socially isolated, he or she relies more on the abuser for care, resulting in a mutual dependency. Such hybrid cases are unique in many ways and tend to have worse outcomes for victims than other kinds of elder abuse, perhaps because the abuse is accompanied by the stress of financial loss.

In 2003 the National Academies Press published *Elder Mistreatment: Abuse, Neglect, and Exploitation in an Aging America*. It defined elder mistreatment as "(a) intentional actions that cause harm or create a serious risk of harm (whether or not harm is intended) to a vulnerable elder by a caregiver or other person who stands in a trust relationship to the elder or (b) failure by a caregiver to satisfy the elder's basic needs or to protect the elder from harm. The term 'mistreatment' is meant to exclude cases of so-called self-neglect—failure of an older person to satisfy his or her own basic needs and to protect himself or herself from harm—and also cases involving victimization of elders by strangers."

The numbers behind this are alarming and disheartening, in part because so much of it is likely going unreported. In 2007 a study of over 7,000 community-residing seniors was conducted by NIJ, and the results were published in *The National Elder Mistreatment Study*. It estimated that approximately 1 in 10 elders have experienced at least one form of elder mistreatment in the past year. There's more.

- Eleven percent of elders reported experiencing at least one form of mistreatment—emotional, physical, sexual, or potential neglect—in the past year.
- Past-year prevalence was 5.1 percent for emotional mistreatment, 1.6 percent for physical mistreatment, 0.6 percent for sexual mistreatment, and 5.1 percent for potential neglect.
- Financial exploitation by a family member in the past year was reported by 5.2 percent of elders.

WARNING SIGNS

The risk of elder mistreatment is higher for individuals with the following characteristics: low household income, unemployed or retired, reporting poor health, having experienced a prior traumatic event, or reporting low levels of social support.

Financial Exploitation

According to the Department of Justice, surprisingly little is known about the financial exploitation of seniors in the United States, as these crimes are difficult to detect, definitions vary, and no national reporting mechanism exists. Such cases are often not reported at all. Adding to the problem, some victims of financial exploitation may be unaware of being exploited owing to cognitive disabilities or dementia. Likewise, dependence on the perpetrator for care or shelter, fear of retaliation, or fear of the loss of independence if their exploitation should become known keeps many elders from reporting financial abuse.

In 2009, 11 percent of older people responding to a phone survey reported experiencing at least one form of mistreatment—emotional, physical, or sexual. (The study did not include any individuals in residential care or with severe cognitive incapacity.) Financial exploitation by a family member was reported by 5.2 percent of older people in one year. Approximately 4.6 percent of adults over age 60 reported experiencing some form of emotional mistreatment in the past year, and only 8 percent of these individuals reported the event to the police.

Based on these results, it is estimated that for every one case of elder abuse, neglect, exploitation, or self-neglect reported to authorities, about five more go unreported.

By now you are probably asking, how is this possible? Well, there are some theories. The reports suggest that criminal justice researchers have generally paid little attention to elder abuse until only recently. As stated before, no uniform reporting system exists, and the available national incidence and prevalence data from administrative records are unreliable due to varying state definitions and reporting mechanisms. Research is still needed to determine the prevalence of elder abuse, neglect, and exploitation among elders with dementia and those residing in residential facilities, to identify risk factors for victimization, and to evaluate the efficacy of interventions.

This lack of research on the forensic aspects of elder mistreatment means that there are no forensic guidelines.

Now, I am no detective. Frankly, I don't even own a trench coat or a pair of gumshoed footwear, but I do know that without those established guidelines, investigations and more importantly prosecutions make it very difficult for law enforcement to proceed.

What I am is a doctor and, frankly, I am ashamed to admit that the medical community, which should have taken a stronger position by now, has not done a good job. At present, the medical community cannot easily distinguish between those types of injuries that indicate abuse or neglect and those that are the natural effects of illness or aging. Remember what I wrote earlier about geriatric specialists and the depressing ratio of caregivers to seniors? Speaking of depression, remember what I wrote about the numbers of geriatric psychiatrists being even worse? Well, after reading this chapter, my guess is you are going to go out and find one.

Anyway, since so few experts are available to testify in court and limited data exist to bolster cases brought into the system, little is often done.

- Advocate. This needs a national movement and the best way to accomplish that is by speaking with a strong voice. Senior advocacy groups, the AMA, commercial and non-governmental organizations will need to take on enterprises of social awareness in ways similar to child abuse awareness campaigns.
- Vote. Identify representatives and candidates who make senior abuse issues a part of their campaign platform. Those that don't better or you could allow them to find another avenue of social expression.

Nursing Home Abuse

One thing that is inevitable is that at some time we will all be vulnerable. Frankly, we all already have been. Unlike the baby crocodile, we don't pop out of the egg ready for aggression and battle. There are rumors among some that I did, but those saying that are lying. It's a well-known fact that I was a forceps delivery, so technically "they" started it first.

The difference is that as babies, we generally had someone looking out for us. Soon enough the day will come for most of us when we can't properly see to all of our needs, and we will be vulnerable again. Remember what I said about hazmat incidents and the buddy system? Well, keep that in mind as we get into the next section because this stuff is really scary.

WHAT YOU CAN DO

It is often tough to determine if a loved one is the victim of abuse, especially if he or she is heavily medicated, has difficulty communicating, or suffers from dementia. Table 11 lists a few things you can look for. If you find any of them, you need to investigate further.

You have rights, you know.

Table 11. Potential Markers to Identify Elder Mistreatment

Physical Condition and Quality of Care
Documented but untreated injuries
Undocumented injuries and fractures
Multiple, untreated, or undocumented pressure sores
Medical orders not followed
Poor oral care, poor hygiene, and lack of cleanliness of resident (e.g., unchanged adult diapers, untrimmed fingernails and toenails)
Malnourished residents that have no documentation for low weight
Bruising on nonambulatory residents; bruising in unusual locations
Statements and facts concerning poor care
Level of care for residents with nonattentive family members

Facility Characteristics
Unchanged linens
Strong odors (urine, feces)
Trash cans that have not been emptied
Food issues (cafeteria smells at all hours; food left on trays)
Past problems

Inconsistencies between
Medical records, statements made by staff members, or what is viewed by investigator
Statements given by different groups
The reported time of death and condition of the body

Staff Behaviors
Staff members who follow the investigator too closely
Lack of knowledge or concern about a resident
Evasiveness, both unintended and purposeful, verbal and nonverbal
Facility's unwillingness to release medical records

THE NURSING HOME REFORM ACT

During the 1980s, reports of nursing home abuse and neglect surfaced in alarming numbers. In an effort to reform nursing home practices and procedures and to set standards for the care rendered to residents of them, Congress passed the Nursing Home Reform Act of 1987. This law was incorporated into the Omnibus Budget Reconciliation Act (OBRA) of 1987, and everything was right with the world. These are both extremely sexy reads, by the way.

Actually, if you are a resident in a nursing home or have a loved one who is, it is important to be familiar with the rights provided by the Nursing

Home Reform Act. The law requires nursing homes to promote and protect the rights of each resident and places a strong emphasis on individual dignity and self-determination. In order to participate in Medicare or Medicaid, nursing homes must meet residents' rights requirements.

Required Resident Services

The Nursing Home Reform Act specifies what services nursing homes must give residents and establishes standards for these services. Required services include periodic assessments for each resident, a comprehensive care plan for each resident, provision of nursing services, social services, rehabilitation services, pharmaceutical services, dietary services, and, if the facility has more than 120 beds, the services of a full-time social worker.

Residents' Bill of Rights

The act is comprehensive and provides numerous rights. Among the more pertinent are these:

- The right to freedom from abuse, mistreatment, and neglect. This includes making independent decisions on clothing and spending free time, choosing your own activities inside and outside the nursing home, participating in a resident council, and selecting your own physician. The nursing home must make reasonable accommodations of a resident's needs and preferences.
- The right to dignity, respect, and freedom from physical restraints. You have the right to be free from abuse, both mental and physical, corporal punishment, involuntary seclusion, and physical and chemical restraints. You also have the right to self-determination.
- The right to privacy. This includes private and unrestricted communication with persons of your choice, private treatment and care of personal needs, and confidentiality regarding medical, personal, and financial affairs.
- The right to accommodation of medical, physical, psychological, and social needs.
- The right to security of possessions. This includes managing your own financial affairs and not being charged for services

covered by Medicare and Medicaid. You have the right to file a complaint if the nursing home is managing your financial affairs in an abusive, neglectful, or inappropriate way.

- You have the right to participate in the review of one's care plan and to be fully informed in advance about any changes in care, treatment, or change of status in the facility.
- The right to voice grievances without discrimination or reprisal. This includes the right to review your medical record and to object if you find something incorrect.
- The right to visits from your personal physician, representatives from the health department and ombudsman programs, and your relatives. All nursing home residents also have the right to reasonable visits by organizations or individuals providing health, social, legal, or other services.
- Residents have rights during transfers and discharges (including the right to a 30-day notice and a safe transfer or discharge with sufficient preparation by the nursing home. Residents also have a right to remain in the nursing facility unless the transfer or discharge is deemed necessary to meet the resident's welfare, required to protect other residents and staff, or a facility charge has not been provided after reasonable notice.

Sounds like I am Mirandizing a little, I know. There's more. The full list of resident rights is provided in 42 C.F.R. §483.10 (http://www.gpo.gov/fdsys/granule/CFR-2011-title42-v015/CFR-2011-title42-v015-sec483–10/content-detail.html).

Restraints: Chemical and Physical

If you walked into an establishment or a private home and found a 15-year-old girl chained, tied, or lashed to a bed or imprisoned in a crawl space, more than likely you would be alarmed and would probably call the authorities to investigate, right? Yet if you walked into a nursing home or even an assisted living setting and you saw an 80-year-old woman like that, would you feel the same way? Would you react the same way? If not, why not?

Now, I'm not picking on you, but therein is the issue, even for some professionals in law enforcement and medicine. It's a subtle form of age-ism, and it facilitates some really bad behaviors.

Now try this one on for size. You walk into a house and see a 15-year-old girl lying on a bed, her head back, eyes almost rolling white, with dried saliva around her mouth. Alarmed? If she were 80, would you have the same reaction?

That scenario actually illustrates the danger with "chemical restraint." Chemical restraint is the use of legal drugs, often by healthcare providers, to render a subject (often known as their patient) controllable. It's actually a fairly common practice, and it is spreading, and not just in the long-term-care environment. Many in the emergency care arena and even in the prehospital setting use it. Now to be fair, it has its place: if the individual is combative and dangerous, the judicious and *temporary* use by an objective, well-trained, licensed physician who "knows" the patient is appropriate. Unfortunately, that is not always the case. Sometimes "chemical restraint" is administered due to staff or provider laziness, to facilitate control, to reduce the irritation of a demanding patient or out of a poor diagnostic ability to recognize a problem by the provider. In those cases it really constitutes a potential assault.

So how do you know and what can you do?

Well, if you are the one being chemically controlled, not much.

This advice really is more for the loved one, advocate, or friend of a senior. If you see a sudden change in cognition, make sure that a physician consultation *of your choosing* takes place.

WHAT YOU CAN DO

Ask specifically for a "medical chart review," again by the healthcare professional of your choice. If you hold the power of attorney or guardianship, you have the same proxy rights for the affected individual's right and may well be the only person advocating on his or her behalf.

Certification

To monitor whether nursing homes meet the Nursing Home Reform Act requirements, the law also established a certification process that requires states to conduct unannounced surveys, including resident interviews, at irregular intervals at least once every 15 months. The federal government did not issue regulations to implement the new survey process until 1995. The surveys generally focus on residents' rights, quality of care, quality of life, and the services provided to residents. Surveyors also conduct more targeted surveys, or complaint investigations, in response to complaints against nursing homes. It is also discoverable, so if you are considering a certain nursing home, query your state department of aging to get the facts.

If the survey reveals that a nursing home is out of compliance, the Nursing Home Reform Act enforcement process begins. The severity of the remedy depends on whether the deficiency puts a resident in immediate jeopardy and whether the deficiency is an isolated incident, part of a pattern, or widespread throughout the facility. For some violations, nursing homes have an opportunity to correct the deficiency before remedies may be imposed. Any or all of the following sanctions can be imposed to enforce compliance with the Nursing Home Reform Act:

- Directed in-service training of staff
- Directed plan of correction
- State monitoring
- Civil monetary penalties
- Denial of payment for all new Medicare or Medicaid admissions
- Denial of payment for all Medicaid or Medicare patients
- Temporary management
- Termination of the provider agreement

Finally, this is again a starting point. More comprehensive reading can be found in the act itself. Enforcement issues are also addressed in the AARP Public Policy Institute's fact sheet, "Federal and State Enforcement of the 1987 Nursing Home Reform Act."*

*www.aarp.org/home-garden/liveable-communities/info-2001/federal_and_state_enforcement_of_the_1987_nursing_home_reform_act.html

Who Regulates the Personnel and the Nursing Home?

There are many agencies involved, and regulation does not just apply to the nursing home. It is also the licensure or certification of the people who may be providing support and care. Some of the governing agencies are federal, and some are run by your state. As I described in my first book, most healthcare or care providers are regulated by state agencies or boards.

In a more general sense, I am offering the following as a starting point:

State Boards of Nursing. The Board of Nursing is a state agency that oversees the nursing profession. Nurses must be licensed to practice their profession, and that licensing is provided separately by each state. The Board of Nursing creates and administers the exam that must be passed for a license. It also sets other standards that nurses must meet to get a license and to renew it. Most states require license renewal every two years, and many require nurses to complete continuing education courses to keep their license active. The board also approves courses that will qualify to meet the continuing education requirement. It is also the agency that certifies schools that train the entry-level licensed practical nurses. State boards also set ethical standards for nurses and take action when those standards are violated.

US Department of Health and Human Services (HHS). HHS is the federal agency designed to protect the health of all American citizens. Programs like Medicare and Medicaid provide health insurance for a large number of people, and through the allocation of funds to pay medical fees, they have a significant impact on the type of care that nurses can provide. HHS is responsible for administering a number of federal laws that have an impact on nursing practices. The Health Insurance Portability and Accountability Act, which protects patient information, is one of those laws, and HHS issues guidelines to help nurses abide by this law. The department also has established health information technology standards that apply to the nursing and medical professions.

State Boards of Physicians and Surgeons or Medical Boards. State medical boards govern physician licensure and make certain that they have maintained appropriate levels of continuing education to keep their credentials. An MD or DO degree is conferred by a medical university, but the ability to practice medicine depends on the maintenance of an active license. These Boards also investigate and act on complaints and address misbehavior. This is different than board certification, which is endowed by a medical specialty organization. Ideally a physician has licensure (required) and board certification (not always required).

US Department of Labor. The Labor Department is another federal agency that plays a role in the practice of providers. It enforces laws that deal with workers' rights as they relate to all sorts of issues, including health care. Some of the department's regulations mandate conditions that must be covered and the types of coverage that must be provided. These regulations include the laws that guarantee people the right to continuing insurance and portability once they leave a job. Since the Labor Department monitors insurance coverage, it has an impact on the medical decisions with which providers are involved.

For more specific information, you will need to contact your state department of health.

Who Is on Your Side?

There are some strong institutions for advocacy for nursing home patients and residents. I have listed a few as follows:

LeadingAge (formerly American Association of Homes and Services for the Aging). LeadingAge seeks to help individuals and their families through its member not-for-profit organizations. There are currently 5,700 member organizations, providing services ranging from adult day care, home health, community services, senior housing, assisted-living residences, and nursing homes. More information can be found at http://www.leadingage.org/.

National Consumer Voice for Quality Long-Term Care (formerly National Citizen's Coalition for Nursing Home Reform). Formed in 1975, the National Consumer Voice for Quality Long-Term Care endeavors to address such issues as inadequate staffing in nursing homes, poor working conditions, maintenance of residents' rights and empowerment of residents, support for family members, and the results of poor care, such as pressure sores, dehydration, incontinence, and contracture of residents' muscles. Local resources, listed by state, can be found at http://theconsumervoice.org/get_help.

Administration on Aging (AoA). Part of the US Department of Health and Human Services, the AoA (http://www.aoa.gov/) has been given the mission of helping elderly individuals "maintain their dignity and independence in their homes and communities through comprehensive, coordinated, and cost effective systems of long-term care, and livable communities across the U.S." One of the programs managed by the AoA is the Long-Term Care Ombudsman Program, which helps fund and train ombudsmen at the state level to serve as advocates for nursing home patients. To find the ombudsman office for your state, go to the website for the National Long-Term Care Ombudsman Resource Center (http://ltcombudsman.org/).

Home Care Attendant Abuse

This is another potentially dangerous area. Many of the people providing home-based care in many places are unregulated. In general, if you can afford to, don't hire unregulated workers, regardless of their credentials and experience. Here are some steps you will want to take.

First, find out if they have some professional credential and determine who regulates them. Technically, in many instances, it's no one.

If they have a professional license, then it will be the respective state board. If they do not, or if they are what is often called "personal care workers in health services" or "unlicensed assistive personnel," there may be no licensure, credential, or regulatory oversight at all. In cases like that, you will want to initiate some background checking of your own like the Better Business Bureau (BBB), criminal records, and more.

CERTIFIED NURSE ASSISTANTS

Certified Nurse Assistant (CNA) credentialing is established by a state. In general, CNAs must pass an accredited course, pass that state's respective CNA exam, pass a practical exam that will monitor the ability to perform basic CNA activities, and have a certain amount of on-duty experience while under supervision, although the amount may vary. They will then have to register within the state in which the exams were performed.

GERIATRIC CARE MANAGERS

You can find geriatric care managers in the phone book or online, usually under listings for social workers, nurses, eldercare, or home health care. Because this service is essentially an unregulated industry, you need to check the prospective geriatric care manager's references, certification, licensure, and experience. Look for individuals who have received certification in the geriatric care management field. There are three basic kinds of certification:

- Care Manager Certified (CMC), awarded by the National Academy of Certified Care Managers
- Certified Case Manager (CCM), given by the Commission for Case Manager Certification
- Certified Advanced Social Worker in Case Management (C-ASWCM) or Certified Social Work Case Manager (C-SWCM), certifications awarded by the National Association of Social Workers (NASW) for *licensed* social workers

---

WHAT YOU CAN DO

First check with your state or local Agency on Aging to determine what the laws are in your state.

You or your loved one probably want to stay in his or her home as long as possible, but he or she could use help with everyday activities. One option is to find someone through an agency. Another is to hire someone yourself. That has risk as I mentioned before.

Finding Candidates

First go watch a rerun of *Whatever Happened to Baby Jane?* That is exactly what you don't want.

- Ask friends, neighbors, co-workers, or other caregivers you know for referrals.
- Post a bulletin board ad at your place of worship, the library, a local recreation center, or at a nearby senior center, adult day center, or hospital.
- Look into a job placement program at a college that has a social work program.
- Run an ad in the newspaper or on a local website. Your ad should describe the job and its duties. Include a phone number or e-mail address, but don't give out your name or other personal information.

Considering Applicants

- Write a detailed job description that you can share with applicants. Include all the tasks you will require, the hours and days of the job, and personal preferences with regard to driving and other transportation options. Also jot down questions you will want to ask to get a sense of the applicants' personality.
- Decide how much you're prepared to pay. If you hire someone directly, you need to look into how you will pay taxes and possibly a Social Security contribution. Check with the Internal Revenue Service for proper tax forms and instructions. For details, see the IRS publications "Hiring Household Employees" (http://www.irs.gov/Businesses/Small-Businesses-%26-Self-Employed/Hiring-Household-Employees) and "Independent Contractor (Self-Employed) or Employee?"(http://www.irs.gov/Businesses/Small-Businesses-%26-Self-Employed/Independent-Contractor-Self-Employed-or-Employee).
- Conduct the initial interview by phone. Ask about work experience, hours of availability, driving experience, and special training with a condition such as Alzheimer's disease.

Conducting an Interview

Ask job candidates to bring a résumé or job history as well as names and telephone numbers for at least two references. If this is for someone you love, make sure your loved one participates in the interview if possible or at least has the opportunity to meet anyone you would like to hire. Describe to applicants your loved one's needs, health concerns, and likes and dislikes. Outline the duties you expect him or her to perform. Be friendly but professional. Stick to questions that will help you determine if this person is a good match for the job—and for your loved one. Make sure to get the person's name, address, telephone number, and Social Security number. Don't be afraid to ask for proof of identity, ideally a Social Security card. If not available, ask to see a driver's license or other photo ID.

You can also ask if he or she has ever been in trouble with the law. Check that—there are hundreds of services where a background check can be performed. Ask if any professional complaints have been lodged. Again, also check with the Better Business Bureau. Find out if he or she has any special training, such as working with clients who have dementia or other conditions. Also ask about his or her work history, including why he or she left the former job. Ask about his or her expectations of this position and why he or she is working in the home care field. Invite the candidate to ask questions about the job and your expectations. Give honest answers. Be clear about salary and benefits, such as vacation and other time off. Head off any misunderstandings by addressing these issues directly.

Checking References

Always call references. A reference can confirm your feelings about a person or give you important information that you missed. If it's a former employer, ask about the candidate's punctuality and attendance as well as the precise nature of his or her work. Find out why the applicant left the position and whether there were any problems. Take notes on each applicant so you can refer to them when making your decision.

I said it before. I'll say it again. Get a *criminal* background check. I mentioned numerous sites, but you can also contact your local law enforcement agency to find out how to do this.

Have a probationary period for the candidate, a one-month trial period before you commit to hiring him or her permanently.

I have a friend who thought this was a good idea for newlyweds, but based on how that went over, I cannot completely endorse that. Explain that this would be an opportunity to see if this is a mutually acceptable arrangement.

Once someone accepts your job offer, put your entire agreement in writing. Include information about the trial period, job duties, salary, pay schedule, time off, start date, and termination policy. Keep copies of this job contract signed by both of you.

For children of seniors, try to be at your loved one's house for the first few days to familiarize the new caregiver with the routine.

HOW TO STAY ON TOP OF THE SITUATION

Conduct unannounced drop-in visits. This is a good rule whether your loved one is in a skilled nursing facility, a nursing home, an assisted living center, or getting home care and assistance. I also like using email, texts, and even video teleconferencing (VTC) to stay abreast. VTC is extremely valuable in that it reveals all the nonverbal cues about how things are going. I don't want to sound overly paranoid, but also consider installation of nanny cams. They are surprisingly affordable and they add a layer of assurance.

Otherwise, in general, you might want to also look for things that signal a decrease in thinking skills or vision and /or the inability to be physically active. Then engage your healthcare provider to assure that the cause is a legitimate one and not the result of clandestine activity. There are other cues that something may be wrong.

Around the House

Is the house more unkempt than usual? In the kitchen, do you see scorched pots and pans? If household bills are piling up and mail is left unopened, it could be a sign that the simple tasks of writing bills, balancing a checkbook, and keeping track of due dates is becoming overwhelming.

In the Fridge

Is the refrigerator well stocked with fresh produce and meats? Do you notice lots of moldy, expired food products? These could be signs that your aging parents are becoming malnourished, especially if they also appear to have lost weight and have little interest in food. Poor diet can exacerbate chronic diseases, lead to a weakened immune system, and increase the risk of dementia.

In the Medicine Cabinet

Is a loved one taking more medications? Are expired pill bottles mixed in with current ones? Are the pills organized to prevent taking the wrong dose or too many? Do they have trouble holding a coherent conversation, often repeating the same story?

Frankly, I do that now, so I have no idea what kind of indicator that will be for me in the future.

Additionally, dizziness, confusion, and signs of dementia can be caused by medications or taking the wrong combination of drugs.

In Their Social Life

When was the last time your parents went out with friends or out to dinner? Do they still do the things they used to enjoy? If you find them reluctant to leave the house, it could be a sign that they're having a hard time driving, moving about, and seeing or hearing, and so they'd rather stay home. This could eventually lead to social isolation, and eventually, loneliness and depression. Try to find out what's causing them to disengage.

Outside the Home

If your loved one is still driving, have them drive you somewhere so that you can assess their driving skills. It's especially important to do this if you notice dents or scratches on their car or if they've recently received speeding or traffic tickets.

Fraud and Electronic Theft

Sadly, many older Americans are the targets of a variety of scams or fraud. Some of the easiest mechanisms for thieves is via information on medical bills, health care documents, and prescriptions. Here are some common scams that target seniors:

Phishing. This is the attempt to acquire sensitive information, such as

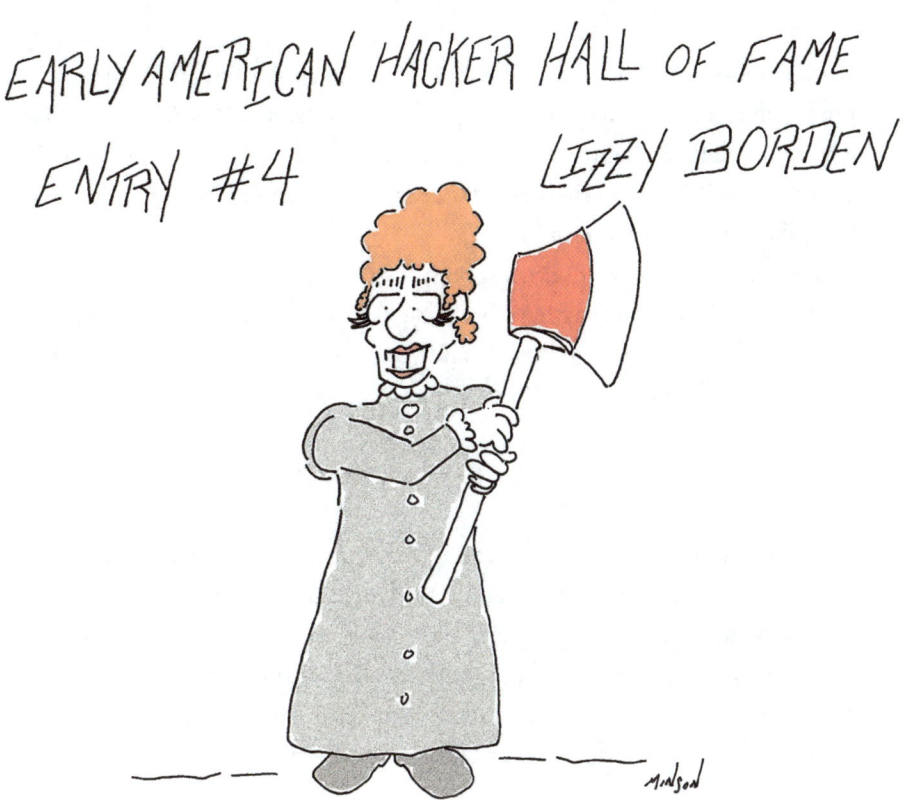

EARLY AMERICAN HACKER HALL OF FAME
ENTRY #4   LIZZY BORDEN

user names, passwords, and credit card details (and sometimes, indirectly, money) by masquerading as a trustworthy entity in an electronic communication. This usually involves a fake web address, but the "page" looks like the real thing. The key thing here is that the scammers generally suggest they are trying to protect as you have already had a scam applied and they want to assure your information.

To protect yourself, always look at the web address. If it looks odd, don't respond. Call your credit card account or bank first to confirm.

Phone scams. These are just what they sound like. Someone calls you asking if you want to donate to a worthy cause or masquerading as a credit protection resource. They just need to confirm some information.

To protect yourself, get their name and number and then call *them* back. In the meantime you can contact your bank, account, or credit card company, or whoever they say they represent, and work it that way.

Hacking. This is basically an Internet break-in. There are whole books written about this. Suffice it to say here that you should invest in some firewall and malware detection and prevention software. If you get an email, especially one requiring *emergency action*, don't react. Contact the organization if it is a service provider or retailer or service, independent from the communication online.

There are a number of services, both for-profit and nonprofit, that can help. If you think you may have been the victim of identity theft, contact your local law enforcement agency and your credit card or insurance companies immediately.

SENIOR CRIMESTOPPERS

There are a bunch of programs bearing this name, the Senior Crimestoppers Program. Some are supported by the banking industry, some by law enforcement. One private program is a collaboration between the banking industry and some federal programs. AARP routinely devotes a great deal of attention to this subject. I like to explain online fraud, scams, and crime, especially identity theft, as a lot like antibiotic therapy applied to bacteria.

Bacteria often develop resistance to antibiotics, and so new medications have to be developed. In a way it is like biological one-upmanship is always going on. Cybercrime and fraudulent scams are a lot like that. You buy anti-malware programs and they develop something new. You buy the antidote to that and they create something else... and on and on it goes. Just remember, offers and programs, charitable enterprises, and appeals for help all can be fronts for attempts to get your information for exploitation.

Oh, and if a member of the Nigerian royal family sends you an email asking for your help in moving millions out of the country . . . don't answer it.

WHAT YOU CAN DO

First, be skeptical.

A deal that sounds too good to be true usually is! Be wary of promises to fix your credit problems, low-interest credit card offers, deals that let you skip credit card payments, work-at-home job opportunities, risk-free investments, and free travel. Don't share personal information with some-one you don't trust. Beware of payday and tax refund loans. Interest rates on these loans are usually excessive. Sometimes you will be asked to enter into legitimate agreements online. While the intent may not be criminal, the risk potential may still be there.

Read and understand any contract, legal document, or terms of ser-vice before you sign or click "I Agree." Do not sign a contract with blank spaces or where the terms are incomplete. Some contracts include a clause that prohibits you from taking legal action and require you to engage in mandatory arbitration with a company in the case of a dispute. Get estimates from several contractors for things like home or car repairs. Make sure the estimates are for the exact same repairs or objectives for a fair comparison. Before you buy anything, make sure you understand and accept the store's refund, return, and early termination/cancellation policies, especially for services that charge monthly fees. When paying for your purchases, double-check the final price. If you think the price that has been charged is incorrect, speak up. Remember, when shopping online, your purchase may include additional fees, such as shipping, han-dling, and convenience fees that are not calculated until you check out. When shopping online, look for the padlock icon in the bottom right-hand corner of your screen or a URL that begins with "https" to ensure that your payment information is transmitted securely. Don't buy under stress. Avoid making big-ticket purchases during times of duress (e.g., coping with a death or debt). If you are having difficulty making pay-ments on loans, notify your lender immediately so that you can work out a payment plan.

Check your bank accounts and bill statements carefully. You can check them online so you can zoom in easily in case you need to make the state-ment larger for easier reading. If you notice unauthorized charges, alert your bank immediately. Do not give your personal information, such as bank account numbers or PINs, to anyone in a phone call, letter, email, fax, or text message.

It is not an option for everyone, but if you have means, set aside some emergency funds (cash) to support yourself and your immediate family for at least six months in case of an emergency. Your banker can help with this. Finally, always get someone you trust to advise you on a financial enterprise.

A second set of objective, *competent*, advocating eyes never hurts.

Oh, and take a lesson from the fine folks at Enron. Remember them? Who could forget, right? Well, if nothing else, they did teach us that having a good shredder is really a good idea.

I'm still working on an after-school special song for shredding personal financial hard copies and bills.

Maybe, "I'm just a bill, yes, I'm only a bill . . . and I get shredded sometimes just for the thrill . . . ? No?

Physical Crime and Safety

Remember John Magruder, the great military faker? Well, here is where his lesson will really apply. How you appear can make all the difference in how a criminal perceives you as a target.

Generally, unless you have a longstanding feud going on, physical crime against seniors is usually about burglary or theft. They want what you have. This is actually known as property crime. Property crime is any crime when money or valuables are damaged or stolen from a person, home, or business without direct personal contact. This includes burglary from a business or residence and auto theft. Victims of property crimes suffer financial losses and may feel violated and continue to feel unsafe thereafter.

MORE THINGS YOU CAN DO

Security Systems

Get a security system. There are many types. The most common is one that allows for some lock integrity that, if breached (think break-in), sets off alarms—either audibly or silently—and that usually triggers a signal to police or a private security center.

It's a lot like a medic alert system that most seniors already know about. The difference obviously is that you activate the medical alert system via a wearable device that patches through to a call center. There are also some systems that incorporate a security or law enforcement component as well. Of course, the vulnerability is that you as the user have to activate the system. If someone breaks in and removes it before you can initiate the alert, well, you get the idea.

Surveillance Systems

These may or may not include other aspects of security systems.

Surveillance systems are just that—electronic video feeds that load to a computer system. It may be hardwired directly, but more and more are becoming purely wireless technologies. A pure surveillance system does not have any built-in alert. Granted, they are kind of expensive, but many are not, and if your children, friends, or loved ones are distant, the video may be transmittable by computer link so they can also check on you.

Now what I am going to relate is not something I recommend, but the story I am about to tell is true. I have an older friend. She is the one that told me about John Bankhead Magruder. She also has a home security system, or so I thought. Everywhere around her home are signs showing the system she uses. There are stickers on her windows with the company's logo. In fact, she even has a small yard placard.

It wasn't until I started researching this book that I learned that she actually doesn't have a system at all. She had just ordered the signage off the Internet. We had a long, long talk when I learned this, and she has actually gotten one since then, but she had for the longest time been pulling a Magruder. She also pointed out that the appearance of invulnerability was as effective a tool at times as the ability to enforce such appearances. In a way she is correct, but if you can afford it, please don't gamble.

Medical Alerts

Most people have heard of these. The television is overwhelmed with advertisements proposing the risks of falls with no communications leading to prolonged agony or even death. I am in favor of preventing that, both the fall and the prolonged agony and death. A medical alert bracelet, amulet, pendant, hairpiece—something—can actually mean the difference in life or death.

Additionally, many such devices now incorporate an all-hazards, two-way response via a dispatcher/service center through the device. That said, I am still in favor of having a security system as well. As I mentioned earlier, if the activation of a response relies on your hitting the button, then a home invasion or break-in may not allow you the time, awareness, or capacity to do it. Door triggers or alarms work even if you are asleep or unable to get to the alert yourself.

Need I even bring this up? Have them. Make sure they work and that the batteries are fresh. If you are not up to physically doing this yourself, ask your local fire department to help. They'll be happy to.

CONFRONTATIONAL SITUATIONS

If you are confronted by someone who tries to rob you, you have two choices: fight or give them the stuff they want to steal. My suggestion?

Give it to them if it is a matter of life and death. Now that does not mean that you should advertise or make it easy for them.

WHAT YOU CAN DO

In a car or a house, always lock doors and close or roll up the windows. Stay alert and check the surroundings constantly.

Secure your car, even if you are parked in your driveway or leaving the car for just a minute. This can be enough to discourage many would-be auto thieves. Before you get out, check the car and the area around it. Most law enforcement agencies and insurance companies recommend you consider installing tracking or security devices on your car as well.

Take part in car theft prevention programs that allow police officers to stop your car if it's being driven during hours when you don't normally drive. Many senior communities have this program.

SHOPPING TIPS

When shopping, empty wallets and purses beforehand of items you won't need. Keep packages out of sight in the car trunk.

Do not walk with your arms full of bundles that limit your line of sight or ability to respond. Keep your wallet in a front pants pocket or inside your coat pocket. Keep purses closed and held snugly near your body. Keep all receipts separate from purchases. That way, if someone steals your goods, you will have the receipts to show what was stolen and to provide for insurance purposes.

AT HOME

At home, set up timed lights and have a trusted neighbor pick up mail and newspapers while you are away. Make sure your windows and house number are visible from the street. Illuminate doorways and walkways. Trim shrubs. Ask the police department to perform a security survey.

SOME GOOD NEWS?

According to the Bureau of Justice Statistics, seniors experience the lowest number of victimizations and the lowest rates of victimizations when compared with the general population.

The violent victimization rate of seniors has declined by more than 22 percent since 2001.

The bad news? It's still an issue.

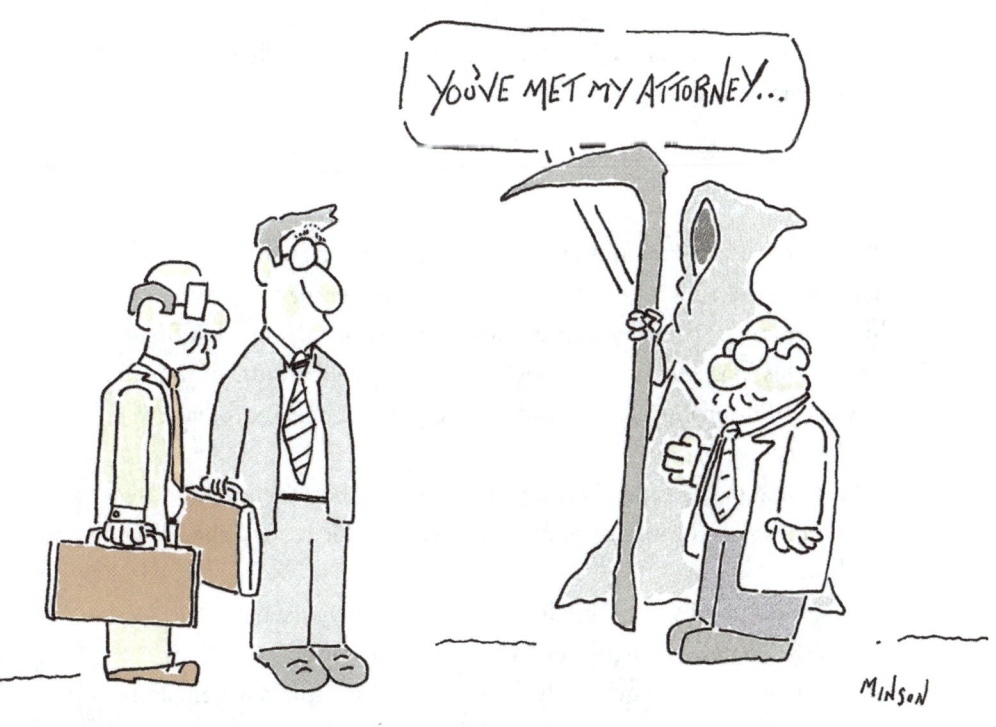

To avoid becoming a violent crime statistic, walk assertively, but not aggressively. Carry only the cash and/or credit cards that are immediately needed. Don't take shortcuts through deserted or dark areas. Stay where there are lights and people. When going outside, go with a friend if possible. When traveling, check with hotel staff about areas that should be avoided.

Remember what I said earlier? If you're confronted by a robber, hand over your money or valuables. They're not worth your life.

A Word about Social Media

I like social media, but unfortunately it is a bonanza for criminals. If you post that you are off to Aruba for Christmas and you won't have computer access for two weeks to gloat, the joke may well be on you. When you get back, your house may look like the second act of *How the Grinch Stole Christmas*. All you may find is a weird little girl with antenna sticking out of her head named Cindy Lou, wondering what the heck. Have no idea what I am talking about? Haven't seen it? Where have you been? Oh yeah, right, Aruba! I read that on your profile.

Anyway, with social media, less is often more. Especially with the bathing suit shots.

Safety

Okay, so this is about common unintended hazards. There is a ton of material on this subject available. That said, I am going to go over some things you might consider to prevent injury and or calamity. I addressed some of this in the discussion about your physical environment, but there are some additional general considerations you might want to have in mind.

According to the Federal Emergency Management Agency, here are some things a senior might want to have in terms of a safety checklist.

- Consider having a medical alert or a buddy system.
- Keep a fire extinguisher and smoke detector on every floor.
- Use extreme caution when smoking. Never smoke when alone or in bed. Better yet, don't smoke at all!

- Always get up slowly after sitting or lying down. Take your time, and make sure you have your balance.
- Wear properly fitting shoes with low heels.
- Use a correctly measured walking aid.
- Remove or tack down all scatter rugs.
- Remove electrical or telephone cords from traffic areas.
- Avoid using slippery wax on floors.
- Wipe up spills promptly.
- Avoid standing on ladders or chairs. Remember Franklin's reaching tool? Well, they still make and sell those.
- Have sturdy rails for all stairs inside and outside the house or, if necessary, purchase a stair lift.
- Use only nonglare 100-watt (or greater) incandescent bulbs (or the fluorescent equivalents).
- Make sure that all stair cases have good lighting with switches at top and bottom.
- Staircase steps should have a nonslip surface.
- Use night lights for floor and surface illumination.
- Use recommended bath aids, securely installed on the walls of the bath/shower stall and on the sides of the toilet.
- Skid-proof the tub and make sure the bath mat has a nonslip bottom.
- To avoid scalds, turn the water heater to 120 degrees Fahrenheit or below.
- Mark cold and hot faucets clearly.
- Use door locks that can be opened from both sides.
- If possible, bathe only when help is available.

IN THE KITCHEN
- Store sharp knives in a rack.
- Use a kettle with an automatic shutoff.
- Store heavier objects at waist level.
- Store hazardous items separate from food.
- Avoid wearing long, loose clothing when cooking over the stove.
- Make sure food is rotated regularly. Check expiration dates.

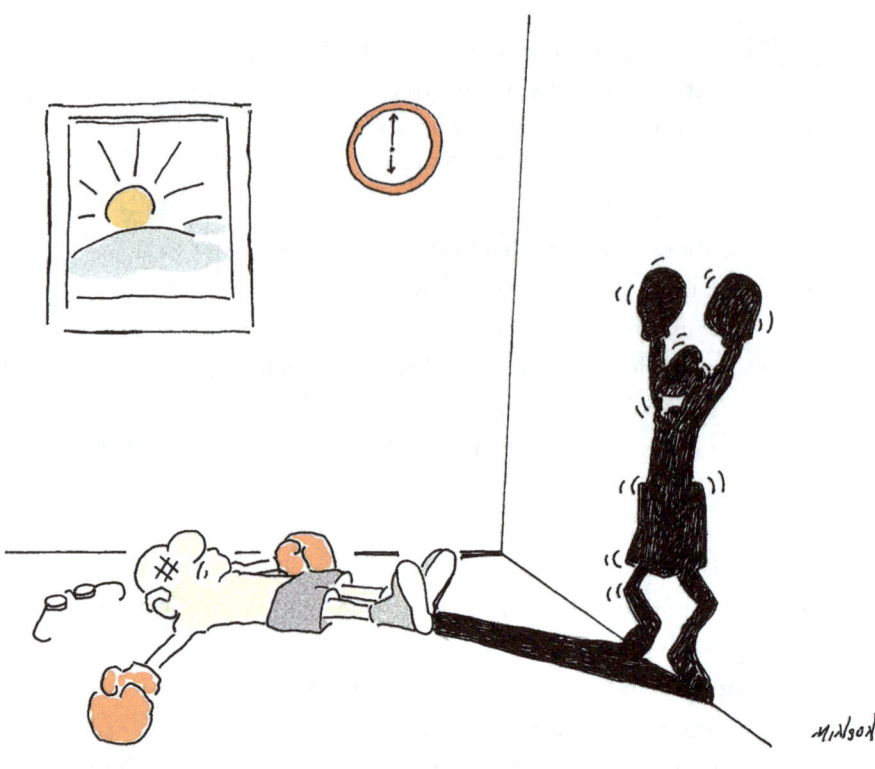

Summary

So there is a lot of heavy stuff in this chapter, I know, but before I close it out, I have an anecdote that I think illustrates the last thing I want to share.

Most people don't know that I had a very brief "career" as a light heavyweight boxer. It was slightly under three months, in fact, but it was highly instructive. Mostly what it taught me was that I had no business being a boxer.

I really didn't even look the part. I was six-three and weighed a 177 pounds. Most of it was in my thighs. I had been a distance runner, so I looked like some kind of living R. Crumb character or spindly new growth coming out of an old tree stump. This actually wasn't as bad as it seems. I had extremely long arms and was deceptively strong for being so spare-looking. In boxing the power to punch doesn't reside in the arms. Like a home-run batter, the power is a whole-body thing. The legs and hips play a huge role. So I looked like that. Most opponents simply thought they could wade in and clobber me. For three whole fights, I used that. I'd sting with a long ropy jab and then when they became frustrated, they would get mad or charge. Then it would happen. I'd crank a tight right uppercut and they would go down.

I learned a couple of things from that. My trainer was an odd old guy who would sometimes really hit me with a flyswatter as I was working the bag to "improve my concentration." Frankly, I think he had come from the how-to-train-your-cat school of boxing, but anyway, he liked to tell me that no matter what happened in a match, I couldn't lose my temper.

Since I was winning, I couldn't really argue, but then something happened. I gained three pounds. Suddenly I was no longer a light heavyweight. I was a heavyweight, which meant I could now fight against people of unlimited size. You can imagine how this worked out.

My one and only heavyweight match was with a guy named Rendell Ledbetter. He was a college football player and a legitimately skilled boxer. He was also 221 pounds. I started the match with the usual optimism that accompanies dreams borne of movies like *Rocky* or *Rudy*, and I went in thinking, "Stay with my skills, keep my objectivity, and I can do this."

It was pretty much a big fat lie.

I jabbed, and at first he even looked a tad impressed. A few seconds later, however, he waded past it. It was just what I was waiting for. I uncranked old faithful, the devastating right uppercut, and it landed, but to my surprise, instead of seeing that slight shocked expression followed by the drop, Rendell just seemed to sort of blink.

It went downhill from there quickly. I made it through the first round and got back to my corner in pretty rugged shape. My trainer looked at the angry expression on my shocked, bruised face and said, "What? It's a fist fight. You were expecting maybe a hug?"

The second round I don't remember at all. I am told that for some reason I kept swinging, unconsciously, admittedly, but I didn't go down. To his credit, my trainer threw in the towel—I suppose to spare me from a life of mandatory nutrition by milkshakes and children's puzzles.

I learned two things from this. I had no business boxing, and when you are in a fight like that, try to keep your objectivity. Also, when it comes to your safety and security, the best thing you can have in your corner is a buddy looking out for you, a plan, and tactical objectivity, also known as a cool head.

To that end, here's a website with a really nice tool that can give you a lot of state-specific resources so you can explore how to assess your safety and security: http://www.ncea.aoa.gov/Stop_Abuse/Get_Help/State/index.aspx.

Good luck.

The Pursuit of Happiness

Look at me, I am old, but I'm happy.

Yusuf Islam (formerly known as Cat Stevens)

If you've ever seen the movie *Dead Poets Society,* you may remember the scene where the boys are reading aloud from their textbooks by J. Evans Prichard, describing how to judge "poetry" by plotting a graph with the score for perfection on the horizontal axis and importance on the vertical. The calculated total area of the poem yielded the measure of the poem's greatness.

This is perfectly summated by Robin Williams's character with one word: "Excrement."

To try to define, quantify, or characterize happiness would be an equally dopey act on my part. So I won't.

Even the Founding Fathers, who went out on a limb with specifics in a lot of other areas, didn't elaborate on what they meant by the phrase "pursuit of happiness," and the ensuing arguments about it have constituted Americans' favorite parlor game ever since.

Oh, I know that the historical progression of the term comes, for many, from an English treatise by John Locke equating property and prosperity, as inherent to a material basis of independence and happiness.

Others claim that Jefferson's intent was more along the lines of Adam Ferguson's *An Essay on the History of Civil Society* which states:

> If, in reality, courage and a heart devoted to the good of mankind are the constituents of human felicity, the kindness which is done infers a happiness in the person from whom it proceeds, not in him on whom it is bestowed; and the greatest good which men possessed of fortitude and generosity can procure to their fellow creatures is a participation of this happy character. If this be the good of the individual, it is likewise that of mankind; and virtue no longer imposes a task by which we are obliged to bestow upon others that good from which we ourselves refrain; but supposes, in the highest degree, as possessed by ourselves, that state of felicity which we are required to promote in the world.

I think that *is* probably closer to what Jefferson was thinking and that the Constitutional Convention's Committee of Detail, or "Committee of Five," knew what they were about when they agreed to the use of the phrase.

Jefferson, you see, was an Epicurean, which as we all know means he could communicate with fish.

I'm lying, of course. I just wanted to see if you were paying attention.

The Epicurean philosophy believes that the pursuit of happiness proposes autarchy, which translates as self-rule, self-sufficiency, or freedom. It also believes that "pleasure" is the greatest good, but the way to attain such pleasure is to live modestly and to gain knowledge of the workings of the world and the limits of one's desires. This leads to tranquility and pleasure as an obliteration of earthly pain.

Sounds kind of Zen-like to me.

Regardless of what they meant, we aren't going to get any further explanation, and that is the beauty of those three words. They are effectively applied to each of us and as unique to us all as a perfectly tailored codpiece.

So what is my point? Well, in thinking about what I could reasonably include under this heading, I had to exercise some subjective bias. I started thinking, what seems to make people happy?

Independence and self-determination are part of it for sure, but there is also pleasure and fulfillment. There is also love and, if you are still even vaguely aware of the physical, sex. Speaking of awareness, how we handle our decline, which is inevitable, can make clear our thoughts and our wishes—our legacy, if you will—and the assurances of our goals.

So suddenly it seemed fairly reasonable to try to address the things I like. That made it easy. So, just as promised, I am going to talk about sex. Admittedly, it is a fairly short chapter, but that should not be interpreted as meaning anything about me at all. Finally, there is one thing we all know we'll be dealing with. Pauper and king, rich or poor, celebrated or obscure, we will all die.

How we prepare for that can make a lot of difference our impact on the happiness of those around us.

Remember the Epicurean principle.

To also be fair, I have asked the printers of this book to leave at least one blank page so you can add in whatever you think I left out that makes you happy.

And as for communicating with fish, if you have a line on that, send me a letter, because my weedless lures just aren't doing the trick anymore.

CHAPTER 9

SEX AND SEXUALITY
THE *SCHOOLHOUSE ROCK* SEGMENT THAT NEVER WAS

"Okay, so let me just get this out of the way up front. There will be no giggling!"

That is how my professor of human sexuality started off our course in college. He meant it, too. I can only imagine what it must have been like for him, year after year, with probably nearly depressing predictability, hearing the snorts, wheezes, guffaws, and occasional heavy breathing that issued from his audience during certain lectures. I think it explained a lot. He always seemed kind of an irritable guy. I always thought it might just be that having to be the constant referee for what everyone else was having a ball over could make you pretty dour. Then again, lifeguards still like the pool, so who knows?

Actually, if you think about it, sex is one of the most polarizing issues, concepts, acts, and enterprises known to mankind. Arguably it is one of the strongest influences on our behavior. It has occupied the fancies and attentions of kings and presidents—if what you read is correct, lots of them—and there is not a single soul on the planet that doesn't have at least some kind of opinion on the subject.

As I think about it, if a giggle is—as John Lennon used to say—what gets you through the night, knock yourself out.

Most people like sex. They certainly like to talk about it—for certain, if it is about someone else. Many times we lie about it. We like getting it, we usually like keeping it under wraps, and almost since the beginning of humankind the libido really hasn't changed all that much.

I mean, remember old Og Mammothtail, the burger-eating cave-dweller? If it hadn't been for sex, that caveman would have been the end of the line, and I would not have written this book, and you wouldn't be reading it. So, it's important, if only from an anecdotal point of view.

The Case for Sex (As If I Really Needed to Write This)

There are a lot of good reasons to have sex. First, there's nothing good on cable. Second, there was something really good on cable and it gave me an idea. Seriously, though, it offers the benefits of the stuff I mentioned in chapter 2, such as increasing blood flow through physical exertion (your results may vary). It also boosts the immune system. It promotes sound sleep. It reduces stress and depression, and it causes the release of beneficial hormones, including endorphins, which can ease certain pain syndromes.

So what's not to love? Which reminds me: it is also an expression of love, sometimes, and can be one of the most delightful human connections.

If, however, this is a subject that makes you uncomfortable then go ahead and skip ahead to the next chapter. It's about death and dying.

Oh, you're still here?

Alternatively, if you end up reading this book in private, under the sheets, with a flashlight for illumination, well, a part of me will be deeply satisfied.

Pardon the Freudian slip there. What I meant to say is that it won't hurt my feelings.

Before I go on, I want to offer that sexuality and sex are a part of our overall happiness. I'm not the only one who thinks so. Former Surgeon General David Satcher described it as part of a healthy personality. According to a survey by AARP, a clear majority of men and women age 45 and up say a satisfying sexual relationship is important to their quality of life. So, it sure sounds like someone besides me is agreeing with Dr. Satcher.

SOME DEFINITIONS

Sex is defined by both the concept and the act. The concept refers to the state of being male or female. Regarding the act, if you don't already have that definition down, you need to be reading a different book.

Sexuality is the dynamic outcome of physical capacity, motivation, attitudes, opportunity for partnership, and sexual conduct.

Sexual mores are concepts and values that include influences like sex outside marriage, not having sex unless in love, and religious beliefs as guiding sexual behavior.

Regardless of the definitions, we as biological creatures need connectivity—social and physical connectivity. That includes and is why this chapter is focused on sex. It can be experienced in many ways, and it can be—at any age—a healthy part of life or a destructive influence. So, with that little sermon and disclaimer out of the way, let's talk *revolutionary* sex.

A Matter of Perspective or Why Franklin Was Celebrated in France and Hamilton Got It Rough in Philadelphia

When people think of the Founding Fathers and sex, most immediately envision Ben Franklin—hopefully not in his Speedo. I mean, Franklin is still widely regarded as something of a sexual wag, mostly for his behavior in France. According to legend, Franklin, as an envoy to the French, became a veritable sympathetic symbol of the American cause and a celebrated, almost worshipped, character. He was kind of like the Jerry Lewis of the 1700s. This was in part a pure accident of his personality meshing with the French sensibility and in part shrewd calculation. He was, in the French mind, alternatively a rustic with his plain attire and beaver cap, which he had actually never worn prior, and a libertine with his appreciation for, pursuit of, and indulgence with the fairer sex. All the more impressive, he did it while suffering from gout and being 70. In many ways this perception and his "relationship" with the French made the birth of the United States possible.

Yes, the *double entendre* was intentional.

Now consider, alternatively, the case of Alexander Hamilton. It was a few years later. The United States was an actual nation, and Hamilton was the head of the national treasury. Unbeknownst to most people at the time, he was also engaged in an adulterous affair with a married woman. When the husband of Hamilton's lover threatened to go to the press and Congress unless Hamilton paid him a thousand dollars a year, Hamilton paid.

The federal government hasn't changed all that much, and despite the hush money, the secret got out. Congress immediately convened and determined that an investigation should be undertaken to determine if Hamilton had used treasury money to pay the bribe. He hadn't, but he was ordered by Congress to come before its members and offer an apology. Thus a fine tradition of American politics was established.

Now, I am guessing right about now you are thinking, "Why wasn't history class this much fun when I took it?"

What can we take from this? That social perspective makes a lot of difference in how sex and sexuality are interpreted. So let's fast-forward a couple of hundred years, and I'll illustrate what I mean by that.

The National Social Life, Health, and Aging Project

In 2005 the National Social Life, Health, and Aging Project was published. This study was designed to examine the relationship between sexual behavior, sexual problems, and healthy sexual activities, attitudes toward sex and sexuality, satisfaction with sex, characteristics of the sexual partners and the quality of the partnership, and nonsexual intimacy among older women and men.

I'm exhausted just reading that.

The method was to compare measures of sexuality for those 57–85 years old, by age and by gender. The investigators and study designers considered sexual mores, sexual interest, and relationship satisfaction and then discussed and analyzed the properties of each.

USING THE STUDY TO UNDERSTAND SENIOR SEXUALITY

If you are interested, you can read the NSHAP and draw your own conclusions about sexuality among older adults. The data contain a good deal of information about marital status, cohabiting, and romantic relationships as well as the links of sexual behavior to certain relationship types. It also contains information on sexual problems experienced by the respondents.

The investigators of the NHSAP asked about sexual histories, preferences, attitudes, relationship status and definitions, and sexual problems that included performance impediments and failures. They also asked about how often sex included intercourse, how often during intercourse they used a condom, how often they participated in oral sex, and how often sex included hugging, kissing, or other ways of associated sexual touching.

Amazingly, not one of the investigators was punched in the nose. Quite to the contrary, the respondents were candid and open.

FINDINGS—OR WHO ARE THESE PEOPLE AND WHAT ARE THEY DOING?

In short, seniors are married, unmarried, monogamous, polyamorous, straight, gay, healthy, and unhealthy. Or, to say it better, they are like everybody else with a few more wrinkles.

Among 45- to 59-year-olds with sexual partners, 56 percent said they had sexual intercourse once a week or more. Among 60- to 70-year-olds with partners, 46 percent of men and 38 percent of women had sex at least once a week, as did 34 percent of those 70 or older.

Similar findings emerged in a survey conducted by the National Council on the Aging (NCOA). The study found that nearly half of all Americans age 60 or over had sex at least once a month and that nearly half also wanted to have sex more frequently. Another finding: people find their mates more physically attractive over time.

So, repeat after me, "Give it time, baby."

The NSHAP survey found that sexuality among older adults tends to vary some with age and gender. At all ages in the study, men were more likely than women to have a partner, more likely to be sexually active with that partner, and tended to have more positive and permissive attitudes toward sex.

Sorry, ladies.

For both sexes the differences in perspectives on sexual partnerships, behaviors, problems, and attitudes all differed substantially by age. There were lots of reasons for that, such as religious beliefs, background, and personal preferences. There was also a difference in the two major demographic blocks within the study.

The youngest NSHAP respondents were part of the baby boom and had experienced the sexual revolution. The oldest respondents were teenagers during the 1940s, a period of more conservative sexual mores, excepting, of course, the work of Henry Miller.

While this difference was not explored in depth, the researchers did offer that certain differences in the responses might be related to these generational-sociological distinctions.

As stated, in each age group, men were more likely to have a current partner than women. This may be related to the higher mortality rate among men and age differences between spouses and thus could have indicated a sociological rather than sexual phenomenon. Also, people in relationships were more likely to have sex in all forms and varieties. Overall, the rate of acquisition of new partners was relatively low. Most reported considering "sex" to include intercourse, and the majority of respondents reported that they were heterosexual. Overall, 4 percent of men and 5 percent of women reported at least one same-sex partnership at some time in their lives. Bear in mind that the data were gathered in 2005. The changing social dynamics and laws regarding same-sex relationships will certainly have an effect on the applicability of similar studies in years to come.

One interesting observation: it appears that at the oldest ages sexual activity consisted *entirely* of kissing, hugging, and sexual touching more often than it did at younger ages.

Respondents also rated their own physical and emotional health and that of their spouse or partner, and they provided ratings of their relationship across a range of dimensions. This rich and detailed information allowed researchers and the respondents to contextualize sexuality at older ages.

Sounds a lot like perception was a major determinant? It was.

DOUBLES—WE'RE NOT TALKING TENNIS HERE

For most older adults, marriage provides the social and emotional context for the vast majority of all sexual activity. According to NHSAP, marriage also provided the predominant opportunity for intimacy and positively affected physical and emotional satisfaction with sex.

That doesn't seem too terribly surprising and reinforces the intimacy, connection, and desire for same that exists no matter the age of a person.

At the younger ages in the survey's range, virtually all married men and women were sexually active, and married people showed substantially higher rates of sexual activity than the unmarried.

This led the investigators to conclude that marriage was an important predictor of physical and mental health for both men and women. Additionally, they pointed out that it seemed to affect financial well-being.

Sounds like the old Certs commercial, huh? "Two, two, two mints in one."

Some Alarming Discoveries

SEXUALLY TRANSMITTED DISEASES (STDs)

According to the Centers for Disease Control and Prevention, between 2007 and 2011 chlamydia infections among Americans 65 and over increased by 31 percent, and syphilis cases increased by 52 percent. Those numbers are similar to STD trends in the 20- to 24-year-old age group, where chlamydia increased by 35 percent and syphilis by 64 percent.

GENITAL HERPES AND HPV

Genital herpes and human papillomavirus (HPV) are the most common infections among older women. According to some studies, genital herpes prevalence among men and women over 70 was 28 percent, and the rate was higher in women than in men. Chlamydia, gonorrhea, and syphilis cases occurred in less than 1 percent of older women, but the percentage is likely an underestimate due to the lack of a uniform tracking system and STDs being overlooked by doctors. High-risk HPV, an important factor in cervical cancer and dysplasia, was found in 6 percent of the women. This is the virus that causes cervical cancer. Cervical cancer is one of the leading causes of female cancer deaths, and 20 percent of cases occur in women over 65. Many of the screening and prevention practices for cervical cancer, including the HPV vaccine, have age-based criteria that exclude older women.

While some of these STDs were contracted in later life, many of the infections likely occurred earlier and have either stayed dormant or persisted through the years. In a recent study of women aged 67 to 99, however, 1 percent were diagnosed with an STD during the nine years of the study, highlighting the fact that older women are still very much at risk for new STDs. Further complicating the diagnosis of STDs in older women is the fact that many can produce symptoms similar to those experienced by postmenopausal women. For example, chlamydia and gonorrhea can present as pelvic pain and pain during intercourse, problems routinely encountered in older women.

My recommendation? Do not ignore pain. If something hurts, stop and see a healthcare provider.

HIV

HIV infections in the United States occur in people over 50, and this number is as high as 17 percent in some population subsets. Almost a third of these new infections are among older women, particularly within minority racial and ethnic groups. The likelihood of receiving an HIV and AIDS diagnosis at the same time increases with age. The CDC estimates that by 2015, half of all people with HIV in the United States will be over 50, and that more than a third will be women. This longer survival of people diagnosed earlier in life probably accounts for the increasing number of older adults with HIV.

WHY THE INCREASE IN STDs?

A lot of reasons are offered for why we are seeing such a rise in STDs among seniors. The first may be that there are increased opportunities for sex among seniors. In the past it was thought that at some point in life sex was no longer an issue or interest for people.

Okay, well, we discounted that already.

Also consider that people are staying healthier longer, that the old sexual mores are being replaced with a different generational expectation of an experience in life (thank you, baby boomers), and that many senior communities are providing greater interaction settings—and you can see what I mean. Now add in the fact that many seniors are not practicing safe sex, and you have a perfect storm brewing for a health crisis for something completely preventable.

According to the NHSAP, more than 90 percent of men over 50 didn't use a condom when having sex with a date or casual acquaintance, and 70 percent didn't do so when they had sex with a stranger. Among women over 50, a majority also reported having sex without a condom. By contrast, in other surveys, 70 to 80 percent of teens say they used a condom during their last sexual encounter. All age groups were more likely to use condoms with casual partners than in monogamous relationships.

So why aren't we protecting ourselves? In some cases it is because of a misperception that since fertility and pregnancy issues no longer apply, it's the Summer of Love time again. As some members of the senior demographic still have their perceptions welded to the pre-safe-sex era, they don't consider this as a priority. Well, guess what? It is! So go see your healthcare provider and protect yourself.

Going Solo—Or Nobody Gets a Bigger Kick Out of Me Than Me!

Seems like the perfect moment to transition to the subject of masturbation or self-love, or, as I used to call it, "How I spent my summer vacation."

Masturbation or self-gratification is often the subject of all kinds of low humor, so maybe I should try to restrain myself. Too late?

It *has* also been considered an indicator of sexual interest. Interestingly enough, the data in the NHSAP indicated substantial differences between the sexes and among age blocks as well when it came to indulging in self-stimulation.

These differences were consistent with previous studies on younger age groups in both the United States and other countries, which suggest that masturbation among seniors does not compensate for the act of "real" sex, with 63 percent of men aged 57–64 years (those with the most partnered sex) reporting some kind of activity in the preceding year, compared with 28 percent of men in the older age groups. Overall, 25 percent of women in an intimate relationship and 23 percent of women not in relationships reported engaging in masturbation.

The conclusion? Again, the differences in groups of seniors may be related to those subjects who came of age before or during the sexual revolution. This suggests that mores and social context rather than biological age are the deciding influence.

Which reminds me of a story.

A man is being interviewed for a sexual survey. The investigator in a white lab coat sits down at his desk facing the participant and asks, "So how often would you say you think about sex?"

The subject sort of startles and says, "Sorry? My mind was somewhere else."

So What's Stopping You? Or, Houston, We Have a Sexual Problem

It's inevitable. At some point, most people will experience a problem with or having sex. There can be many reasons for that.

REASONS FOR NOT HAVING SEX

Some seniors report diminished or no sexual activity. In the NHSAP, sexual inactivity was not generally related to age. There's another myth we can get rid of. The most common reasons cited among seniors are declining vitality or health issues, physical issues related specifically to sex, lack of interest, and lack of opportunity.

According to the survey, for women lacking a partner, there was a reported, progressive lack of interest. This was generally ascribed to a lack of opportunity and not having met the right person. Sounds familiar, huh?

Among men, not having met the right person was a less a reason for decreasing interest. In other words, a woman's lack of a partner seems to influence a lowering of her sexual interest, whereas a man's similar lack of an intimate partner did not lower his interest in finding one. No judgments here.

Physical and Psychological Issues

If the research has told us anything about how we age, a decrease in sexual activity will probably be due to ill health, an injury, or the onset of a new disease or condition. In other words, for many women and men, when "age" does influence sexual inactivity at all, it is through declining physical capacity—whether your own or a partner's.

It may also be psychological, as in cases involving the loss of a partner, either through disability or death. That makes it no less relevant or real since, in any age group, sex and sexuality are as much a state of mind as a physical act.

In the NHSAP study if a respondent reported a problem, he or she was asked the extent to which he or she was bothered by it and if it meant the end of sexual activity. The reasons given by seniors were similar to a lot of other previous findings.

In elderly men, the most common physical sexual problem was erectile difficulty. I think it is important to reflect a moment on some misused verbiage. Erectile dissatisfaction is not the same thing as erectile dysfunction—though, certainly, erectile dysfunction will amount to dissatisfaction. According to the American Urological Association, erectile dysfunction is defined as "the inability to achieve or maintain an erection sufficient for satisfactory sexual performance."

The one thing that a man experiencing a less than satisfactory erection should not do is panic. If there is a medical cause, get help. Remember, 15 to 25 percent of American men over 65 have experienced impotence or erectile dysfunction (ED) on occasion. In older men ED usually has a physical cause—heart disease, high blood pressure, or diabetes—or is a side effect of medication. The good news is that treatment is available. Just let your healthcare provider know what's going on and ask why. If the answer is something patronizing or unsatisfactory, get another opinion and maybe another provider.

Other common sexual problems for men were premature climax and lack of interest in sex. If it is a matter of technique, well, it can actually be kind of fun working through the issue. At the very least, it would make a novel icebreaker. If a sudden lack of sexual interest occurs, it may be due to a psychological or neurological condition. Again, see your healthcare provider.

Lack of Interest

For women, the most common sexual problem was lack of interest in sex, which was not significantly correlated with age. Up to 49 percent reported this as a problem. Physically, both failure to lubricate and inability to climax were also common physically related problems. As with men's erectile problems, women's difficulties with lubrication appeared to level off with age, indicating perhaps a "ceiling"—whether biological or sociological.

In contrast, inorgasmia increased dramatically with age. (For some reason that always sounds to me like a suburb in Portland, as in "Oh yeah, me and the wife got a bungalow over to central inorgasmia. It's close to the park and shopping, don't ya know.")

Those who reported at least one sexual problem were asked if they ever avoided sex because of the problem. Between 23 percent and 34 percent of sexually active women said that they had avoided sex. Comparable figures for men were 22–30 percent, with age not a significant factor in either case. The solution? As above, make sure it is not medically related first.

Nonsexual Intimacy

If there is one thing that everybody from Kinsey to Masters and Johnson have taught us, it is that there is no such thing as normal. Average, maybe, but normal, nope. It's what is legal and mutual that you need to worry about, not "normal." Similarly, a lot of people get caught up in the idea of the end point of sex—orgasms. Those are pretty nice, I'll admit, but, to quote an old needlepoint philosophy I once saw, "It's more about the journey than the destination." And the journey is all about intimacy.

Want to know something really interesting about intimacy and morbidity (health issues and deteriorating health quality of life) and mortality (being dead) in seniors? Both sexual *and* nonsexual interactions with others have a demonstrable positive effect on elderly individuals' mortality and morbidity. Those who had it did better. Those who didn't, did not. So when someone says they were going at it like their lives depended on it… well… maybe they were.

THE CASE FOR CUDDLING

This makes a lot of sense when you think about it. I don't know if you recall the baby monkey pictures from the Harry Harlow studies in the 1950s. They were also known as the "monkey love" experiments. Dr. Harlow was interested in examining the relationship between maternal deprivation and emotional injury. I am not espousing, championing, defending, or even discussing that here. What I remember about the study was a picture in a textbook that I saw as a kid. It showed a small rhesus monkey baby preferentially clutching a cloth-covered surrogate "mother" even though food was offered if the monkey would transfer to a bare wire-frame mother.

It said to me, without a degree in psychology, mind you, that warm, nurturing contact is important. It's a fundamental need, as necessary as eating. True, it made a difference in emotional development with the young, but I think we never shake that need. The maintenance and improvements in senior health in the studies supports that thinking, too. I'll take contact one step further.

This can include a number of activities like petting or touching a dog, cat, or other pet or greeting someone with an embrace, kiss, or pat on the back. It can involve playing or cuddling with a grandchild. Or perhaps it is hugging, kissing, caressing, or other close physical contact with a partner. For that matter, it could be hugging, kissing, caressing, or other close physical contact with any other adult.

Mind you, you might want to make sure it is okay with the other person first. Otherwise, it can get you kicked off public transit. I gauge a lot by the acceptable nature of behavior on public transit, I know.

Regardless, close physical contact with others is a useful indicator of overall intimacy and a really healthy act.

So for the "what you can do" piece to this, you might consider the expression of kindness and affection. Just, you know, be careful about doing it with a partner made of chicken wire. If Harlow is right, it won't be that much fun.

What Are We to Make of This, Professor?

So what does all this really mean? I think it means that good sex is important no matter the age. It's also really about the human connection and a reinforcement of some of the pleasures of life. Of course, as you just read, "good sex" is very much in the eye of the beholder.

Additionally, I am reminded of an older patient, a reviewer of this book, who said to me, "But you know, Doc, even bad sex is better than no sex."

I consider him a single data point.

The Talk

So we've all heard it, that most uncomfortable of conversations. Generally it sort of starts off with a parent saying, "I know you are coming into that time in life when your body is starting to change. You are probably experiencing some sensations that are confusing and maybe even a little frightening. I just want you know that what you are going through is normal."

I know what you are thinking: it's the sex talk everyone had to endure as a wretchedly embarrassed teenager or deliver as the parent, but hang on. While it may be completely accurate and applicable to a teenager, the very same conversation could apply to an aging parent, an aging peer, your image in the mirror, or even a newly indoctrinated werewolf.

If I could offer one thing here, it would be this. If you have a loved one, parent, peer, or friend, don't shy away from having this conversation. Also one of the biggest deterrents to senior sex is the opposition by younger family members stemming from their discomfort with the idea of a senior parent as a sexual being. If you think about it, this is really a kind of ageism. You've already read about the benefits of good sex and intimacy. As we will get into soon, it could actually be a matter of life and death.

So with that in mind, we have come to that time in a book's life when it starts to encounter subjects that can be confusing and even at times frightening. It's probably long overdue, but I think we need to have a talk about the changes and those funny feelings that you're experiencing.

Sexual Health

As you already know, I am a big advocate of getting regular checkups and engaging in good health maintenance and disease prevention activities. This includes getting checkups to make sure you are healthy enough for sexual activity. For men that includes a physical and a prostate evaluation.

Now bend over and repeat after me: "Mooooon River . . ."

You'll thank me, maybe not right away, but eventually.

For women, it includes a physical examination and may or may not include a pelvic examination. You need to talk this over with your practitioner, as this is an area of considerable discussion in the medical community. Just make sure you have that talk.

I touched on this earlier, but it's a sad fact that very few of us can count on physical performance like we experienced when we were in our 20s. The same is true for sex and sexuality. When it becomes a concern, however, is when the changes are sudden or there is pain, bleeding, or other physical evidence that something is wrong. The good news is that for most, sex can still be satisfying and rewarding well into later years.

Go slow. Someone, probably someone French, is supposed to have said that the act of love should be a banquet, not a fast-food experience. I'd take that to heart. In a peripheral consideration, I'm suddenly experiencing a craving.

Honestly though, as you get older, it may take a while for both you and your partner to get up and going during intercourse. Let foreplay take as long as you need, and you'll cut down on the risk of injury. Remember what I wrote earlier about exercise and physical activity? Well . . .

Besides, you'll also enjoy the experience more as you both build up together.

Experiment more often. This sounds like I am talking about science lab and, in a way, I am. Biology and chemistry, at least, and maybe physics. That said, just like in science class, if you are going to experiment, do the required reading and, for crying out loud, wear your protective equipment, and maybe wait an hour after you eat. I'm just saying....

In that same spirit, you might also want to vary your routine. Sex doesn't have to be a nighttime-only activity. You may actually have more energy earlier in the day, so morning sex may be better for both of you. Also, don't be afraid to try new positions. Some are specifically designed for people with arthritis, back pain, or other conditions that may make traditional positions hard or painful. Just get that checkup first.

Have I made my point about getting a checkup? Good.

For Women

As we have seen by the statistics, women can expect to be sexually active throughout their senior years. Without the concern about potential pregnancy, many postmenopausal women find they enjoy sex more. Here are suggestions for enjoying sex in this new chapter of your life.

WHAT YOU CAN DO

• Pay attention to hygiene issues. We already know that seniors' immune systems are not as vigorous as when they were younger. Because vaginal pH rises with the decrease in estrogen associated with menopause, your chances for infections increase.

• Don't use soap to wash your vagina. Look for a cleanser that has the same pH as a healthy vagina instead. Also, from a purely medical standpoint, you might want to be sure to urinate after sex. This practice can help prevent urinary tract infections.

• Lube, glorious lube. With apologies to the creators of the musical *Oliver*, this is a really important point. Lower hormone levels can leave vaginal tissue thin and dry. As a result, sex may become uncomfortable and undesirable. For many women lubricant will help, but others may find that vaginal estrogen is more effective in relieving dryness and other symptoms. Vaginal estrogen can be administered in tablet form, in an insertable ring, or in a cream.

Aside from entering a monastery, the surest way to avoid contracting a sexually transmitted disease is to insist that your male partner uses a male condom.

Just remember to use *water-based lubricants*. It's important to remember that condoms, which are made of latex, can only be used with water-based lubricants. This is something like K-Y Jelly or other lubricants that have "water-based" on the label. Oil-based lubricants like petroleum jelly can break down the latex and the material of the condom and cause them to fail. It's messy and it's dangerous. If you are not sure, ask the pharmacist.

If you are embarrassed, you can say something like, "Say, is this water-based?"

If the answer is yes, then assume a puzzled expression and say, "Well then, I can't use it to caulk the bathroom."

They'll never even suspect.

• As with the men, get a checkup. I mean, think about it: if you were going out for a high school sport, you'd get a physical, right? Well, think of this as a prerequisite for the world's greatest gym class.

The Largest Sex Organ in the Body

Here is a fun question. Who said that the brain is the largest sex organ in the human body? A lot of people think it was Sigmund Freud. Others say it was Oscar Wilde. I spent way too much time researching this one point, and all I could come up with is that I'm pretty sure it was not just some guy named Eddie.

No matter the original author, the fact is that it is true. As you have seen, normal and average are nonexistent concepts when it comes to matters of sex among seniors. In that way not much has changed.

It is all pretty individualized and subjective, which brings to mind the first time I went on a school field trip. It was to the museum of art. I think I was like eight years old or so. Our teacher asked us if we knew what art was. Then after a bunch of us gave our answers, she told us that art was whatever we thought it was. I was never sure if that meant we were right in the first place or not.

One thing I do know: when it comes to good sex or what is sexy, it's what *you* think it is.

Connectivity and Fulfillment

Granted, this chapter started off about sex, but happiness, while certainly enhanced by it, is related to a lot more.

LOVE

With all the talk about biology and anatomy and the physical aspects of the expression of love, I'll bet you thought I was going to leave the real thing out. Well, I'm not. I will, however, concede that there have been about a million books written about this subject, so it would be ridiculous for me to try to take it on in a single chapter. Even for those works of literature that don't overtly admit it, love is the basic reason for and highest aspiration of everything human. It is the greatest force in the world and the most sublime connection of the universe. If there is one thing, only one, that I could hope you take away from this book, it would be this.

If you really want fulfillment, at any age, do your dead level best to find love. The really weird thing about it, at least in my experience, is that the best way to find it is to bestow it. Maybe it will be in passion. Maybe it will be in fraternity. Maybe it will be in service and kindness. In any case, like with the world's biggest magnifying glass or a telescope turned around backward or a metaphysical savings and loan, it pays you back with interest.

I wish you luck. I really mean it.

OTHER LIFE FORMS

Now this is definitely not for everyone, but for some seniors the presence of a pet in their lives provides a wonderful source of affection and joy. Oh . . . I'm no longer talking about sex. My editor felt I should clarify that!

If having a pet is something you think you might like, consider adopting an animal. There are lots of services and experts associated with your local animal shelter who can advise you on the proper type, breed, and temperament of pet for you. I went through this. I had put off getting a dog for years while I was going through internship and residency because I didn't feel it would be fair to the animal. When I did go to the shelter, I started out looking at puppies, but then I realized that if I really wanted to do something good, I should consider an adult dog. They were much less likely to get a home, and if I could provide it, I'd feel good. It turned out to be a fantastic decision.

His name was Henry, and everyone who knew him will tell you that there has never been a greater quadruped. Not Rin Tin Tin, not Lassie, not Old Yeller. No dog had anything on Henry. He was a great, powerful-looking thing with a temperament like the Dali Lama. He was that pacific, smart, and gentle. There was something about that dog that connected with everyone, and I was much richer for having known him. Now, I know not every story is like that, but if you think you might have a place in your life for a pet, consider an adoption. Just do your research, ask questions, and take your time.

OTHER PURSUITS

For many seniors, the latter years provide new opportunities that might not have been possible at other times in life. Without the distractions of career and associated obligations, the possibilities of exploring new educational, vocational, and social pursuits provide wonderful opportunities. Here's what I am talking about.

First, Get Connected

If I were going to offer one thing to a senior, in order to maintain the proper stimulation and interaction necessary to maintain a vital mind and fulfilling life, it would be to get connected. I am talking about social connection as well as awareness of the world. If only for self-preservation, making sure you don't become socially isolated can prevent being caught by surprise in the event of a crisis or emergency. I mean, you want to know if there is a twister coming—or a plague of frogs, right? I mean, especially if you are French!

So maintain some kind of current event connection. Get online. Regardless of how you feel about it, the world operates via information technology. Your doctor's office, your friends, the media—it is all based on communication technology. If this is intimidating, go to your local senior center and get help. There are also free computer programs through many community colleges and universities.

Even if you cannot afford a computer or don't have one, you can be connected. You can use the computer at your senior center or local library. Just because the computer isn't yours doesn't mean you can't have a free email account through Yahoo, Gmail, or whatever. Just remember, if you use any public computer, close your email out and, for crying out loud, don't autosave your password. Additionally, if you have a smartphone, most are little computers. Get someone to set up your email. You can at least access it that way.

Now, I have recently had an experience with the indoctrination of information technology. My mother was resisting getting a computer. The conversation had even gotten to the point that it was a little strident. When we presented her with a laptop at Christmas, I also included, as part of the gift, my own limited tech services. Now this is not self-deprecating, but my tech support skills are limited!

Even so, I do know how to turn it on and how and why to shut off or allow certain things, like firewalls to prevent hacking and malware. So I sat down with her, and we went through the most common things she would need: surfing the web, accessing email, creating little checklists. I am happy to say she can use it at will, and she's got a lot more control. More importantly, she is intellectually connected.

Make sure you take precautions and be careful about your personal information, but to deny the value of this venue is pointless. Resistance is futile. Luddites, get with it.

So once you are online, you can start to search for opportunities, programs, jobs, and educational and entertainment seminars. Maybe you always wanted to watch that show *Lost*. Well, now you can, in one sitting if you have a good cushion. Not to ruin it for you, but I doubt you will be happy with the ending.

The Internet can open the world to you. You can pursue hobbies with like-minded folks, pursue a passion, and indulge in a veritable unlimited library of information. Once you have that in hand, then you can indulge any number of intellectual pursuits to your heart's content.

Hobbies

For many, advancing age presents opportunities of interest. We tend to have had more life experience, and we know what we like. If you need a little priming for some ideas of leisure activity, well, take the words of John Adams to heart.

Remember when pushed by the French about his tastes in music and art, he replied that he did not really have any. He explained it further saying "I must study politics and war that my sons may have liberty to study mathematics and philosophy, geography, natural history, naval architecture, navigation, commerce, and agriculture, in order to give their children a right to study painting, poetry, music, architecture, statuary, tapestry, and porcelain."

In many ways that is how it is with us as we make our living and live our lives. We often put off those elevated pursuits until, at some point in our lives, we can indulge the things that enrich our souls. So if you are at that point, maybe you can:

- Join a book club.
- Join a gym, health club, or recreation center.
- Take up hiking or backpacking.

- Play tennis, golf, swim, ride horses, fish, or ski.
- Join a local theater group.
- Join a senior softball league.
- Learn pottery, weaving, or stained glass.
- Take up gardening.
- Learn to play chess or bridge.
- Learn ballroom dancing, country dancing, or square dancing.
- Learn new board games or online games.

Education

I don't know how many times a day I hear busy people express with longing, "Boy, I really would like to go back to school," or "Man, I wish I had the time to get that taxidermy course under my belt. I've been meaning to stuff my beloved pet Holstein, but it's just that I am so busy at work."

Well, now may be your chance. This doesn't mean you have to head up to Harvard for that advanced degree in taxidermy. In fact, there are many good opportunities all around. Maybe you don't want a degree. Maybe you just want to audit a course.

Here's what I am talking about. I have a friend who likes history, but she had dedicated her life to the service of her country and the protection of its citizens through her service in the US Public Health Service. In fact, I found in her someone who enjoyed the same sort of strange historical anecdotes that I use to pepper this book. One thing she was always talking about was how much she wished she had studied history more in school, so when she retired, I suggested she look into the course offerings at the local university. It proved an incredibly enriching experience.

Teach

"But I don't want to stuff owls, beavers, and roadkill of the great Southwest," you might be saying. Okay, well, maybe taking a class isn't your thing. Maybe teaching one is.

Chances are pretty good that you know how to do something. You are probably very good at it, maybe even the best, as in, "I am one of the world's greatest compost pilers" or "Nobody can tan iguana hides like me!"

Well, if that is the case, use it. I am talking about teaching. Nothing can validate a personality and restore a mind like imparting the experience and knowledge of decades of activity to receptive minds. It doesn't even have to be in a formal educational setting. Senior centers are always looking for experts to lead learning endeavors. Museums need docents. Nuclear power plants need people to say, "Don't push *that* button."

What I am getting at is this: don't be constrained by traditional educational settings.

Volunteer

If you have the good fortune of health and some discretionary time, you might consider volunteering and helping others. This could include other seniors or young people. It is amazing how rewarding mentoring or contributing to the well-being of a young person can be.

Here are some things you might find interesting:

- Medical organizations. In addition to the American Red Cross, local hospitals, nursing homes, or mental health clinics, you can also volunteer for hospice care at www.growthhouse.org. This is an organization for more than 150 organizations that provide free service for those needing care for the dying.
- Environmental—Earthwatch, Audubon Society, Sierra Club, Greenpeace, and Nature Conservancy.
- Adult literacy—Proliteracy Worldwide (www.proliteracy.org).
- Helping children. Mentor a young person through Big Brothers Big Sisters (www.bbbs.org) or through the National Mentoring Network (www.mentoring.org). Represent neglected and abused children during judicial proceedings (www.seniorcorps.org). Join the Foster Grandparent Program (www.seniorcorps.org).
- Help the elderly and homebound. Help deliver meals with your local Meals on Wheels, church, community group, or charities.
- Consider volunteering or even becoming a docent at a museum.
- Habitat for Humanity. Work to build affordable housing for those in need (www.habitat.org). Or volunteer to help provide help for the homeless. This is usually done through local churches and civic organizations.

This doesn't have to be the grand trek around the world. If you have the means, well, you certainly have the time. If you don't, however, you might consider subsidizing your trip. If money is tight but you would still like to travel, consider getting a seasonal job. For example, work at a ski lodge, summer camp, or a casino. Just pick a city and check out available seasonal jobs. Many of these jobs will offer you room and board plus a small salary.

Here's what I am talking about. When I was in my internship, I didn't have much money. I had a week coming up for a vacation and I wanted to do something interesting. As it happened, I had been reading a copy of *Travels with Charley* by John Steinbeck. It starts off with him almost dying in a storm and getting a diagnosis of heart disease. So what does he do? He decides he hasn't been as acquainted lately with his country like he used to be, and he packs up his standard poodle, Charley, and takes a slow drive across America.

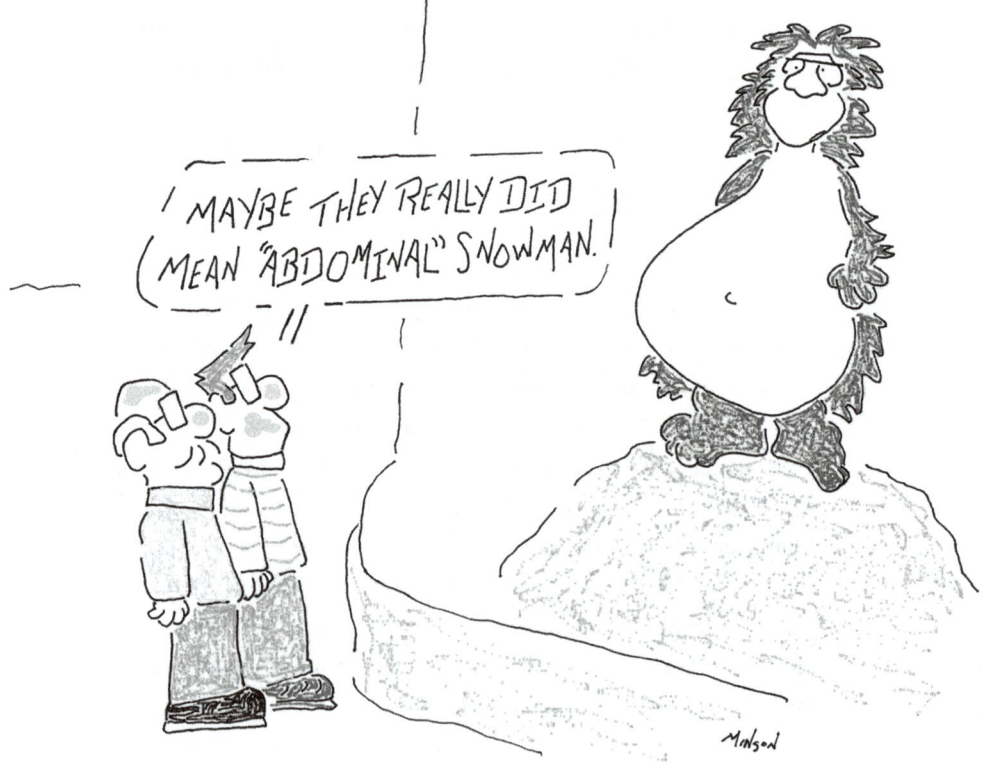

Now I didn't have time to cross the country, or a poodle for that matter, but I liked the idea. So I booked an ultracheap flight, rented a Rambler at the local Rent-A-Wreck, and drove un-agendaed and un-itineraried around the Midwest. It was a great trip. A complete adventure. The only caveat now is that if you do make such a trip, make sure someone knows how, when, and where you are going, just in case.

Fitness

I've been harping about health throughout this book. I am a physician, after all. If you have the inclination, your senior years provide the perfect opportunity to indulge in some fitness goals. If you always wanted to train for a marathon, swim the English Channel, throw the javelin, it really doesn't matter—just make sure you are cleared by your healthcare provider and get going. (If you choose the javelin, maybe make sure you have a little bit of room.)

Your ideas should be limitless! Decide what you would like to accomplish in your remaining life. Set goals for learning, travel, and social interaction and go after it.

This is your time of choice, your time to do what you want to do, your time for self-renewal. In any case, don't be constrained by conventional thinking. Be bold!

What Makes Me Happy

Remember poor Alexander Hamilton and his apology to Congress? Well, in case you were wondering why he isn't predominantly known for his sexual peccadilloes, it's because something even more notorious occurred that became his signature entry in history. It was right after the election of 1800. Vice President Aaron Burr—no, not the guy in the wheelchair—responded to what he considered attacks upon his character by Hamilton and challenged the secretary of the treasury to a duel.

The two men met at the base of some cliffs in Weehawken, New Jersey, and though the details of the exchange of gunfire are sketchy and debated, the result was that Hamilton died. For that reason, Hamilton is remembered more for his dying in New Jersey than for his sexual dalliance.

A reviewer/editor of this book did comment that perhaps dying in New

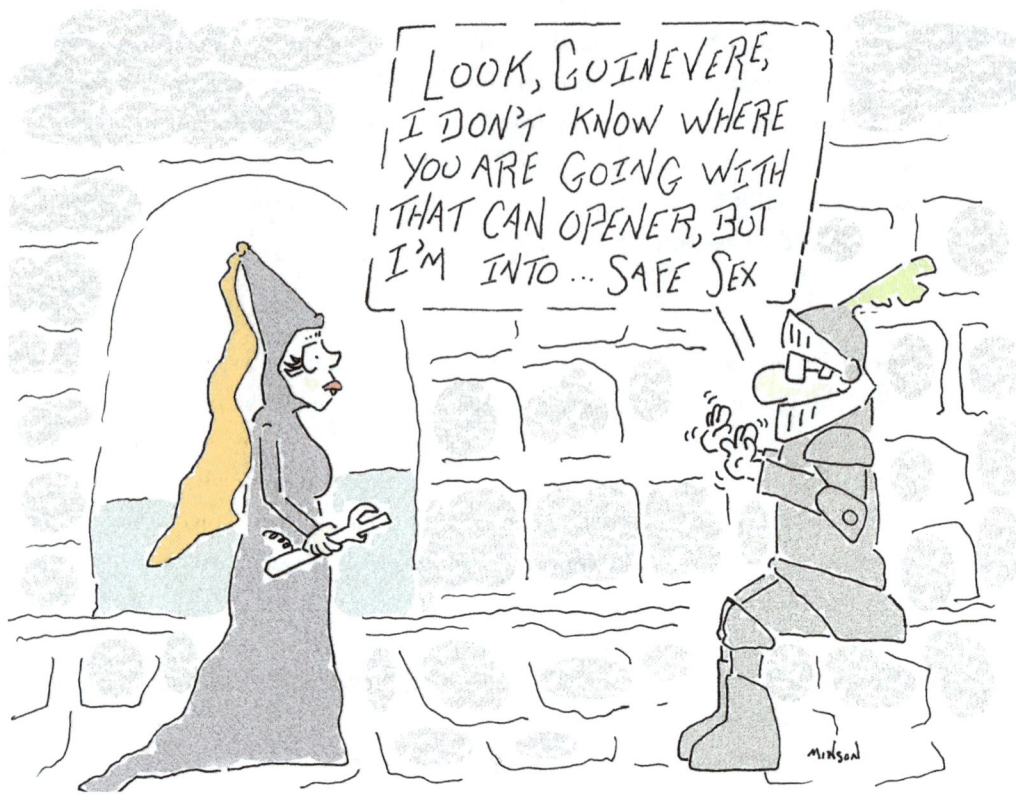

Jersey was redundant. I reserve my judgments on that. I will say it provides a perfect segue to the final chapter on death and dying.

Oh, and if any of you noticed that my chapter on sex is actually the shortest in the book, I defy you to draw any conclusions from that.

WHAT MAKES ME HAPPY

_____

_____

_____

_____

_____

_____

_____

_____

_____

_____

_____

_____

_____

_____

_____

_____

_____

_____

_____

_____

_____

_____

_____

_____

_____

_____

_____

_____

CHAPTER 10

END OF LIFE
I AM NOT COUNTING ON A SEQUEL

*"There is no lion on the Serengeti
that knows its good end."*
African proverb

With respect to Mel Brooks, it really isn't easy being king. It may be good, but it isn't easy.

Consider the king of the beasts. A male lion starts out as a cub, with a bunch of other males cubs that are there in such great numbers only because their mortality rate is so high. At the age of two (that is, in lion years, so they are really adolescents) they are kicked out of the pride by the reigning male. Subsequently, they go off to young lion indoctrination training, also known as surviving on the plain, where they deal with hunters, starvation issues, and a lot more. Then when they think they are ready, or are just sick of doing what they have been doing, they have to fight to get a pride of their own. It's super dangerous and violent and often to the death. Oh, and there are no guarantees they will be successful.

So it's all good times and gravy when they make it, right?

Sort of. It has its benefits: reproduction, meals delivered by lionesses, lots of naps. But here's the downside. The average male lion's tenure over a pride is roughly two years.

That is one term in Congress! And you know how it ends? The male lion is generally defeated in a brutal battle that often leaves him dead or acutely crippled and debilitated. From that point on, he can look forward to death from infection, starvation (because he can't catch game due to his injuries), or predation by others. Nice, huh?

What is my point with this happy story? It's that if the noble lion can't expect any better, why are we so arrogant?

Actually, there is a slightly more pleasant lesson I like to take from this. It is that we all have a pretty limited time being vertical and we really should make the most of it because eventually—I don't want to ruin the ending for you here—but as in every biography I have ever read, the story ends with us dying.

Sorry for the spoiler.

Some Lessons from the Deaths of the Founding Fathers

Death can teach us a lot if we have to courage to learn. I'll offer the following as examples.

You already know how Hamilton died.

Washington, they think, died of an airway restriction, basically an infectious laryngitis, although there is a lot of speculation that his physicians didn't help the situation much and may have contributed to his end.

Ben Franklin did not die from an STD. I am not sure where I first heard that, but when I was in high school the rumor was that Ben Franklin, maybe because of his French proclivities, had contracted a disease that killed him.

Wait, let me clarify. That passage makes it sound like I was in high school *when* Franklin died. I wasn't. I was in high school when disco was at its height, so I was just there for the death of good taste.

Jefferson died of complications due to prostate cancer. So remember what I wrote in the last chapter… guys, get checked!

Adams died of congestive heart failure. Same admonition!

Here's something I found really interesting. James Monroe died of a heart attack while moving furniture for a family member. Now this was a guy who had survived malaria, a gunshot wound, and tuberculosis. So maybe if you want to get out of helping someone move, say, "Oh, hey, I would love to, but you know what happened to James Monroe."

Then hand them this book and run away.

Alzheimer's

Some of you have gotten to this point in the book and you are thinking, "How is it that this book is about aging and there has been no mention of Alzheimer's?"

Well, it is interesting. Of course, I was planning on getting to the subject much earlier, but during the course of researching this book, I realized something. The process and the effects of Alzheimer's on the brain—but, more importantly, on the *mind*—is really much more suited to a discussion of death.

The death of the mind.

I got this phrase from a really sad and beautiful online essay, "Alzheimer's: A Slow Death of Mind and Humanity," written by Clive Donegal (a pen name, as I understand it) about his interactions with his mother during her decline due to the disease. It is raw, disturbing, and doesn't have a satisfyingly happy ending. That is what makes it so effective and so good in my opinion. It also affected me to the point that I thought it belonged here as we talk about our death. After all, what we really are is a mental force, a personality and spirit housed in a really goofy physical contraption called the human body.

There have been almost as many books written about Alzheimer's as there have been about love, so rather than try to arrogantly offer a comprehensively neat and tidy entry here, I'm going to touch briefly on the clinical considerations and provide resources for you to learn more. I'll start be delineating dementia and Alzheimer's, two terms that unfortunately are used interchangeably.

DEMENTIA

Dementia is a syndrome characterized by dysfunction in the cerebral cortex, the part of the brain that controls perception, memory, thoughts, language, and consciousness. Depending on the cause, sometimes, dementia can be stopped or reversed.

Impairment in Memory

This is not just forgetfulness. This is the loss of foundational and inherent memory. It's the difference between "Hey, where did I put my sandwich?" and "What is a sandwich?"

I'm going to offer a story here. It's kind of sad, but every year during college football season, I remember an episode with my grandmother when she was starting to have issues with her short-term memory. I could focus on it, I suppose, with sadness or melancholy, but that would not do her justice. Throughout her life she was always kind of whimsical and, frankly, had a kind of Lucille Ball quality. For that reason, I think she'd be okay with my telling this.

We were watching the OU Sooners play. My grandmother, a lifelong Oklahoman, loved the Sooners. It was during the era of the wishbone, and the Sooners ran a kind of high-octane option offense that scored and fumbled a lot. Anyway, they were scoring on these big long, dramatic runs. The thing is, every time they showed a replay, my grandmother would yell, "Good Lord, they are scoring again."

Now this went on for a while. The team would score. We'd celebrate. Then when the replay started, I would explain that they weren't getting *another* touchdown. It was just the replay.

Then it hit me. What was I doing? In comparison, the game *she* was watching was a whole lot more exciting than the one I was seeing. I mean, by her count, it was the greatest offensive performance in history: 60 touchdowns and about a million yards rushing. So I decided to go with it. She was providing one more lesson, I think, whether she knew it or not.

I remember it fondly every fall.

Impairment in Cognition

Cognition is the ability to organize thoughts and reason, the ability to use language, or the ability to accurately "see" the world (and not because of eye disease), and these impairments are severe enough to cause a decline in the usual level of function.

Although some kinds of memory loss are normal parts of aging, the changes due to aging are not normally severe enough to interfere with the level of function. Many different diseases can cause dementia, but Alzheimer's is one of the most common throughout the world. Other causes can include but are not limited to: depression, adverse effects of drugs, drug or alcohol abuse, space-occupying lesions, strokes, normal pressure hydrocephalus, and metabolic conditions and endocrine conditions like hypothyroidism and nutritional conditions.

ALZHEIMER'S DISEASE

Alzheimer's disease is a slowly progressive disease of the brain that is characterized by impairment of memory and eventually by disturbances in reasoning, planning, language, and perception. Many scientists believe that Alzheimer's disease results from an increase in the production or accumulation of a specific protein (beta-amyloid protein) in the brain that leads to nerve cell death.

The likelihood of having Alzheimer's disease increases substantially after the age of 70 and may affect around 50 percent of persons over the age of 85. Nonetheless, Alzheimer's disease is not a normal part of aging and is not something that inevitably happens in later life. Associated factors include the following:

- Age
- Low mental ability in early life
- Reduced mental and physical activity in late life
- Head injuries
- Vascular diseases, such as hypertension and atherosclerosis, smoking, obesity, and diabetes
- Decreased reserve capacity of the brain
- Reduced brain size
- Low educational and occupational status
- Down's syndrome or other forms of mental retardation

How It Kills

At some point as the disease progresses, patients lose the ability to coordinate basic motor skills, such as swallowing, walking, or controlling their bladder or bowels. Difficulty swallowing can cause food to be inhaled, which can result in pneumonia. Inability to walk can lead to bedsores. Incontinence can result in bladder infections. The lack of awareness and

Table 12. The Main Stages of Alzheimer's Disease

MILD OR EARLY-STAGE	Memory loss and other early cognitive impairments are minor but become progressively apparent. The individual can compensate and function independently.
MODERATE OR MID-STAGE	Changes become more obvious and disabling. Mental abilities decline, personality changes, and physical problems develop. The individual requires caregiver support for some or many daily activities.
SEVERE OR LATE-STAGE	Personality deteriorates. Physical problems are greater with loss of control over bodily functions. The individual is completely dependent on others for the most basic activities.

disorientation can lead to falls, injuries, and the like. These physical issues often lead to further complications and death because Alzheimer's patients are unable to understand and participate in their own treatment.

Table 12 summarizes the different stages of Alzheimer's disease.

Causes: Genetics and Other Health Factors

The mechanisms of Alzheimer's are still a subject of research, research that will hopefully someday lead to more effective treatments and cures. What we currently know is that the disease has both genetic and contributory factors. The genes linked to the disease can be associated as familial or sporadic and can be linked to certain proteins.

Other potentially predisposing risk factors for Alzheimer's disease include high blood pressure (hypertension), coronary artery disease, diabetes, and possibly elevated blood cholesterol. Individuals who have completed less than eight years of education also have an increased risk for Alzheimer's disease. These factors increase the risk of Alzheimer's disease, but by no means do they mean that Alzheimer's disease is inevitable in persons with these factors.

Diagnosing Alzheimer's

No specific blood test or imaging test exists for the diagnosis of Alzheimer's disease. Alzheimer's disease is diagnosed when: a person has sufficient cognitive decline to meet criteria for dementia, the clinical course is consistent with that of Alzheimer's disease, and no other brain diseases or other processes are better explanations for the dementia.

As I wrote earlier, healthcare providers may look for certain genes called apogenes (the protein markers), but these are really more to fulfill the clinical picture than to diagnose.

Treatment

Currently, two different classes of pharmaceuticals are approved by the FDA for treating Alzheimer's disease: cholinesterase inhibitors and partial glutamate antagonists. Understand that they don't cure the disease or actually stop its progress, but they do alleviate some of the effects of the disease for some people.

Other symptoms of Alzheimer's disease include agitation, depression, hallucinations, anxiety, and sleep disorders. Standard psychiatric drugs are widely used to treat these symptoms, although none of these drugs have been *specifically* approved by the FDA for treating these symptoms in patients with Alzheimer's disease. If these behaviors are infrequent or mild, they often do not require treatment with medication. Nonpharmacologic measures such as therapy and psychosocial tools like music and activities can be very useful.

In many ways, the concepts of palliative care come into play here like nowhere else.

Alzheimer's disease varies in its effect on patients and on their capacity to cope with it and may depend on such factors as a patient's lifelong personality patterns and the nature and severity of stress in the immediate environment. Depression, severe uneasiness, paranoia, or delusions may accompany or result from the disease, but these conditions can often be improved by appropriate treatments. As stated before, although there is no cure for Alzheimer's disease, treatments are available to alleviate many of the symptoms that cause suffering.

Here are some additional resources for Alzheimer's patients and their families:
• The Alzheimer's Association's helpline (1–800–272–3900) and lists of local chapters (www.alz.org/chapter/)
• The National Institute on Aging's "Alzheimer's Disease Fact Sheet" (http://www.nia.nih.gov/alzheimers/publication/alzheimers-disease-fact-sheet)
• The CDC's article on Alzheimer's disease (http://www.cdc.gov/aging/aginginfo/alzheimers.htm)

- Alzheimer's Disease Education and Referral (ADEAR) Center (www
.nia.nih.gov/alzheimers)

The National Institute on Aging's ADEAR Center offers information
and publications for families, caregivers, and professionals on diagnosis,
treatment, patient care, caregiver needs, long-term care, education and
training, and research related to Alzheimer's disease. Staff members answer
telephone, e-mail, and written requests and make referrals to local and
national resources. Visit the ADEAR website to learn more about Alzheimer's and other dementias, find clinical trials, and sign up for email updates.
- Alzheimer's Association (toll-free: 1–866–403–3013 or www.alz.org)
- Alzheimer's Foundation of America (toll-free: 1–866–232–8484 or
www.alzfdn.org)
- Eldercare Locator (toll-free: 1–800–677–1116 or www.eldercare.gov)
- Family Caregiver Alliance (toll-free: 1–800–445–8106 or www
.caregiver.org)
- NIH SeniorHealth (www.nihseniorhealth.gov/alzheimersdisease/toc
.html)

Living Wills, Powers of Attorney, and Advanced Directives

While I have already discussed these to some degree with regard to an
individual's finances, there are some end-of-life particulars that warrant
additional consideration. With the concept of diminished decision-
making already in mind, I'd like to dedicate a little discussion to making
sure your wishes are met during the final stages of life. This includes the
kind of medical care would you want if you were too ill or hurt to express
your intentions.

LIVING WILLS

A living will tells which treatments you want if you are dying or permanently unconscious. You can accept or refuse medical care. You might
want to include instructions on the use of dialysis and ventilators (breathing machines), whether you want to be resuscitated if your breathing
or heartbeat stops, whether you want tube feedings, and your decisions
about organ or tissue donation.

I covered this earlier, but one aspect of it is worth going over again because it has relevance when someone is anticipating a decline in cognition and health.

A durable power of attorney (DPA) for health care is a document that names your healthcare proxy without a specific expiration date. Your proxy or agent is someone you trust to make health decisions for you if you are unable to do so. It becomes active anytime you are unconscious or unable to make medical decisions. Living wills and DPAs are legal in most states.

Even if these advance directives aren't officially recognized by the law in your state, they can still guide your loved ones and doctor if you are unable to make decisions about your medical care. Ask your doctor, lawyer, or state representative about the law in your state.

ADVANCE DIRECTIVES

An advance directive tells your physician and healthcare providers what kind of care you would like to have if you become unable to make medical decisions. It goes hand in hand with some other subjects we have covered, like the Responsible Payee for Social Security and the authorized person for sharing medical information with Medicare. Advance directives are, however, distinct legal documents that allow you to spell out your decisions about end-of-life care ahead of time. They give you a way to tell your wishes to family, friends, and healthcare professionals and to avoid confusion later on.

If you are admitted to the hospital, the hospital staff will probably talk to you about advance directives. This is especially true if you anticipate potential debility or have a progressively debilitating disease.

A good advance directive has a sliding scale of care, meaning it describes the kind of treatment you would want depending on how sick you are. Advance directives usually tell your doctor that you don't want certain kinds of treatment. However, they can also say that you do or don't want a certain treatment no matter how ill you are.

Advance directives can take many forms. Laws about advance directives are different in each state. Check with your attorney general's office or the state department of health.

Advance directives and living wills do not have to be complicated legal documents. They can be short, simple statements about what you want done or not done if and when you can't speak for yourself. Remember, anything you write by yourself or with a computer software package should follow your state laws and needs some validation. You should have what you write reviewed by your doctor and a lawyer to make sure your directives are understood exactly as you intend. When you are satisfied with your directives, the orders should be notarized, if possible, and copies should be given to your family and your healthcare provider.

Can I Change My Advance Directive?

You may change or cancel your advance directive at any time, as long as you are considered of sound mind to do so. Being of sound mind means that you are still able to think rationally and communicate your wishes in a clear manner (remember our competency definitions). Again, your changes must be made, signed, and notarized according to the laws in your state. Make sure that your healthcare provider and any family members who knew about your directives are also aware that you have changed them.

If you do not have time to put your changes in writing, you can make them known while you are in the hospital. Tell your doctor and any family or friends present exactly what you want to happen. Usually, wishes that are made in person will be followed in place of the ones made earlier in writing. Just be sure your instructions are clearly understood by everyone.

THE DO NOT RESUSCITATE ORDER

A Do Not Resuscitate (DNR) order is a kind of advance directive. A DNR is a request not to have cardiopulmonary resuscitation (CPR) if your heart stops or if you stop breathing. Unless given other instructions, hospital staff will try to help any patient who experiences that. You can use an advance directive form or tell your healthcare providers that you don't want to be resuscitated. Your admitting doctor will put the DNR order in your medical chart. Make sure he or she does. That will be where a resuscitation team looks if you go into cardiopulmonary arrest. Likely they won't already know you, so having the DNR there will be hugely important. Doctors and hospitals in all states accept DNR orders.

Here are some good resources for information provided by the US National Library of Medicine (http://www.nlm.nih.gov/medlineplus/advancedirectives.html) and the American Academy of Family Physicians (http://familydoctor.org/familydoctor/en/healthcare-management/end-of -life-issues/advance-directives-and-do-not-resuscitate-orders.printerview .all.html).

Hospice

Hospice care for the purpose of this book is end-of-life care. A team of health care professionals and volunteers provides it. They give medical, psychological, and spiritual support. The goal of this care is to help people who are dying have peace, comfort, and dignity. The caregivers try to control pain and other symptoms so a person can remain as comfortable as possible while remaining alert. Hospice programs also provide services to support a patient's family.

Usually, a hospice patient is expected to live six months or less. Hospice care can take place in various settings:

- At home
- At a hospice center
- In a hospital
- In a skilled nursing facility

Hospice care is extremely nuanced and specific to the individual patient, but you can find some great resources at the following websites of the US Administration on Aging's Eldercare Locator (http://www.eldercare.gov/ELDERCARE.NET/Public/Resources/Factsheets/Hospice_Care.aspx) and of the National Hospice and Palliative Care Organization (http://www.nhpco.org/about/hospice-care).

Physical Death

YOUR LEGACY AND MAKING YOUR WISHES KNOWN

I have gone into great examination of various aspects of the Founding Fathers lives, many of whom became presidents. If anything, presidents, at least after a second term is secured, become obsessed about their legacies. Your legacy is no less important.

Estate Planning

It's unfortunate how many people believe that estate planning is only for wealthy people. The truth is that people at all economic levels benefit from some kind of estate planning. Shoot, if all you have is a giant ball of string, there is probably someone you want to have it, or if you don't, there are probably a bunch of cats at a shelter that would go nuts with the benevolent donation. Upon death, an estate plan legally protects and distributes your property based on your wishes and the needs of your family and/or survivors with as little tax penalty as possible.

As covered earlier, a will is the most basic and practical first step in estate planning. It makes clear how you want your property to be distributed after you die. Otherwise, the aftermath of a funeral can resemble the combative interlude of a hockey game.

Writing a will can be as simple as typing out how you want your assets to be transferred to loved ones or charitable organizations after your death. If you don't have a will when you die (known as dying *intestate*), your estate will be handled in probate, and your property could be distributed differently than what you would like. If I can offer one thing here it would be this: get some sort of official validation. This can be as basic as a witness or it can include a notary endorsement—or even better, you can consult an attorney. That, actually, is probably the best.

Legal Requirements

In order to create a will in most states, you must be 18 years of age or older. A will must be written in sound judgment and mental capacity to be valid. I have a million goofy things that come to mind here but I'm not indulging a single one. The document must clearly state that it is your will. An executor of your will must also be named. More on that later.

It is not necessary to notarize or record your will, but these can safeguard against any claims that your will is invalid. To be valid, you *must* sign a will in the presence of at least two witnesses.

The Executor

In England this is a big guy with a huge axe and a hood. No, I'm kidding. An executor is the person who is responsible for settling the estate after death and who ensures that your estate is distributed according to your wishes. Duties of an executor include the following:

- Taking inventory of property and belongings
- Appraising and distributing assets
- Paying taxes
- Settling debts owed by the deceased

Most importantly, the executor is legally obligated to act in the interests of the deceased, following the wishes provided by the will. Here again, it could be helpful to consult an attorney to help with the probate process or offer legal guidance; however, any person over the age of 18 who hasn't been convicted of a felony can be named executor of a will. Some people choose a lawyer, accountant, or financial consultant based on their experience. Others choose a spouse, adult child, relative, or friend. Since the role of executor can be demanding, it's often a good idea to ask the person being named in a will if he or she is willing to serve. It is also courteous to offer some kind of compensation. Hey, maybe that big ball of string!

A tip: if you've been named executor in someone's will but are not able or do not want to serve, you need to file a declination, which is a legal document that declines your designation as an executor. The contingent executor named in the will then assumes responsibility. If no contingent executor is named, the court will appoint one.

Who Gets What

Again, this is a starting point, and I wrote this only to show how complex this issue is. Get to a real attorney, as opposed to all the amateur ones that seem to populate my life. In advance of that, here are some things you might want to be thinking about. Primary beneficiaries are your first choice to receive your assets. You should also consider choosing secondary or contingent beneficiaries. If your primary beneficiary dies before you do or does not meet a condition (such as age) for inheritance, your secondary beneficiaries will receive all your assets. Designating a secondary beneficiary can also prevent your loved ones from going through a probate battle, which can be time-consuming and expensive. Just remember to use specific names instead of broad categories like "niece" and "nephew" when naming beneficiaries in your will.

You should also add primary and secondary beneficiaries on your individual bank accounts, deeds to your home and car, contents of your safe deposit boxes, investments, and insurance policies to make it easier to transfer the assets. Also remember that granting someone a power of attorney does not automatically make this person a beneficiary of your assets. After you die, this person will not have the right to the money or to even access your account. If you want this person to be a beneficiary, you must state it in your will.

Finally, and I say this because I advocated that you adopt a pet in the last chapter, make sure to account for your non-human charges. You can address the standards and the disposition of your "best friend" so that the rest of his or her days are assured in a manner you would want.

Keeping It Fresh

It's a good idea to review estate plans and wills from time to time. Consider changes in these situations:

- The value of your assets change
- You marry, divorce, or remarry
- You have a child
- You move to a different state
- The executor of your will dies or becomes incapacitated or your relationship changes
- One of your heirs dies
- The laws affecting your estate change

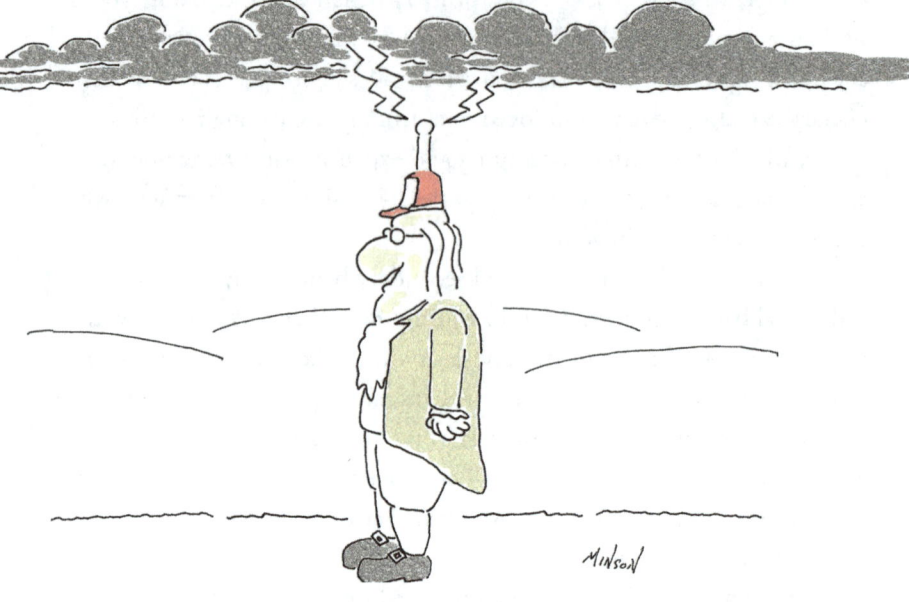

BEN FRANKLIN'S LESS CELEBRATED BROTHER, IRVING, INVENTOR OF THE LIGHTNING ROD HAT.

The Social Media Will

Social media are a part of daily life, so what happens to the online content that you created once you die? If you are active online, you should consider creating a statement of how you would like your online identity to be handled—like a social media will. This can impact your reputation, can serve as an adjunct notice of your death, and can also have applications to intellectual property or creative enterprises. Just as I discussed earlier, you should appoint someone you trust as an online executor. This person will be responsible for the closure of your e-mail addresses, social media profiles, and blogs after you are deceased. You might also take the following steps to help you write a social media will.

Review the privacy policies and the terms and conditions of each website where you have a presence. State how you would like your profiles to be handled. You may want to completely cancel your profile or keep it up for friends and family to visit. Some sites allow users to create a memorial profile where other users can still see your profile but can't post anything new. Give the social media executor a document that lists all the sites where you have a profile, along with your usernames and passwords. Stipulate in your will that the online executor should have a copy of your death certificate. The online executor may need this as proof in order for websites to take any actions on your behalf. Check to see if the social media platforms have account management features to let you proactively manage what happens to your accounts after you die.

DISPOSITION OF MORTAL REMAINS

If you are good at shopping for and dealing with this subject already, you have my sympathies. This is one of those things that you don't think about until you have to, and then it is very difficult to be an informed consumer.

Know the Laws

No kidding, laws vary state by state. In some states you *have* to purchase certain things for burial. I used to have an older relative who loved to say, "Just put me in a pine box and plant me in the pasture."

Well, with respect to how it was back on the old Oregon Trail, that may not be possible. In fact, I am pretty sure it isn't.

Consumerism

You don't have to buy everything they offer. The rules for funeral service and decedent professionals are dictated by your state. When you are being offered an array of services, like outer casket shells, embalming, and more, get everything in writing. Make sure you review that list before you pay.

Okay, so bear with me here. If you ever saw *The Big Lebowski*, you know that when the Dude and Walter are discussing the container for the cremated remains of their bowling buddy Donny, they suddenly realize they are being pressured to buy an expensive vessel and decide on an alternate plan. Their option: a Folgers coffee can.

Now, I am not going that far in recommending that here, but if you are considering buying an urn or container, just know you do not have to buy one at the funeral home. You can provide one of your choosing. As for me, my wife knows that, given my tastes, I should be in a Café Bustelo can.

In all seriousness, containers for the dead include urns for the cremated, pressboard, unfinished wood, fiberboard, or other material. Caskets are rigid containers made of higher-grade wood or metal designed to hold remains.

On that note, I have left instructions that I be cremated and put on the flower bed. As I think about it, that sounds kind of Buddhist in a way, or maybe it's more like botany. Anyway, I hope to come back some day as one fierce daisy.

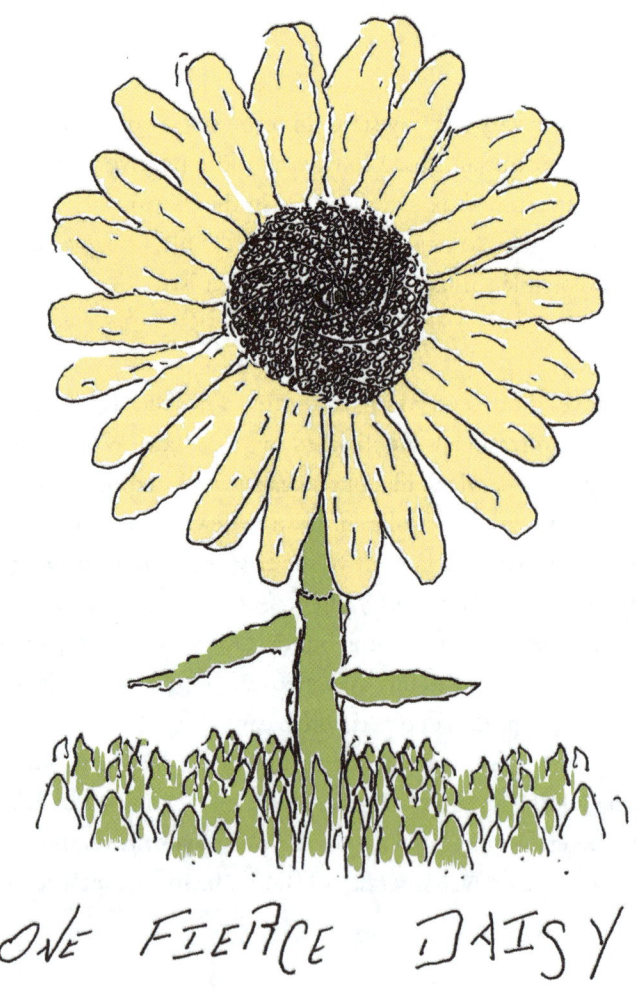

ONE FIERCE DAISY

Embalming

Most people think embalming is required. It isn't. You really don't have to do this unless there will be an interval between death and burial. Then it is a determination of law.

Types of Funerals

This really is pretty individualized, with some reasonable constraints, of course. This may include a service at a church, home, or public location. It may also—but, again, may not—include graveside services and memorial services, which are ceremonies of remembrance without the body present. And if you are a Viking, then you should be reading this book in some Old Norse text and you probably already know you'll need a boat, fire, and an accurate archer.

Cemeteries

Most cemeteries will have some rules about the terms of their lots. When considering a cemetery, think about things like religious considerations, location, and whether certain costs like grave maintenance are included.

National Cemeteries

All military veterans are entitled to a free burial in a national cemetery and a grave marker. This eligibility extends to some civilians who provided military-related service and some Public Health Service personnel. For more information, visit the Department of Veterans Affairs. To reach the regional Veterans Affairs office in your area, call 1–800–827–1000.

Finally, if this part of the book prompts you to look into some of this in advance, well then, I have done my job. The Federal Trade Commission publication Shopping for Funeral Services (http://publications.usa.gov/USAPubs.php?PubID=3028) is a great source of additional material. Again, just don't wait until . . . well, you know.

For a period of time the subject of how Americans with terminal illnesses could influence or even act in terms of the circumstances of their death was a part of the popular dialogue. This was due in part because of the controversy surrounding the philosophy and actions of Dr. Jack Kevorkian.

On its face value, this self-determination seems, depending on the person, to be as distinct a right as choosing one's course in life. On the other, it is a very individualized consideration that, if attempted in a sort of one-size-fits-all fashion, can lead to nothing less than a nightmare.

According to two US Supreme Court decisions in 1997, *Vacco, Attorney General of New York, et al. v. Quill et al.* and *Washington v. Glucksberg*, there is no constitutional right to die nor is there a fundamental liberty interest in a right to assisted suicide that is protected by the due process clause. Moreover, the ban on assisted suicide, as set forth in Washington's law, was rationally related to legitimate government interests. Those government interests include the following:

- To preserve life
- To prevent suicide
- To avoid the involvement of third parties and the use of arbitrary, unfair, or undue influence
- To protect the integrity of the medical profession
- To avoid future movement toward euthanasia and other abuses

The Supreme Court did not, however, ban assisted suicide. The opinion recognized the right of states to engage "in serious, thoughtful examinations of physician-assisted suicide." That is what I hope happens.

I am going to make a prediction. This issue *is* going to be revisited. The volume and impact of the advancing demographic of seniors and the issues that age and end of life carry with it will make the discussion necessary. I'm sort of optimistic about this because of some precedent social occurrences. The baby boomers, despite what anyone may think of them, have been the biggest social force—adjusting mores, viewpoints, and social attitudes—in history. They have—because of their social and political mass—the potential to make this dialogue happen. If they don't, it will be to their detriment, and likely they will suffer for it.

Again, if you think this issue isn't going to have to be addressed, I'll offer this. It already is. Unfortunately, it being done in a piecemeal fashion and in the shadows, and that really isn't right.

Here is what I don't want to see happen. I don't want the subject to be decided based on money. Or staffing requirements. Or space availability. My guess is neither do you.

SAYING GOOD-BYE

I got nothing here, so I am going to let a patient of mine address this. He was dying. He had a debilitating illness, and he was aware that eventually he would be at the mercy of a machine to "keeping his biology going." He had written down everything he wanted. He had addressed his legacy, his wishes for the disposition of his remains—he wanted his ashes to be poured into the cement of a building on his property—and he had addressed the advanced directive in a very specific way. Still, he also knew that he couldn't anticipate everything and there would probably be unforeseen issues. He called his children and loved ones around, and he offered a very simple sentiment.

He said, "I am sure it will turn out that you may have to agree when the doctor comes in and says that Dad has reached this point and we need to quit.

So, let's get this out of the way now.

I forgive you.

Okay? Just get on with it, and then get on with being happy. I'll be fine."

Pretty good.

A Final Thought before I Go

I know this may seem like a really depressing way to end this book, but there was no real way to sugarcoat it. I also think that there is a lot you can do to make sure that despite the inevitable (for all of us)—that we are going to die—there is a lot you can do to make sure it is on your terms.

One of the overriding themes of this book (and also of my first one) is that I really want to help equip people with the tools and concepts necessary to live their lives on their own terms. It's a pretty attractive concept and, in my opinion, the most satisfying way to get through life.

I've never liked bullies or having to concede to others' concepts of the quality or worth of my life, and as I start heading into my own senior years, I don't think that will change.

So what can you do? Well, here's a pretty interesting piece of information for you to chew on, assuming of course that you still have teeth. We, the old, are the largest growing population demographic, and through 2040 our numbers will just get bigger. Know what that means? That means political power. As a friend of mine likes to say, "I'm old, I read, I vote—and, oh yeah, I have the time to call up and make my opinions known to my political representatives. In short, I am a voice."

That baby, (baby boomers) equates to power. You've lived a long time. You've the benefit of experience: mistakes and successes, trial and error, and you're still here, for at least a while. Use that time well. Get connected, read, write, and make yourself heard. It is one last shot at changing the world. I, for one, will be glad you did.

Be well.

REFERENCES

Administration on Aging. 2001. *Older Adults and Mental Health: Issues and Opportunities*. Washington, DC: US Department of Health and Human Services.

Administration on Aging, Administration for Community Living. 2013. *A Profile of Older Americans*. Washington, DC: US Department of Health and Human Services. http://www.aoa.gov/Aging_Statistics/Profile/2013/docs/2013_Profile.pdf.

Alzheimer's Association. 2010. *Alzheimer's Disease Facts and Figures*. http://www.alz.org/documents_custom/report_alzfactsfigures2010.pdf.

Alzheimer's Association. 2012. *2012 Alzheimer's Disease Facts and Figures*. http://www.alz.org/utah/documents/2012_facts_and_figures.pdf.

American Bar Association Commission on Law and Aging and American Psychological Association. 2008. *Assessment of Older Adults with Diminished Capacity: A Handbook for Psychologists*. http://www.apa.org/pi/aging/programs/assessment/capacity-psychologist-handbook.pdf.

American Psychological Association. 2008. *Survey of Psychology Health Service Providers*. http://www.apa.org/workforce/publications/08-hsp/report.pdf.

American Psychological Association, Committee on Aging. 2009. *Multicultural Competency in Geropsychology*. http://www.apa.org/pi/aging/programs/pipeline/multicultural-geropsychology.aspx.

American Psychological Association, Government Relations Office. *Growing Mental and Behavioral Health Concerns Facing Older Americans*. http://www.apa.org/about/gr/issues/aging/growing-concerns.aspx.

American Psychological Association, Office on Aging. 2005. *Psychology and Aging: Addressing Mental Health Needs of Older Adults*. http://www.apa.org/pi/aging/resources/guides/aging.pdf.

Areán, P. A., J. Alvidrez, A. Barrera, G. S. Robinson, and S. Hicks. 2002. "Would Older Medical Patients Use Psychological Services? *Gerontologist* 42:392–98.

Areán, P.A., P. Raue, R. S. Mackin, D. Kanellopoulos, C. McCulloch, and G. Alexopoulos. 2010. "Problem-Solving Therapy and Supportive Therapy in Older Adults with Major Depression and Executive Dysfunction. *American Journal of Psychiatry* 167:1391–98.

Australian Government, Department of Health and Ageing. 2008. *Functional Incontinence*. Archived from the original on 2008–07–23. Retrieved 2008–08–29.

Barnes, D. E., and K. Yaffe. 2011. "The Projected Effect of Risk Factor Reduction on Alzheimer's Disease Prevalence." *Lancet Neurology* 10:819–28.

Bartels, S. J., F. C. Blow, L. M. Brockmann, and A. D. Van Citters. 2005. *Substance Abuse and Mental Health Care among Older Americans: The State of the Knowledge and Future Directions.* Rockville, MD: American Psychological Association. http://www.apa.org/about/gr/issues/aging/mental-health.aspx.

Braithwaite, D. O. 1993. "'Isn't It Great That People Like You Get Out?': The Process of Adjusting to Disability." In *Case Studies in Health Communication*, ed. E. B. Ray, 149–60. Hillsdale, NJ: Lawrence Erlbaum Associates.

Braveman, P.A. 2003. "Monitoring Equity in Health and Healthcare: A Conceptual Framework." *Journal of Health, Population, and Nutrition* 21 (3): 181.

Budnitz, D. S., N. Shehab, S. R. Kegler, and C. L. Richards. 2007. "Medication Use Leading to Emergency Department Visits for Adverse Drug Events in Older Adults." *Annals of Internal Medicine* 147(11): 755–65.

Burgio, K. L., J. L. Locher, P. S. Goode et al. "Behavioral vs. Drug Treatment for Urge Urinary Incontinence in Older Women: A Randomized Controlled Trial." *JAMA* 280:1995–2000.

Burt, C. W., and E. Hing. 2005. "Use of Computerized Clinical Support Systems in Medical Settings: United States, 2001–03." *Advance Data from Vital and Health Statistics* 353:1–8.

Chun-Ju Hsiao, Ph.D.; Paul C. Beatty, Ph.D. Burt, C. W., E. Hing, and D. Woodwell. 2005; CDC: 2009. "Electronic Medical Record Use by Office-Based Physicians: United States." NCHS Health E-stats. http://www.cdc.gov/nchs/data/hestat/emr_ehr/emr_ehr.pdf.

Burt, C. W., and J. E. Sisk. 2005. "Which Physicians and Practices Are Using Electronic Medical Records?" Health Aff (Millwood) 24 (5): 1334–43.

Centers for Disease Control and Prevention. 2015. "National Study of Long-Term Care Providers." http://www.cdc.gov/nchs/nsltcp.htm.

Centers for Disease Control and Prevention. 2015. "National Survey of Residential Care Facilities." Rev. ed. http://www.cdc.gov/nchs/nsrcf/about_nsrcf.htm.

Centers for Disease Control and Prevention. 2010. "Attitudes Toward Mental Illness—35 States, District of Columbia, and Puerto Rico, 2007." *MMWR* 59 (20): 619–25. http://www.cdc.gov/mmwr/preview/mmwrhtml/mm5920a3.htm.

Centers for Disease Control and Prevention. 2010. "Potentially Preventable Emergency Department Visits by Nursing Home Residents: United States, 2004." NCHS Data Brief, no. 33. http://www.cdc.gov/nchs/data/databriefs/db33.htm.

Centers for Disease Control and Prevention, National Center for Injury Prevention and Control. 2006. *Web-Based Injury Statistics Query and Reporting System (WISQARS).* http://www.cdc.gov/ncipc/wisqars.

Centers for Disease Control and Prevention and US Department of Housing and Urban Development. 2008. *Healthy Housing Inspection Manual.* Atlanta: US Department of Health and Human Services.

Chapman, D. P. "National Sleep Awareness Week—March 5–11, 2012." 2012. *MMWR* 61 (8): 147. http://www.cdc.gov/mmwr/pdf/wk/mm6108.pdf.

Chapman, D. P., L. R. Presley-Cantrell, Y. Liu, G. S. Perry, A. G. Wheaton, and J. B. Croft. "Frequent Insufficient Sleep, Anxiety, and Depressive Disorders in U.S.

Community Dwellers: 20 States, 2010." 2013. *Psychiatric Services* 64:385.

Chapman, D. P., A. G. Wheaton, G. S. Perry, S. L. Sturgis, T. W. Strine, and J. B. Croft. 2012. "Household Demographics and Perceived Insufficient Sleep among U.S. Adults." *Journal of Community Health* 37 (2): 344–49.

Ciechanowski, P., N. Chaytor, J. Miller, R. Fraser, J. Russo, J. Unutzer, and F. Gilliam. 2010. PEARLS Depression Treatment for Individuals with Epilepsy: A Randomized Controlled Trial. *Epilepsy & Behavior* 19 (3): 225–31.

Ciechanowski, P., E. Wagner, K. Schmaling, S. Schwartz , B. Williams, P. Diehr, et al. 2004. "Community-Integrated Home-Based Depression Treatment in Older Adults: A Randomized Controlled Trial." *JAMA* 291 (13): 1569–77.

Crimmins, E. M., S. H. Preston, and B. Cohen (eds.); Panel on Understanding Divergent Trends in Longevity in High-Income Countries. 2011. *Explaining Divergent Levels of Longevity in High-Income Countries*. Washington, DC: National Academies Press.

Decker, F. H. 2006. "Nursing Staff and the Outcomes of Nursing Home Stays." *Medical Care* 44 (9): 812–21.

Dittmann, Melissa. "Fighting Ageism: Geropsychologists Are Striving to Stop Negative Age Stereotypes and Meet the Growing Mental Health Needs of Older Adults." 2003. *Monitor on Psychology* 34 (5). http://www.apa.org/monitor/may03/fighting.aspx.

Donegal, Clive. 2012. "Alzheimer's: A Slow Death of Mind and Humanity." http://clive-donegal.hubpages.com/hub/Old-timers-disease-I-can-live-without-it-Please

Dufour, M., and R. K. Fuller. 1995. "Alcohol in the Elderly." *Annual Review of Medicine* 46:123–32.

Fang, J., A. G. Wheaton, N. Keenan, K. J. Greenlund, G. S. Perry, and J. B. Croft. 2012. "Association of Sleep Duration and Hypertension among U.S. Adults Varies by Age and Sex. *American Journal of Hypertension*. 25 (3): 335–341.

Federal Interagency Forum on Aging-Related Statistics. 2008. *Older Americans 2008: Key Indicators of Well-Being*. Washington, DC: US Government Printing Office.

Federal Trade Commission. 2013. *Shopping for Funeral Services*. Washington, DC: Federal Trade Commission.

Gabrel, C., and A. Jones. 2000. *The National Nursing Home Survey: 1997 Summary*. Vital and Health Statistics, series 13, no. 147. Washington, DC: National Center for Health Statistics.

Gfroerer, J., M. Penne, M. Pemberton, and R. Folsom. 2003. "Substance Abuse Treatment Need among Older Adults in 2020: The Impact of the Aging Baby-Boom Cohort." *Drug and Alcohol Dependence* 69 (2): 127–35.

Guberman, Nancy, Jean-Pierre Lavoie, Laure Blein, and Ignace Olazabal. "Baby Boom Caregivers: Care in the Age of Individualization." *Gerontologist* 52 (2): 210–18.

Harris-Kojetin, L., M. Sengupta, E. Park-Lee, and R. Valverde. *Long-Term Care Services in the United States: 2013 Overview*. Vital and Health Statistics, series 3; Analytical and Epidemiological Studies 37. Hyattsville, MD: US Department of Health and Human Services, National Center for Health Statistics. http://www.cdc.gov/nchs/data/nsltcp/long_term_care_services_2013.pdf.

Hing, E., and C. W. Burt. 2007. "Office-Based Medical Practices: Methods and Estimates from the National Ambulatory Medical Care Survey." *Advance Data from Vital and Health Statistics* 383:1–15.

Hing, E. S., C. W. Burt, and D. A. Woodwell. 2007. "Electronic Medical Record Use by Office-Based Physicians and Their Practices: United States, 2006." *Advance Data from Vital and Health Statistics* 393:1–7.

Houser, A., W. Fox-Grage, and M. J. Gibson. 2006. *Across the States: Profiles of Long-Term Care and Independent Living.* Washington, DC: AARP Public Policy Institute.

Hoyert, D. L., and J. Q. Xu. *Deaths: Preliminary Data for 2011.* 2012. National Vital Statistics Reports 61 (6). Hyattsville, MD. National Center for Health Statistics.

Institute of Medicine. 2012. *The Mental Health and Substance Use Workforce for Older Adults: In Whose Hands?* http://www.iom.edu/Reports/2012/The-Mental-Health-and-Substance-Use-Workforce-for-Older-Adults.aspx.

Jones, Adrienne L., Abigail J. Moss, and Lauren D. Harris-Kojetin. 2011. *Use of Advance Directives in Long-term Care Populations.* NCHS Data Brief 54. Washington, DC: US Department of Health and Human Services, Centers for Disease Control and Prevention.

Karel, M. J., M. Gatz, and M. Smyer. 2012. "Aging and Mental Health in the Decade Ahead: What Psychologists Need to Know." *American Psychologist* 67:184–98.

Kawachi, I. 2002. "A Glossary for Health Inequalities." *Journal of Epidemiology and Community Health* 56 (9): 647.

Koh, S., K. Blank, C. I. Cohen, G. Cohen, W. Faison, G. Kennedy, et al. 2010. "Public's View of Mental Health Services for the Elderly: Responses to Dear Abby." *Psychiatric Services* 61 (11): 1146–49.

Let's Eat for the Health of It. 2010. USDA Home and Garden Bulletin, no. 232-CP; HHS Publication, no. HHS-ODPHP-2010–01-DGA-B. Washington, DC: US Department of Agriculture, US Department of Health and Human Services.

Linder, J. A., J. Ma, D. W. Bates, B. Middleton, and R. S. Stafford. 2007. "Electronic Health Record Use and the Quality of Ambulatory Care in the United States." *Archives of Internal Medicine* 167 (13): 1400–5.

Link, B. G., and J. C. Phelan. "Conceptualizing Stigma." *Annual Review of Sociology* 27:363–85.

Liu, Y., L. R. McKnight-Eily, T. W. Strine, M. M. Zack, D. P. Chapman, A. G. Wheaton, G. S. Perry, and J. B. Croft. 2013. "The Association between Perceived Insufficient Sleep, Frequent Mental Distress, Obesity, and Chronic Diseases." *BMC Public Health* 13:84.

McCracken, Harry, and Lev Grossman. 2013. "Can Google Solve Death?" in "Google vs. Death." Special issue, *Time,* Sept. 30.

McCurry, S. M., R. G. Logsdon, L. Teri, and M. V. Vitiello. 2007. "Evidence-Based Psychological Treatments for Insomnia in Older Adults." *Psychology and Aging* 22 (1): 18–27.

Meyer, Julie. 2012. *Centenarians: 2010*. 2010 Census Special Reports, C2010SR-03. Washington, DC: US Department of Commerce, US Census Bureau.

Mickus, M., C. C. Colenda, and A. J. Hogan. 2000. "Knowledge of Mental Health Benefits and Preferences for Type of Mental Health Providers among the General Public." *Psychiatric Services* 51:199–202.

Moss, Michael. 2013. *Salt Sugar Fat: How the Food Giants Hooked Us*. New York: Random House.

National Alliance on Mental Illness. 2009. *Depression in Older Persons: Fact Sheet*. http://www.nami.org/Template.cfm?Section=Depression&Template=/ContentManagement/ContentDisplay.cfm&ContentID=88876.

National Center for Health Statistics. 2007. *Health, United States, 2007*. Hyattsville, MD: US Government Printing Office.

National Center for Health Statistics. 2012. *Healthy People, 2010: Final Review*. DHHS Publication, no. (PHS)2012–1038). Washington, DC: US Government Printing Office.

National Heart, Lung, and Blood Institute. 2011. *Your Guide to Healthy Sleep*. Rev. ed. NIH Publication, no. 11–5271. https://www.nhlbi.nih.gov/health/resources/sleep/healthy-sleep.

National Institute of Mental Health. 2007. *Older Adults: Depression and Suicide Facts*. http://www.nimh.nih.gov/health/publications/older-adults-depression-and-suicide-facts-fact-sheet/index.shtml.

National Institute on Aging. 2015. "Healthy Eating after 50." http://www.nia.nih.gov/health/publication/healthy-eating-after-50.

National Prescribing Service. Managing Urinary Incontinence." http://www.nps.org.au/health_professionals/publications/nps_news/current/nps_news_66_managing_urinary_incontinence_in_primary_care.

National Vital Statistics Reports, Vol 61 No 6. Hyattsville, MD: 2012. National Research Council, Crimmins EM, Preston SH, Cohen B, editors.

Paraprofessional Healthcare Institute. 2011. "PHI Facts: Who Are Direct-Care Workers? http://www.phinational.org/sites/phinational.org/files/clearinghouse/NCDCW%20Fact%20Sheet-1.pdf.

Pearson, W. S., and A. R. Bercovitz. 2006. "Use of Computerized Medical Records in Home Health and Hospice Agencies: United States, 2000." *Vital and Health Statistics* 13 (161): 1–14.

"Prevalence of Urinary Incontinence in Men: Results From the National Health and Nutrition Examination Survey." Alayne D. Parkland, Patricia S. Goode, David T. Redden, Lori G. Borrud, Kathryn L. Burgio. *The Journal of Urology*, September 2010, 184 (3): 1022–27.

Qualls, S. H., D. L. Segal, S. Norman, G. Niederehe, and D. Gallagher-Thompson. 2002. "Psychologists in Practice with Older Adults: Current Patterns, Sources of Training, and Need for Continuing Education." *Professional Psychology: Research and Practice* 33 (5): 5435–42.

Robert Wood Johnson Foundation. 2010. *Chronic Conditions: Making the Case for Ongoing Care*. www.rwjf.org/files/research/50968chronic.care.chartbook.ppt.

Short, Kathleen. 2012. *The Research Supplemental Poverty Measure: 2011*. Current Population Reports. Washington, DC: US Department of Commerce, US Census Bureau. https://www.census.gov/prod/2012pubs/p60–244.pdf.

Speer, D. C., and M. G. Schneider. 2003. "Mental Health Needs of Older Adults and Primary Care: Opportunities for Interdisciplinary Geriatric Team Practice." *Clinical Psychology: Science and Practice* 10 (1): 85–101.

St-Onge, Marie-Pierre, and Dympna Gallagher. 2010. "Body Composition Changes with Aging: The Cause or the Result of Alterations in Metabolic Rate and Macronutrient Oxidation." *Nutrition* 26 (2): 152–56.

Substance Abuse and Mental Health Services Administration. 2007. *An Action Plan for Behavioral Health Workforce Development*. http://www.samhsa.gov/Workforce/Annapolis/WorkforceActionPlan.pdf.

Substance Abuse and Mental Health Services Administration. 2011. *Promoting Emotional Health and Preventing Suicide: A Toolkit for Senior Living Communities*. HHS Publication SMA 4515, CMHS-NSPL-0197. Rockville, MD: Center for Mental Health Services, Substance Abuse and Mental Health Services Administration.

Substance Abuse and Mental Health Services Administration, Center for Substance Abuse Treatment. 2008. *Substance Abuse among Older Adults*. Treatment Improvement Protocols (TIP) 26. Rockville, MD: US Department of Health and Human Services.

The Gerontologist (Vol. 41, No. 5) Laurence G. Branch, Ph.D., Gerontological Society of America (2001)

Unutzer, J. 2007. "Clinical Practice: Late-Life Depression." *New England Journal of Medicine* 357:2269–76.

US Department of Agriculture. 2008. "Nutrition Information for You: Life Stages—Seniors." http://www.nutrition.gov/life-stages/seniors.

US Department of Health and Human Services. 2000. *Healthy People 2010: Understanding and Improving Health*. Washington, DC: US Government Printing Office.

US Department of Health and Human Services. 2006. *Healthy People 2010: Midcourse Review*. Washington, DC: US Government Printing Office.

US Department of Health and Human Services. 2009. *Healthy People 2020: Draft*. Washington, DC: US Government Printing Office.

US Department of Health and Human Services, Substance Abuse and Mental Health Services Administration. 2001. *Promoting Emotional Health and Preventing Suicide: A Toolkit for Senior Living Communities*. Washington, DC: US Government Printing Office.

Vogeli, C., A. E. Shields, T. A. Lee, T. B. Gibson, W. D. Marder, K. B. Weiss, and D. Blumenthal. 2007. "Multiple Chronic Conditions: Prevalence, Health Consequences, and Implications for Quality, Care Management, and Costs." *Journal of General Internal Medicine* 22 (suppl. 3): 391–95.

Walid, M. S., and R. L. Heaton. 2009. "Stepwise Multimodal Treatment of Mixed Urinary Incontinence with Voiding Problems in a Patient with Prolapse." *Journal of Gynecologic Surgery* 25 (3): 121–27. doi:10.1089/gyn.2009.0014.

Wheaton, A. G., G. S. Perry, D. P. Chapman, and J. B. Croft. 2012. "Sleep-Disordered Breathing and Depression among U.S. Adults—National Health and Nutrition Examination Survey, 2005–2008." *Sleep* 35 (4): 461–67.

Whitehead, M. 1991. "The Concepts and Principles of Equity and Health." *Health Promotion International* 6 (3): 217–228.

Wiseman, Suzi, Preston S. Wildon, and Frank Sepulveda. 2014. "What Does a Rhino Hear, and Why Do We Care?" Paper presented at the 167th Meeting of the Acoustical Society of America, Providence, RI.

World Health Organization. 1948. Preamble to the Constitution of the World Health Organization. *Official Records of the World Health Organization* 2:100.

Zhan, C., R. Correa-de-Araujo, A. S. Bierman, J. Sangl, M. R. Miller, S. W. Wickizer, and D. Stryer. 2005. "Suboptimal Prescribing in Elderly Outpatients: Potentially Harmful Drug-Drug and Drug-Disease Combinations." *Journal of the American Geriatric Society* 53 (2): 262–67.

INDEX

Note: Page numbers in *italics* refer to illustrations.

abuse of seniors, 264–95; and advocacy, 271, 278–79; definitions of, 267, 268–69; and demographics of aging Americans, 267; emotional mistreatment, 270; financial exploitation, 268, 269–71; and home health care, 279–84; neglect, 268; in nursing homes, 271–78; physical abuse, 268, 270; prevalence of, 269; prevention of, 283–84; under-reporting of, 270; and restraints, 274–75; signs of, 269, *272*

acetaminophen, 173
acetone, 126
acetylcholine, 96
Adams, John: on the arts, 3, 319; death of, 327; on exercise, 56
addictions, 169, 173
additives, 81
adenosine, 98
adipose (body fat), 19–20, *45*, 45
Administration on Aging (AoA), 278–79
adrenal gland, *45*
adrenalin, 44
advance directives, 334–35
advocates, 236–41; choosing, 236–37, 240–41; guardianship, 237–39, *240*; power of attorney, 228–29, 237, 239–41, *240*, 334
African-Americans, 185
Agency for Healthcare Research and Quality, 75
agents (power of attorney), *240*
aging-in-place, 251
aging-in-place specialists, 123–25
air quality, 112–13, 115–16
Alaska Natives, 185
alcohol, 94–95; and aging physiology, 176; and alcoholism diagnoses, 176–77; and blood pressure management, 199; growing problem of, 146–47; guidelines for,

87; and incontinence, 197; risks associated with, 176; and sleep issues, 102
aldosterone, 46
alkylphenol ethoxylates (APEs), 125
alprazolam, 173, 174
alveoli, 36–37
"Alzheimer's" A Slow Death of Mind and Humanity" (Donegal), 328
Alzheimer's disease, 330–33; causes of, 331; characteristics of, 330; death resulting from, 330–31; and dementia, 328–29; diagnosing, 331–32; and exercise, 61, 62; factors associated with, 330; resources for, 332–33; stages of, *331*; treatment of, 332
Ambien, 174
American Association of Homes and Services for the Aging (now LeadingAge), 278
American Association of Retired People (AARP): and driving cessation, 259; and financial resources, 257; and Nursing Home Reform Act of 1987, 276; and Senior Crimestoppers, 286; and senior-friendly communities, 137; on sexuality of seniors, 301
American Geriatric Society (AGS), 183
American Indians, 185
American National Standards Institute (ANSI), 143
American Recovery and Reinvestment Act (ARRA), 180
American Urological Association, 310
amitriptyline, 166
amnesia, 175
amygdala, 155
amylase, 40, 41, 42
androgens, 44
animal companions, 249, 317, 339
antidepressants, 165
antioxidants, 94–95
apoptosis, 13
appendix, 39

appetite, 45, 160, 163

Area Agency on Aging: and abuse of seniors, 280; and animal companions, 249; and food programs for seniors, 248; and resources for seniors, 256; and transportation services, 259, 260, 261

Aristotle, 12, 202

arrhythmia, 16

art, 156

arteries, 32, *33*, 34–35

arterioles, 32, *33*

arthritis, 185–89; and environmental concerns, 111; management of, 187–88; prevalence of, 185; and shoe selection, 73; tools for, 188–89

Arthritis Foundation, 188

asbestos, 134–35

Asians, 185

assisted living, 230–31, 251

assisted suicide, 344

asthma, 116, 132

astigmatisms, 21

atherosclerosis, 16, 31, 32, 34, 330

Ativan, 174

attorneys: and estate planning, 338; low-cost legal advice, 237, 256

audiograms, 121

autonomic nervous system, 25

bacon, 87

bacteremia, 204

bacterial meningitis, 204

bacteria of the digestive system, 42, 43, 116

bad fats, 11

balance training, 64

bank accounts, 245–46

Bargh, John A., 157

B complex vitamins, 42

beef fat, *93*

behavioral issues, 100

behavior as determinant of health, 10. *See also* exercise and activity; nutrition; sleep

benzodiazepines, 174

"best if used by" date, 81

Bifidobacterium, 42

biking, 67

bile, 41

biofeedback, 202

biology of aging adults, 11–54; and cardio-

vascular system, 31–36; as determinant of health, 10; and digestive system, 38–43; and ears and hearing, 22–24; and endocrine system, 44–46; and eyes and eyesight, 20–22; and genitourinary system, 47–50; and immune system, 50–52; and metabolism, 12–17; and musculoskeletal system, 17–20; and nervous system, 24–28; and pulmonary system, 36–38; and racial inheritance, 11; and the skin, 52–54; and slowing the aging process, 15; and teeth/gums, 28–31

black outs, 35

bladder, 47, 48, 49, 50

blood cells, 44

blood pressure: and Alzheimer's disease, 330, 331; awareness of, 200; drops in, 35; and exercise, 61; low blood pressure, 16; management of, 199–200; prevalence of, 185; and salt intake, 28; treatment of, *198*

blood sugar, 58, 91, 190

body burden of environmental contaminants, 113

body fat (adipose), 19–20, *45*, 45

bolus, 40–41

bones, 17–18, 61

bottled water, 142–45

Bottled Water Basics (EPA), 142

Bowman's capsule, 48

bradycardia, 16

brain: and benefits of exercise, 58; and brain plasticity sleep theory, 97; cells of, 13, 17, 27; and depression, 150; effect of aging on, 28; and eyes, 21–22; ischemic areas in, 150, 164; and low blood pressure, 16; and nervous system, 25, 27; and neurotoxins, 125; and sleep, 96, 97

breath, holding, 35

breathing during exercise, 68

buddy system. *See* advocates, choosing

Bureau of Justice Statistics, 291

burglary, 288

Burr, Aaron, 323

butane, 126

butter, *93*

caffeine, 98, 197

calcium, 19–20, 44

hypertension, 197–200; and Alzheimer's disease, 330, 331; and depression, 150; prevalence of, 185; and salt intake, 28
hypoperfusion, 16
hypothalamus, 44, *45*

ileum, 39
imipramine, 166
immune system, 50–52; and exercise, 61; and intestines, 42; and teeth/gums, 30
impotence, 310
inactivity sleep theory, 96–97
incompetence, 237
incontinence, 49, 190, 192–97
Independent Autonomous Living (IAL), 251
inflammation: and arthritis, 185; and circulatory system, 33; and injuries, 20; and teeth/gums, 30
influenza shots, 52, 203, 204
injuries: and abuse of seniors, 270; and exercise, 62, 68, 71–72, 73; and inflammation, 19–20
insomnia, 100
Institute of Medicine (IOM), 77, 132
Institutional Review Board (IRB), 207
insular cortex, 157
insulin, 44, 45, 46
insurance policies, 225–27, 253–54
intercostal muscle cells, 13
International Symposium on Environmental Factors and Seniors as a Vulnerable Population, 111
Internet access, 318–19
intestines, 38–39, 42
intimacy, nonsexual, 311–12
introverts, 153
Investigational Device Exemption (IDE), 207
Iowa State University, 94, 248
irradiated foods, 81
irritability, 76, 100
ischemia, 150, 164
Islam, Yusuf, 297
isolation, social, 150
Israel, Toby, 153

Jefferson, Thomas: death of, 327; and environmental adaptations, *118*, 119; on ex-

ercise, 56–57; and pursuit of happiness, 298; on remaining well informed, 215
jejunum, 39
Johnston, Joe, 265–66
joint pain, 187
Journal of Personality and Social Psychology, 156
Journal of the American Geriatrics Society, 148

Kennedy, John F., 55
keratinocytes, 53
Kevorkian, Jack, 344
kidneys: and aldosterone, 46; and atherosclerosis, 16; effect of aging on, 49; hormones secreted by, 44, *45*; role of, 48; and urinary system, 47
Kintz, Jarod, 19
kitchen, safety precautions in, 293
Klonopin, 174

Lactobacillus, 42
lactose intolerance, 43, 89
laundry detergents, 125
laxatives, 192
lead, *134*, 134
LeadingAge (formerly American Association of Homes and Services for the Aging), 278
legal resources, 237, 256
legumes, 89
leptin, *45*
leukocytes, 51
Levinson, Arthur D., 14
liberty, 211–15
Lifeline, 258
ligaments, 18, 64
Lincoln, Abraham, 264
lipase, 41, 42
lipids, 34
living trusts, 244
living wills, 333
Locke, John, 2, 298
long-term care, 252–54
long-term-care insurance, 253–54
Long-Term Care Ombudsman Program, 279
lorazepam, 174
love, 316–17

National Commission on Sleep Disorders Research, 100

National Committee for Quality Assurance (NCQA), 225

National Consumer Voice for Quality Long-Term Care, 278

National Council for Community Behavioral Healthcare, 169

National Council on Aging (NCOA), 218, 250, 304

The National Elder Mistreatment Study (National Institute of Justice), 269

National Heart, Lung, and Blood Institute, 103–4

National Highway Transportation Safety Administration, 259

National Institute of Justice (NIJ), 267–68, 269

National Institute of Mental Health (NIMH), 169

National Institute on Aging (NIA): on activity and exercise, 59, 60; on Alzheimer's disease, 333; and depression, 148; on nutritional strategies, 88, 90; and Safety Data Sheets (SDS), 127

National Institutes of Health (NIH), 22, 100

National Interview Health Survey (NHIS), 203

National Oceanic and Atmospheric Administration (NOAA), 140–41

National Research Council, 267

National Science Foundation (NSF), 143

National Sleep Foundation, 100

National Social Life, Health, and Aging Project (NHSAP), 303–5, 308, 309, 310

Natural Resources Defense Council (NRDC), 144

nerves, 28, 54

nervous system, 24–28, 174

neuroendocrine system, 28, 96

neurotoxins, 125

neurotransmitters, 96

New Drug Application (IND), 207

Niebuhr, Reinhold, 17

nose, 28

nursing homes, 252; and abuse of seniors, 271–78, *272*; and certification, 275–76; and guardianship questions, 254–56;

Nursing Home Reform Act of 1987, 272–73, 275–76; regulation of, 276–78; and Residents' Bill of Rights, 273–74; and restraints, 274–75

nutrition, 78–95; and additives, 81, 82; and alcohol, 94–95; and blood pressure management, 199; economical nutrition plans, 94; and fiber, 90–91, 191–92; and food industry, 86; and food labeling, 82–86, *84*, *85*; and genetically engineered foods, 81; guidelines for, 88–94; and irradiated foods, 81; and Minson's Most Wanted foods, 86–88; and pain management, 202–3; and processed foods, 79–82, 92; and salt intake, 91–93; and serving sizes, 84; and teeth/gums, 30; and washing produce, 82; and *What's on Your Plate?* guidelines, 90

Obamacare, 219

obesity, 61, 330

obstructive sleep apnea, 101

Occupational Health and Safety Administration (OSHA), 127

"off-label" prescription drugs, 207

oils, 90

Older Americans Act, 253

olive oil, *93*

omega-3 fatty acids, 187

Omnibus Budget Reconciliation Act (OBRA), 272

opioid painkillers, 173

opioids, 173–74

organochlorines (OCs), 126

orthostatic hypotension, 35

osteoarthritis, 185, *186*

osteoporosis, 17–18, 61

ovaries, 45, 49, 50

oxycodone, 173

OxyContin, 173

Page, Larry, 14

pain and pain management, 200–203; and biofeedback, 202; and exercise, 71, 201; joint pain, 187; and massage, 202; and nutrition, 202–3; relaxation techniques and meditation, 200–201; as risk factor for depression, 150; and sex, 301, 314; and signs of increasing fitness, 71; and smoking, 201; and support groups, 201; and symptoms of depression, 163; tracking, 202

Paine, Thomas, 2

palate, 28

palm oil/palm kernel oils, *93*

pancreas, 40, 41, 44, *45*, 46

parasympathetic nervous system, 25–27, 102

parathyroid, 44, *45*

Parkinson's disease, 164

partial glutamate antagonists, 332

partially hydrogenated oil, *93*

pasteurization, 81

Patient Protection and Affordable Care Act (ACA), 219

payday loans, 286

peanut oil, *93*

pelvic floor exercises, 195–96

pensions, 218

pepsin, 40

Percocet, 173

peripheral nervous system, 25

peristalsis, 40

persistent organic pollutants (POPs), 116

pesticides, 125

pets, 249, 317, 339

pharmacists, 206–7

phishing, 284

phone scams, 284–85

phone service assistance, 258

phthalates, 126

physical therapists, 188

pickles, 87

pill splitting, 208–9

pineal gland, 44, *45*

pituitary gland, 44, *45*

planting zones, changes in, 140–41, *141*

plaque, arterial, 33, 34

pneumococcus diseases and vaccination, 204–5

pneumonia, 37, 204

political power of aging Americans, 346

Pollack, Jackson, 156

polyuria, 195

pool therapy, 69–70

pork fat, *93*

postural hypotension, 166

pot pies, 87

poverty levels, 234–35, *235*

power of attorney, 228–29, 239–41, *240*, 334

preferred provider organizations (PPOs), 225

Prepare to Defend Yourself . . . How to Navigate the Healthcare System & Escape with Your Life (Minson), 1, 178, 179

presbycusis, 24

presbyopia, 21

prescription drugs, 146–47

Prevention Research Center (PRC), 168

probiotic flora of intestines, 42, 43

processed foods, 79–82, 92

Profile of Older Americans, 2013, 183

progesterone, 49

Program of All-Inclusive Care for the Elderly (PACE), 232

Program to Encourage Active, Rewarding Lives (PEARLS), 168–69

propane, 126

property crime, 288–91

prostate, 50, 195

prostate cancer, 195, 327

protease, 40

proteins, 89

psychiatrists, geriatric, 184

psychology and mental health issues, 146–77; and alcohol, 176–77; and art, 156; and color psychology, 154; depression, 147–49; and design psychology, 153; and effect of environment on mental health, 150–53; and exercise, 62; and expectations for happiness, 161–62; and Fêng shui, 154–55; and risk factors, 150–51, 158; and stigma concerns, 149–50; and suicides/suicide attempts, 148, 150, 158, 164–65; and temperature, 156–58. *See also* depression; substance abuse

Psychology of Aesthetics, Creativity and the Art, 156

Psychology Today, 153

psychotherapy, 165

puberty, 54

pulmonary system, 36–38

purified water, 144

pus, 51

pyloric sphincter, 41